AF615141

# The Biomedical Laser:
## Technology and Clinical Applications

# The Biomedical Laser: Technology and Clinical Applications

Edited by

*Leon Goldman*

Director, Laser Laboratory
University of Cincinnati Medical Center

With 165 Illustrations

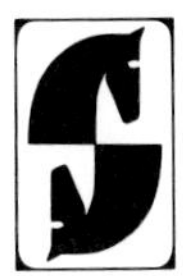

Springer-Verlag
New York Heidelberg Berlin

Leon Goldman, M.D.
Director, Laser Laboratory
University of Cincinnati Medical Center
231 Bethesda Avenue
Cincinnati, Ohio, 45267, U. S. A.

Sponsoring Editor: Chester Van Wert
Production: Abe Krieger

Library of Congress Cataloging in Publication Data
Main entry under title:
The Biomedical lasers, technology and clinical
applications.
Bibliography: p.
Includes index.
1. Lasers in medicine. 2. Lasers in surgery.
3. Lasers in biology. I. Goldman, Leon, 1905-
[DNLM: 1. Lasers. WB 117 B615]
R857.L37B56 610′.28 81-5720
AACR2



Printed in the United States of America

9 8 7 6 5 4 3 2 1

ISBN 0-387-**90571-5** Springer-Verlag New York Heidelberg Berlin
ISBN 3-540-**90571-5** Springer-Verlag Berlin Heidelberg New York

# Contents

# Preface

The laser's range of application is extraordinary. Arthur Schawlow says, "What instrument can shuck a bucket of oysters, correct typing errors, fuse atoms, lay a straight line for a garden bed, repair detached retinas, and drill holes in diamonds?"* The laser's specifically biomedical uses cover a similarly broad and interesting spectrum. In this book, I have endeavored to convey some of the fascination that the laser has long held for me. It is my hope that both clinicians and researchers in the various medical and surgical specialties will find the book a useful introduction. Biologists, particularly molecular biologists, should also find a great deal of relevant information herein.

This volume's distinguished contributors provide admirably lucid discussions of laser principles, instrumentation, and current practice in their respective specialties. Safety, design, capabilities, and costs of various lasers are also reviewed. We have aimed to create a practical text that is comprehensive but not exhaustive. Our emphasis on the practical, rather than the esoteric, is dictated not only by the short history of biomedical laser use, but by the extent of the community to which this information will appeal.

Because of its unique properties and the diversity of its uses, one is apt to forget that the laser employs a special form of light. In studying the laser as a medical, surgical, or biological tool, some understanding of light and its electric effects is required. This is particularly important in surgery, where for the first time the physician has an instrument that does not touch the tissue it cuts. The laser operates with lower hemorrhage rates than the traditional scalpel, the high-frequency electrosurgical unit, the plasma torch, or cryosurgery. Indeed, one type of laser can coagulate bleeding vessels 3–4 mm in diameter. Therefore, appropriate discussion

*Personal communication, 1978.

has been included of the special properties of laser light and its effects on living tissue. Although much is known, many challenges remain in developing the laser's full potential in these areas. Investigations in molecular biology, immunobiology, analytical spectroscopy, phototherapy, photochemotherapy, imaging, laser surgery, and the biomedical aspects of laser communication and information handling are all progressing rapidly, while laser dentistry and laser veterinary medicine are developing more slowly. This book will serve to orient us as we look ahead to new technological developments and to refinements in surgical, diagnostic, and therapeutic techniques.

*Leon Goldman*

# Contributors

Alessandra M. Andreoni, Ph.D., Professor of Physical Technology, University of Milan; Researcher, National Research Council, Istituto di Fisica del Politecnico, 32-20133 Milano, Italy, *Chapter 7*

Billie L. Aronoff, M.D., Director of Surgical Oncology, Charles A. Sammons Cancer Center; Professor of Surgery (Clinical), Southwestern Medical School, University of Texas, Dallas, Texas 75246, U.S.A., *Chapter 19*

Peter Wolf Ascher, M.D., Universitäts Dozent, Neurochirurgische Klinik, Karl Franzens Universität Graz; Director, Neurochirurgischen Universitäts Klinik, Graz, Austria, *Chapter 17*

Michael W. Berns, Ph.D., Professor of Biological Sciences, Developmental and Cell Biology, University of California, Irvine, California 92717, U.S.A., *Chapter 6*

Sari Brenner, M.S., Department of Developmental and Cell Biology, University of California, Irvine, California 92717, U.S.A., *Chapter 6*

Janis Burt, Ph.D., Graduate student, Department of Developmental and Cell Biology, University of California, Irvine, California 92717, U.S.A., *Chapter 6*

L. Karen Chong, B.S., Department of Developmental and Cell Biology, University of California, Irvine, California, 92717, U.S.A., *Chapter 6*

Richard M. Dwyer, M.D., Assistant Clinical Professor of Medicine, UCLA/Harbor General Hospital; Senior Research Scientist, Center for Laser Studies, School of

Engineering, University of Southern California, Los Angeles, California 90007, U.S.A., *Chapter 20*

Gilbert T. Feke, Ph.D., Associate Scientist, Eye Research Institute of Retina Foundation, 20 Staniford Street, Boston, Massachusetts 02114, U.S.A., *Chapter 13*

James P. Fidler, M.D., Associate Professor of Surgery, College of Medicine, University of Cincinnati, Cincinnati, Ohio 45267, U.S.A., *Chapter 16*

Nikolai F. Gamaleya, Ph.D., Professor of Biophysics; Chief, Department of Laser Biology, Kavetski Institute for Oncology Problems, Kiev, U.S.S.R., *Chapter 21*

John A. Goldman, M.D., Associate Professor, Rheumatology and Immunology, Emory School of Medicine, Atlanta, Georgia 39303, U.S.A., *Chapter 23*

Leon Goldman, M.D., Director, Laser Laboratory, University of Cincinnati Medical Center, 231 Bethesda Ave., Cincinnati, Ohio 45267, U.S.A., *Chapters 1, 2, 4, 8, 18, 25*

David B. Greenberg, Ph.D., Head, Department of Chemical & Nuclear Engineering, College of Engineering, University of Cincinnati, Cincinnati, Ohio 45221, U.S.A., *Chapter 22*

Marie J. Hammer-Wilson, M.S., Staff Research Associate III, Department of Developmental and Cell Biology, University of California, Irvine, California 92717, U.S.A., *Chapter 6*

F. Heppner, M.D., Clinical Professor of Neurosurgery, School of Medicine, University of Graz, Graz, Austria, *Chapter 17*

Geza J. Jako, M.D., Research Professor of Otolaryngology, Boston University School of Medicine, Boston, Massachusetts 02118, U.S.A., *Chapter 15*

Isaac Kaplan, M.D., Professor of Surgery, Medical School, Tel Aviv University; Head, Department of Plastic Surgery, Beilinson Hospital, Petah-Tiqwa, Israel, *Chapter 9*

Margarita C. Kitzes, Ph.D., Associate Specialist, Department of Developmental and Cell Biology, University of California, Irvine, California 92717, U.S.A., *Chapter 6*

Maurice B. Landers, III, M.D., Professor of Ophthalmology, Duke University Medical Center, Durham, North Carolina 27710, U.S.A., *Chapter 12*

Lih-Huei L. Liaw, M.S., Staff Research Associate, Department of Developmental and Cell Biology, University of California, Irvine, California 92717, U.S.A., *Chapter 6*

A. Longoni, Ph.D., Professor of Electronics, Istituto di Fisica del Politecnico, 32-20133 Milano, Italy, *Chapter 7*

Byron J. Masterson, M.D., Professor and Chief, Section Gynecologic Oncology, The University of Kansas College of Health Sciences; Director, Section Gynecologic Oncology, Truman Medical Center, Kansas City, Missouri 66103, U.S.A., *Chapter 11*

Patricia A. McNeill, Ph.D., Lecturer, Department of Developmental and Cell Biology, University of California, Irvine, California, U.S.A., *Chapter 6*

Myron C. Muckerheide, Vice President, Research, Mark Laser Systems, Inc., Wausau, Wisconsin 54401, U.S.A., *Chapter 24*

Edward Perry, Engineer and Safety Officer, Laser Laboratory, College of Medicine, University of Cincinnati, Cincinnati, Ohio 45267, U.S.A., *Chapter 8*

Scott P. Peterson, Ph.D., Department of Developmental and Cell Biology, University of California, Irvine, California 92717, U.S.A., *Chapter 6*

Joshua Raif, M.Sc., Vice President Research & Development, Laser Industries Ltd., Tel-Aviv, Israel, *Chapter 9*

Jerome B. Rattner, Ph.D., Researcher, Department of Developmental and Cell Biology, University of California, Irvine, California 92717, U.S.A., *Chapter 6*

Charles E. Riva, D.Sc., Associate Professor of Ophthalmology, Biochemistry and Biophysics, University of Pennsylvania, Philadelphia, Pennsylvania 19104, U.S.A., *Chapter 13*

C. A. Sacchi, Ph.D., Professor of Physics, Istituto di Fisica Politecnico, 32-20133 Milano, Italy, *Chapter 7*

Gary C. Salzman, Ph.D., Biophysics Group, University of California, Los Alamos Scientific Laboratory, Los Alamos, New Mexico 87545, U.S.A., *Chapter 5*

Helmut Schellhas, M.D., Associate Professor of Obstetrics and Gynecology and Radiation Oncology; Director, Gynecologic Oncology, University of Cincinnati Medical Center, Cincinnati, Ohio 45267, U.S.A., *Chapter 10*

Ann Siemens, B.S., Staff Research Associate, Department of Developmental and Cell Biology, University of California, Irvine, California 92717, U.S.A., *Chapter 6*

David H. Sliney, M.Sc., Instructor, Department of Military Medicine and History, Uniformed Services University of the Health Sciences; Chief, Laser Branch, Laser Microwave Division, U.S. Army Environmental Hygiene Agency, Aberdeen Proving Ground, Maryland 21010, U.S.A., *Chapter 3*

Kenneth Strahs, Ph.D., Postdoctoral Researcher, Department of Developmental and Cell Biology, University of California, Irvine, California 92717, U.S.A., *Chapter 6*

Orazio Svelto, Ph.D., Professor of Quantum Electronics, Instituto di Fisica del Politecnico, 32-20133 Milano, Italy, *Chapter 7*

Michael D. Tribbe, Project Engineer, Procter & Gamble Co., Cincinnati, Ohio 45267, U.S.A., *Chapter 22*

Rene C. J. Verschueren, M.D., Ph.D., Department of Surgical Oncology, University Hospital Groningen, 9700 RB Groningen, The Netherlands, *Chapter 14*

Myron L. Wolbarsht, Ph.D., Professor of Ophthalmology and Biomedical Engineering, Duke University Medical Center, Durham, North Carolina 27710, U.S.A., *Chapter 12*

# 1

# Introduction to the Laser in Medicine

*Leon Goldman*

## THE NEED FOR THE DEVELOPMENT OF SPECIAL INSTRUMENTS FOR THE LASER IN MEDICINE

The central problem confronting the laser researcher today in clinical medicine is laser safety. To enhance safety for both the patient and the operator, the flexibility of the laser beam must be increased. All forms of optics have been tested: prisms, lenses, windows, rods, and more recently, fiber optics. Optical fibers of quartz, capable of transmitting laser beams through internal reflection (Fig. 1.1), are proving to be useful in medicine. Quartz fibers are widely used in laser communications, information handling, and computer technology. Current developments include fiber-optics systems for the far-infrared $CO_2$ laser (Fig. 1.2). Other new combinations of special fibers, lens systems, mirrors, and prisms will extend the flexibility of fiber-optic transmission to new areas of treatment.

The safety of the laser for surgical use can also be enhanced by improving its coagulation capabilities. Quartz and sapphire cutting scalpels and transmission probes use transparent blades, with the laser coagulating blood as the incision is made. The optic wave is omitted near the cutting edge of the blade surface, increasing coagulation. For this blade, the argon laser is usually the source of laser radiation because its wavelengths are absorbed by red hemoglobin (Fig. 1.3). A type of photocoagulating scalpel has been developed by Auth (personal communication).

Reductions in the sizes and weights of the operating probes and precision focusing all make for more precise instruments. For lasers in the infrared spectrum, a beam of low-output HeNe laser is often used to outline target areas because

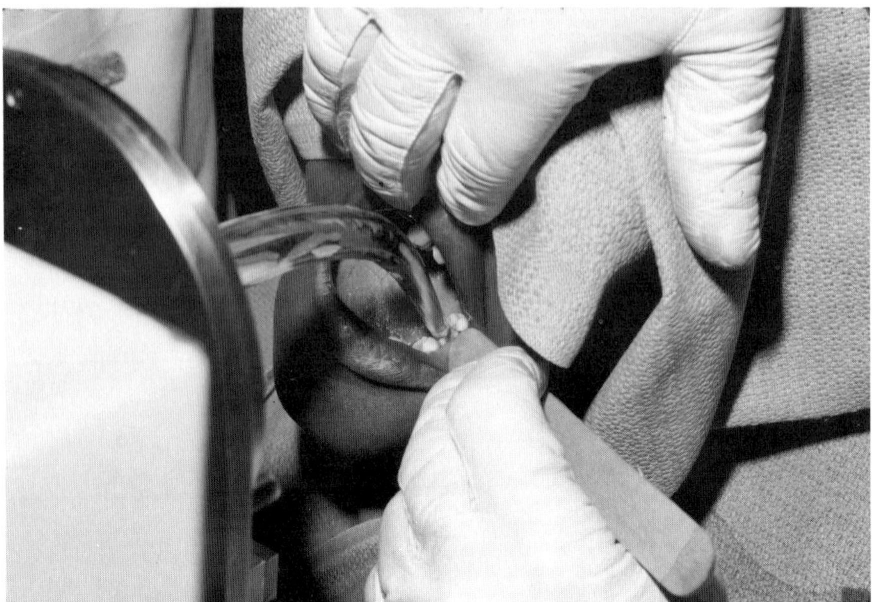

**Fig. 1.1.** Transmission of pulsed ruby laser through tapered quartz rod for treatment of dental caries.

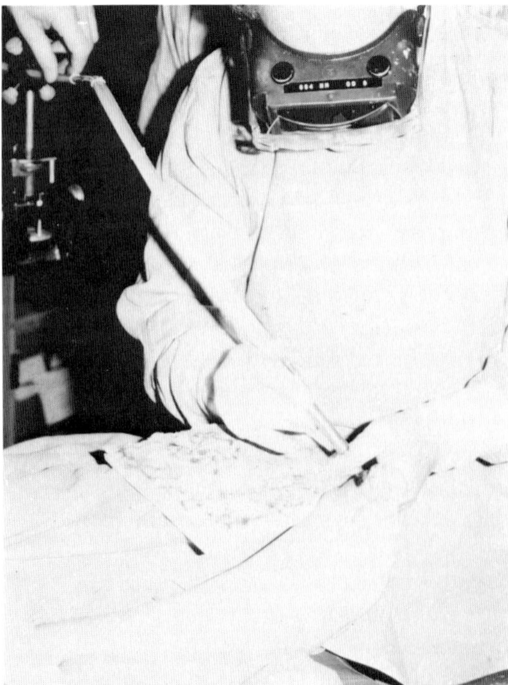

**Fig. 1.2.** Effective treatment of skin cancer of the toe by means of CW Nd laser, 300 W output, transmitted through Nath quartz fiber.

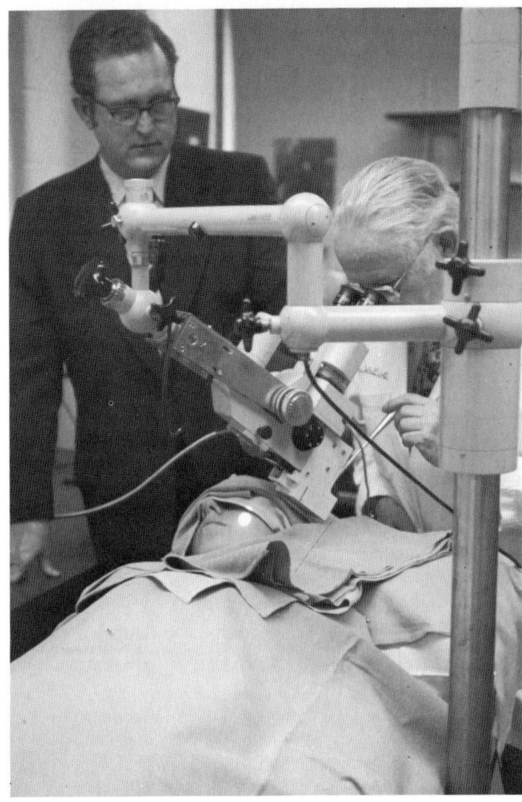

**Fig. 1.3.** Microirradiation with argon laser for small areas residual after laser treatment of vascular lesions of the face. The laser was attached with fiber-optics transmission to an operating microscope.

infrared is invisible, making targeting difficult. Self-contained water cooling will also make the $CO_2$ laser unit more flexible.

## PARAMETERS FOR THE MEASUREMENT OF THE LASER BEAM

For laser scientists to communicate, precise characteristics of each beam must be known. These standard terms will be used frequently in the following chapters:

1. Wavelength, in nanometers
2. Total pulse duration—duration of burst of energy
3. Energy and power densities in joules per square centimeter
4. Irradiance—watts per square centimeter
5. Beam divergence—spread of beam
6. Mode content—single or multiple

The pulse duration of the laser may be expressed in terms of continuous wave (CW); normal mode in milliseconds, or Q-switched. The term Q is carried over from radio- and microwave terminology and identifies the so-called quality factor of a resonating system. It is expressed in nanoseconds.

## TYPES OF LASERS

Ten lasers are now in use in medicine, surgery, and biology (specific details will be described elsewhere):

1. Helium-neon (HeNe) (632.3 nm)
2. Ruby (694.3 nm)
3. Argon (476.5–514.5 nm)
4. Krypton ion (476.1–647 nm)
5. Neodymium (Nd) (near infrared 1060 nm)
6. Neodymium and yttrium aluminum garnet (YAG) (1060 nm)
7. Carbon dioxide ($CO_2$) (10,600 nm infrared)
8. Helium cadmium (325–441.6 nm)
9. Nitrogen (337 nm)
10. Dye

New lasers are being investigated for surgery at the present time, including the carbon monoxide (CO) laser, the holmium (2065 nm), and the R. F. and D. C. wave guide $CO_2$.

## LASER SAFETY

The operator of lasers has a great responsibility for laser safety. Detailed literature on laser measurement devices should be consulted by those responsible for controlling output of laser radiation. The American National Standards Institute (ANSI) has a special committee on laser radiation measurement, and the data are available from them. Measuring instruments are available to measure the output of laser equipment. These devices are essentially absorbent devices that convert the laser beam into heat and measure the change produced. Special devices are available for ultra-fast measurements, such as the 2-photon-absorption fluorescence devices. When continuous wave power measurement is needed, thermal power collimators may be used. Power densities are also measured. Power density is the time rate by which energy is emitted and is usually measured in watts or joules per second. For pulsed lasers, the capacity is measured as joules per centimeter squared of the output of the laser.

### A Special Note of Caution

The American National Standards Institute has issued the following warning in regard to laser measurements.

Measurements should only be attempted by persons trained or experienced in laser technology and radiometry. Routine survey measurements of lasers or laser systems are neither required nor advisable when laser classifications are known and the appropriate control measures implemented. (ANSI, 1979)

## SUMMARY

Developments in the use of the laser beam are proceeding rapidly. New approaches to medical and surgical care with the laser are a major part of this advancement. Although these developments are welcome, improvements in instrumentation, increased knowledge on the part of the user, and extreme caution are highly essential to assure the safety of both the patients and of those who use the equipment.

## REFERENCE

American National Standards Institute Inc (ANSI). Committee on the Safe Use of Lasers. Z136.1—1979, New York.

# 2

# Basic Reactions in Tissue

*Leon Goldman*

The development of instruments for use in medicine has not been as rapid as that in other fields of laser technology because of the following special requirements:

1. Safety for the operator and the patient
2. Flexibility of application
3. Reliability of output
4. Continuing definitions of indications for diagnostic and therapeutic laser use
5. Instrument costs

## OPTICAL CHARACTERISTICS

When a laser is directed at tissues, the basic reaction is one of destruction of tissue, called *photocoagulation necrosis*. This reaction is similar to the tissue changes induced by electrical burns. Laser energy absorption with lasers in the visible light range varies with the optical characteristics of the target tissue and is greater with darker or pigmented tissues. Hence, the operator must know the optical characteristics of the target tissue as well as the quality of the beam that is being directed at that tissue.

The IDL color eye, 400–700 nm, is a spectrophotometer used to determine the optical characteristics of tissues. This is particularly important in the treatment of port-wine marks. As tissues are not homogeneous, the optical quality of each structure produces a varying absorption of laser energy. For thermal reactions of lasers in tissues, the intensity depends on (1) the absorption, reflection, and transmission of the tissues at the laser wavelength; (2) the power density of the laser beam; (3) the speed of incision or time of exposure; (4) the volume and the flow velocity of local blood vessels; and (5) the degree of tension at the area of incision when cutting is used.

With pulsed laser systems, nonthermal reactions may occur, such as the following:

1. Pressure and elastic recoil.
2. Second harmonic generations.
3. Stimulated Raman and Brillouin scattering—of significance in laser diagnostic spectroscopy
4. Inverse Bremstrahlung, in which "loosely bound electrons are accelerated by the strong electric field associated with the laser pulse. Collisions with neighboring atoms and molecules can then result in local thermal effects" (Goldman and Rockwell, 1971).
5. Double-photon absorption, which may produce a transitory excited state or cellular death.
6. Free-radical formation.

## ANALYSIS OF THE REACTIONS

Tissue reactions may be observed with the naked eye and photographed either by photographic techniques including stereophotomicrography or by scanning electron microscopy (SEM) (Fig. 2.1). Temperature changes may be measured by thermistors, by the application of liquid crystals, or by infrared thermography. The reactions in tissues have also been studied by histopathologic, histochemical (including enzyme and biochemical studies), transmission electron microscopy (TEM), and scanning electron microscopy (SEM) techniques.

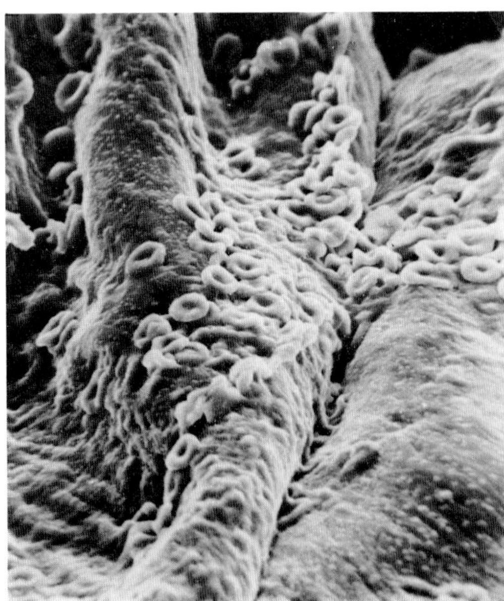

**Fig. 2.1.** Scanning electron microscopy used to study intravascular effects of laser impact on blood vessel. (Courtesy of Johanna Vahl.)

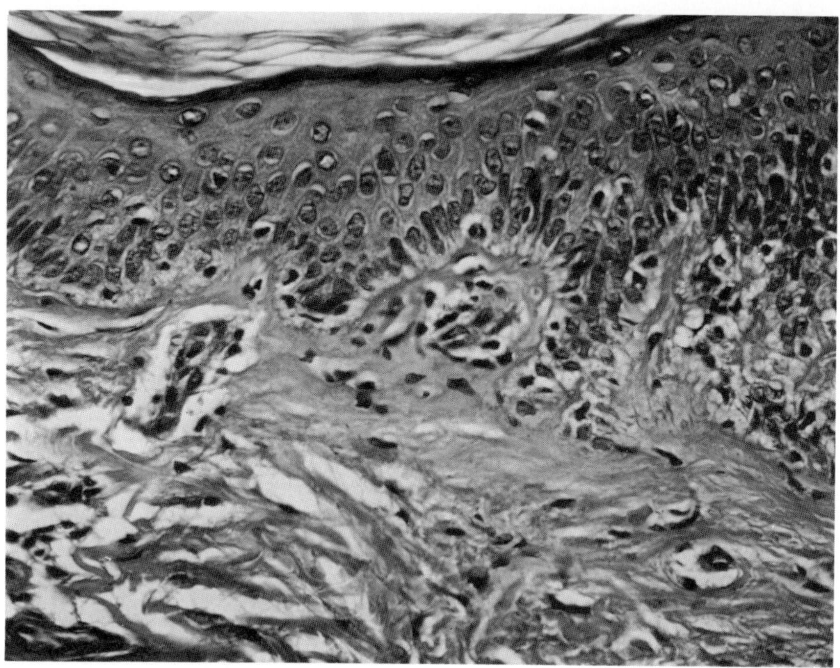

**Fig. 2.2.** Skin of back of hand of elderly male with chronic sun exposure examined after 80 impacts of pulsed ruby laser (20 $J/cm^2$) over a period of months. Minimal changes in epidermis and dermis are same as those in control area (not shown) on the same hand. There is no evidence of precancerous or cancerous change (H&E ×160).

The tissue effects of lasers have been observed in model test systems. The effects of microirradiation on cells in tissue culture have been monitored. Controlled experiments have been performed on animals, and patients have been treated. Controlled studies are under way in many institutions around the world to clarify further the effects of lasers on tissues. Thus far there is no evidence that laser residues have any carcinogenic properties (Figs. 2.2 and 2.3). It is not known whether this will be true with the use and abuse of ultraviolet (UV), vacuum ultraviolet (VUV), and x-ray lasers. For sensitive individuals, incoherent UV irradiation also may be carcinogenic.

## IMPLEMENTATION OF A NEW LASER SYSTEM

The implementation of laser systems follows the basic pattern seen in the adoption of other medical techniques. Initially, a group of people interested in the new technique is established and begins to work separately. Safety requirements for the operator and for experimental animals are developed. Tissue effects are determined, and experimental pathologic studies are conducted to ascertain whether the new technology is effective in human disease. Laser has progressed through

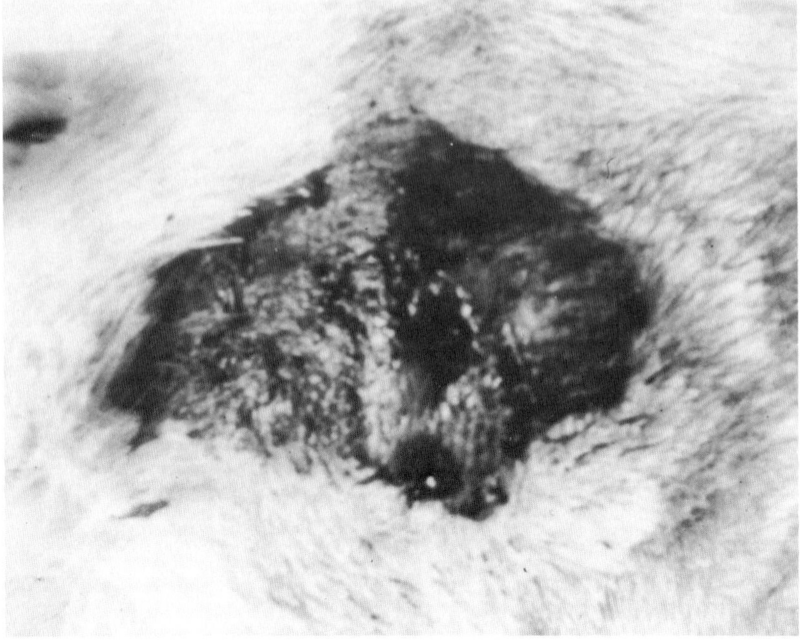

**Fig. 2.3.** Malignant vascular tumor induced in animal by Thorotrast to study laser impact on angiosarcoma.

these various phases and is now in the broad phase of adaptation to the control of human disease states.

The continuing development of smaller, more flexible, and less costly devices with more adaptable beams and greater ease of application will make the laser even safer and more effective in the future.

## SUMMARY

Although the laser holds great promise for future use in medicine and surgery, its use at present is restricted by such limitations as lack of communications, inadequate safety measures, lack of flexibility in application, insufficient knowledge of probable reactions and suitable indications, inadequate controls, and cost. It is anticipated that these handicaps will be overcome as understanding of, and experience in, the use of the laser increase.

## REFERENCE

Goldman L, Rockwell RJ Jr. (1971) Lasers in Medicine. Gordon and Breach, New York, p. 207.

# 3

# Safety with Biomedical Lasers

*David H. Sliney*

Today, despite the wide use of lasers in industry, the potential for hazardous exposure to laser radiation is still probably greatest for the laser research worker and for biomedical personnel engaged in using lasers in surgical applications. This risk is due to the need for flexibility in the arrangement of laser-beam delivery systems (see Chapter 1) and to the requirements for unenclosed, high-power laser beams in these specialized applications.

In most industrial production utilizing medium-power and high-power lasers, engineering control measures (e.g., enclosures) are employed to prevent exposure of workers in the vicinity of the equipment. In the operating room and biomedical research laboratory, in contrast, administrative safety measures are emphasized. Few scientists and engineers consider the installation of permanent beam enclosures, interlocks, and similar fixtures since optical-beam paths can change daily, if not hourly. Laser surgical procedures cannot be accomplished within enclosures. Under these laser-operating conditions, eye protection and protective clothing are normally worn despite the associated reduction in visual capabilities and the possible discomfort.

These generalities do not apply to many of the laser devices used in commercial instruments. For example, the lasers employed in specialized holographic instruments, laser-particle–sizing instruments, and Raman spectrometers are generally well-enclosed, and there is no risk to the user. These products, like other complete laser systems, normally include sufficient engineering controls to preclude any risk. However, unenclosed lasers, originally used as tools in research, are finding their way into some biophysics laboratories for basic studies in photobiology and photochemistry. These latter applications often require open-beam laboratory arrangements and, therefore, the many control measures mentioned in the foregoing paragraph.

## HAZARD ANALYSIS AND LASER CLASSIFICATION

There are three criteria for evaluating laser hazards: (1) the laser itself and its inherent dangers; (2) the environment in which the laser is used (i.e., indoors, outdoors, etc.); and (3) the people who may potentially be exposed to laser radiation, and the people who operate the laser. The first situation is dealt with by using a laser hazard classification scheme that is now almost universally accepted. The latter two hazards may have to be considered if the laser is not in a fail-safe enclosure. Experience and judgment must be exercised by the user or a laser safety officer (LSO).

Safety standards for lasers aid considerably in hazard analysis and controls. The most prominent standard was first produced in 1973 and has since been revised: American National Standards Institute (ANSI, 1976), Safe Use of Lasers. A new edition of the ANSI standard was approved in 1980. Several other organizations have followed suit with safety standards that are comparable: the American Conference of Governmental Industrial Hygienists (AGGIH, 1976), the World Health Organization, and the International Electrotechnical Commission. More importantly, the Food and Drug Administration's Bureau of Radiological Health (BRH) now regulates the manufacture and sale of laser products in the United States (US Department of Health, Education, and Welfare, 1979). This regulation requires that the manufacturer must classify the laser product and thereby greatly aids the user in determining what control measures, if any, are necessary.

The basic concept of the classification schemes of ANSI, ACGIH, WHO, IEC, and BRH is as follows:

Class I laser products are essentially safe and are typically enclosed systems which do not emit hazardous levels.

Class II laser products are limited to visible lasers that are safe for momentary viewing but should not be stared into continuously unless the exposure is within the recommended ocular exposure limits (ELs); the dazzle of the brilliant visible light source would normally preclude staring into the source.

Class III laser products are not safe even for momentary viewing, and procedural controls and protective equipment are normally required with their use.

Class IV laser products are normally considered much more hazardous than class III devices since they may represent a significant fire hazard or skin hazard and may also produce hazardous diffuse reflections. Hazardous diffuse reflections are of particular concern because the probability of hazardous retinal exposure (if the laser operates between 400 and 1400 nm) is far greater than if the exposure were possible only from specular reflections.

General concepts of laser safety are dealt with quite adequately in the aforementioned standards and elsewhere (e.g., Sliney and Wolbarsht, 1980) and will not be discussed further here. The hazard classification of the lasers most commonly encountered in biomedical applications is presented in Table 3.1.

In contrast to laser classification limits, ELs are probably used far less frequently. This is due to the fact that in most applications there is no intentional exposure of

**Table 3.1.** Hazard Classification of Some Representative Lasers*

| Laser type | Wavelength(s) | BRH and ANSI Z-136.1 classification |
|---|---|---|
| Argon, CW | 488 nm, 514 nm | Class I if power output $\Phi < 0.4\ \mu W$, class II if $\leqslant$ to 1 mW; class III up to 0.5 W; and class IV above 0.5 W |
| Helium-neon, CW | 632.8 nm | BRH classification is same as for argon laser; ANSI classification is same except that upper limit of class I is 6.5 $\mu$W |
| Neodymium-YAG, CW | 1064 nm | Class I if power output $\Phi < 0.62$ mW; no class II; class III up to 0.5 W; Class IV for $\Phi > 0.5$W |
| Neodymium-YAG, Q-switched, 10-ns pulse | 1064 nm | Class I if single pulse, and energy $< 2\ \mu J$; no class II: class III if above class I and radiant exposure at output $< 0.34\ J/cm^2$; class IV if radiant exposure is $> 0.34\ J/cm^2$ |
| Carbon dioxide, CW | 10.6 $\mu$m | Class I if output power does not exceed 0.8 mW; no class II; class III if $<$ 0.5 W; class IV if $>$ 0.5 W |
| Gallium-arsenide, CW or PRF $>$ 10 kHz | 910 nm | Class I if power $< 10\ \mu W$ (BRH) or $<$ 0.31 mW (ANSI); no class II; class III if power $>$ class I and $\leq$ 0.5 W; class IV if output power $>$ 0.5 W |

*The values apply only to single-mode lasers or lasers that are nearly "point" sources. These conditions are typical of most of the lasers listed.

personnel. Of course, in some biomedical applications this is not the case, and ELs must be determined. Furthermore, the applicability of the EL to the patient must be considered in both diagnostic and therapeutic applications. The ELs for some of the most common laser exposure conditions of interest to biomedical personnel are presented in Table 3.2. It is emphasized that the ELs were based upon the premise that the potentially exposed individual is awake and not restrained or under medication or anesthesia. There is typically a factor of 3–10 between the EL and the level that produces a clearly visible reaction in tissue. The limits were designed to be sufficiently low to preclude adverse functional or any delayed effects. The limits cannot be considered as fine lines between safe and dangerous conditions. If exposure of patients occurs at levels above the EL, a benefit-vs-risk judgment is clearly required. If the eye is exposed to laser radiation under conditions in which ordinary pupil reactions and eye movement would not take place, the ELs would not be sufficiently conservative to preclude a risk of injury. Likewise, if the skin is exposed to ultraviolet or visible radiation at levels above the applicable EL following the administration of photosensitizing drugs, the EL may not be sufficiently conservative. To analyze the risk of unintentional injury of tissue under these conditions, it may be necessary to review reports on laser bioeffects studies (Goldman and Rockwell, 1971; Sliney and Wolbarsht, 1980; Wolbarsht, 1972).

**Table 3.2.** Exposure Limits[a] of Some Representative Lasers

| Laser type | Wavelength(s) | Ocular exposure limit | Skin exposure limit |
|---|---|---|---|
| Argon | 488 nm, 514.5 nm | 0.5 $\mu$J/cm$^2$ for 1 ns to 18 $\mu$s; 1.8 $t^{3/4}$ mJ/cm$^2$ from 18 $\mu$s to 10 s; 10 mJ/cm$^2$ from 10 s to 10,000 s; and 1 $\mu$W/cm$^2$ for greater durations | 0.02 J/cm$^2$ for 1 ns to 100 ns; 1.1 $t^{1/4}$J/cm$^2$ for 100 ns to 10 s; 0.2 W/cm$^2$ for greater durations |
| Helium-neon | 632.8 nm | 0.5 $\mu$J/cm$^2$ for 1 ns to 18 $\mu$s; 1.8 $t^{3/4}$ mJ/cm$^2$ from 18 $\mu$s to 450 s; 170 mJ/cm$^2$ from 10 s to 10,000 s; and 17 $\mu$W/cm$^2$ for greater durations | Same as for argon laser |
| Neodymium-YAG | 1064 nm | 5 $\mu$J/cm$^2$ for 1 ns to 50 $\mu$s; 9 $t^{3/4}$ mJ/cm$^2$ from 50 $\mu$s to 1000 s; and 1.6 mW/cm$^2$ for greater durations | 0.1 J/cm$^2$ for 1 ns to 100 ns; 5.5 $t^{1/4}$ J/cm$^2$ for 100 ns to 10 s; 1.0 W/cm$^2$ for greater durations |
| Gallium-arsenide | 910 nm | 1.3 $\mu$J/cm$^2$ for 1 ns to 18 $\mu$s; 4.5 $t^{3/4}$ mJ/cm$^2$ from 18 $\mu$s to 1000 s; 0.8 mW/cm$^2$ for greater durations | 0.05 J/cm$^2$ for 1 ns to 100 ns; 2.8 $t^{1/4}$ J/cm$^2$ for 100 ns to 10 s; 0.5 W/cm$^2$ for greater exposure durations |
| Carbon dioxide | 10.6 $\mu$m | 10 mJ/cm$^2$ for 1 ns to 100 ns; 0.56 $t^{1/4}$ J/cm$^2$ for 100 ns to 10 s; and 0.1 W/cm$^2$ for greater exposure durations | Same as ocular EL values |

[a] The exposure limit is averaged over a 7-mm aperture for wavelengths between 400 and 1400 nm for the eye limits only. The other exposure limits are defined for a 1-mm measuring aperture. Repetitive pulses at rates less than 1 pulse per second were assumed for any repetitive exposures. Higher repetition rates require more adjustments of exposure limits.

## ENCLOSED LASERS AND ENCLOSED FACILITIES

Clearly the soundest and safest laser applications are those in which the laser and hazardous beam paths are completely enclosed. As previously noted, this approach may not be possible in all biomedical applications. When the laser of class III or class IV is used in the open, the laser operation should be carried out in a completely enclosed facility. This is not to say that the facility must be airtight and "light tight." So long as there is no direct beam path outside the facility there should be no problem. The use of diffusing baffles, door interlocks, and opaque window shades is called for in most situations. It is not necessary to seal light leaks at the bottom of doors or at vents well above eye level.

## OPEN-BEAM PATHS IN EXPERIMENTAL ARRANGEMENTS

Several general safety procedures have been employed with great success when open beams are being used. Open beams are necessary in surgery and in situations requiring that optical elements along the path be continuously adjusted. The output power of the laser should first be optimized by placing a calorimeter or other radiometric instrument as close to the beam exit as possible. This should enclose the beam path where feasible. Once the laser output has been optimized, a variable-output device can be installed—again, as close to the beam port as possible. For CW laser power outputs of less than 1 W, polarizing elements can be rotated in the normally polarized laser beam to serve as a variable attenuator. Variable-reflectance beam splitters may also serve in this role if the unused secondary beam is terminated in a beam trap. Variable attenuators are most valuable when adjustment of electrical power to the laser alters the beam or is otherwise unacceptable. In essence, the laser safety filter is placed over the beam instead of over the eyes. If the beam remains static during the experiment, it may be not be necessary to wear eye protection, particularly if it is not necessary to view the beam path once the experimental setup has been aligned.

A common complaint of research workers who have used argon lasers is that the commercially available eye-protection filters have such enormous optical densities that the beam is not only safe but also invisible. In many of these instances, the installation of a fixed or variable attenuator to reduce the laser-beam power to 1 mW reduces the risk of eye injury from momentary viewing, while still permitting visibility of the beam. An alternative method for visualizing the position of the

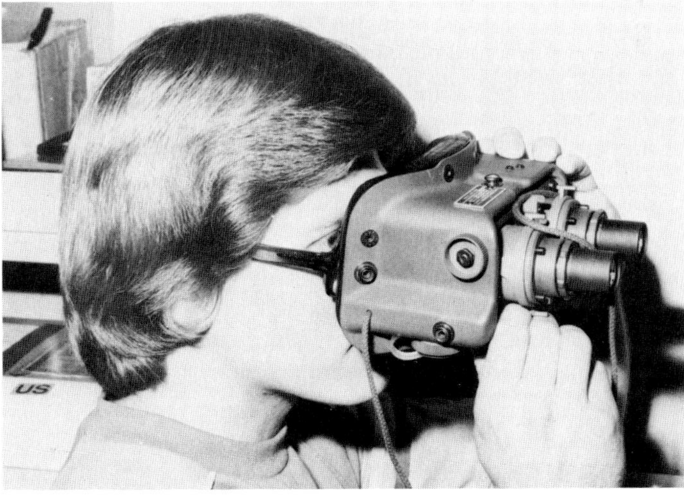

**Fig. 3.1.** Image-converter goggles or image-converter monoculars may be used to visualize laser beams while also protecting eyes from injury.

beam through eye protectors makes use of a fluorescent card. The longer-wavelength fluorescence of the card can be seen through the protective filter. Image-converter monoculars or goggles (Fig. 3.1) may also permit safe viewing of the beam's location and may even render normally invisible ultraviolet or near-infrared beams visible. Studies performed by Lyon at the US Army Environmental Hygiene Agency have demonstrated that modern image-converter tubes sometimes transmit a small fraction of incident laser radiation, but this is insignificant and not hazardous (Sliney and Wolbarsht, 1980). The disadvantages of image converters—or for that matter, of closed-circuit television systems—are some loss of detail, a limited field of view, and a monochrome presentation. Vidicons and image-converter tubes may also be damaged by direct laser exposure at levels comparable to retinal damage levels, and this factor must be considered prior to use if direct intrabeam illumination of the tube is expected. Such television and converter systems are becoming more common when tunable dye lasers are in use. On the other hand, the use of a single dye does not always require such an approach since each dye has a limited spectral range.

## CONTROLLED ENTRY TO FACILITIES

For open-beam class IV laser operations (and even some higher-power class III operations), it is often customary during the laser firing to limit entry to only those persons actually engaged in laser research. When this approach is followed, the laboratory is termed a "controlled area" (ANSI, 1976). This approach is advisable when eye protection is not the principal control measure and when the laboratory personnel require instruction in basic laser safety procedures and are well-familiarized with the experimental arrangement and potentially dangerous conditions (Burch and Gates, 1967). At one time this practice was more common when such a restriction was necessary to limit those requiring eye examinations. In any case, a laboratory director is often receptive to such a policy for no other reason than to keep away the curious.

Entry restrictions are administrative and enforced through the use of signs, special door latches, and interlocks. Class IV laser installations should have door interlocks that are connected to the remote control connector required by the BRH Laser Product Performance Standard. Such a system precludes accidental injury of unprotected personnel entering the laser facility during laser operation; the laser beam is either blocked or shut off when the door is opened. This may be undesirable during use of a surgical laser, and entry control and barriers between the laser and the entrance may be alternative control methods.

## MEDICAL LASERS—SPECIAL CONSIDERATIONS

Many of the safety problems common to the research laboratory apply to the clinical setting as well. Although clinical studies of laser applications in medicine have seldom emphasized the collection of minimal biologic threshold data, clinical experience has produced most of the evidence to support the extrapolation of animal tissue reaction thresholds to human subjects. This is particularly true for skin exposure limits (Goldman and Rockwell, 1971; Rockwell and Goldman, 1974). Studies directed toward better understanding of tissue injury mechanisms have also had a direct impact on safety limits as well as on clinical applications.

The application of specific laser laboratory precautions to the clinical setting is often difficult. Problems arise because the object of the medical application is often to destroy or coagulate tissue, whereas the aim of the safety rules is to minimize or prevent human exposure to hazardous levels. All user safety standards include a clause that excludes irrelevant restrictions on the medical exposure of humans to laser radiation. The primary requirement for safe laser cutting or coagulation of tissue is adequate training of the personnel administering treatment. In the United States, the BRH has set rules that exclude the requirement for a marking of the exit port of a medical laser with a warning label (USDHEW, 1979), but the BRH regulations do require other special features for medical laser products:

1040.11 Specific Purpose Laser Products

(a) Medical laser products. Each medical laser product shall comply with all of the applicable requirements of 1040.10 for laser products of its class. In addition, the manufacturer shall:

(1) Incorporate in each Class III or IV medical laser product a means for the measurement of the level of that laser radiation intended for irradiation of the human body with an error in measurement of no more than $\pm 20$ percent when calibrated in accordance with paragraph (a)(2) of this section. Indication of the measurement shall be in International System Units.

(2) Supply with each Class III or IV medical laser product instructions specifying a procedure and schedule for calibration of the measurement system required by paragraph (a)(1) of this section.

(3) Affix to each medical laser product, in close proximity to each aperture through which is emitted accessible laser radiation in excess of the emission limits of Class I, a label bearing the wording: "Laser aperture."

In addition to the BRH safety requirements, the Bureau of Medical Devices, also of the Food and Drug Administration, requires that the device be registered. A medical device classification is then applied by that organization.

One of the best safety design strategies for laser surgical devices is the use of a short-focal-length lens in the beam-delivery system. Although not always feasible, this feature should dramatically reduce the probability of a very hazardous exposure of personnel in the vicinity of the laser device. The use of fiber-optical light guides of high numerical aperture will also produce a rapidly diverging beam of laser radiation and reduce the chance of unintended hazardous exposure. Positive-action exposure switches, beam shutters, and key-lock master control switches are all features that provide additional safety for the user and the patient. It is generally agreed that only class I or class II lasers should be used in diagnostic instruments unless the actual patient exposure is otherwise ensured to be below the applicable ELs.

## SURGICAL LASERS

With the development of modern portable surgical lasers, the designation of a specific operating room for laser surgery has become less common. During the development of surgical lasers, such specialized facilities were designed (e.g., Goldman and Rockwell, 1971; Goldman and Hornby, 1965; Goldman, 1967; Riggle et al. 1971; Gamaleya, 1977). Today, three types of lasers are most commonly employed in surgical procedures utilizing lasers: the argon laser (488 nm and 514.5 nm), the neodymium laser (1064 nm), and the carbon dioxide laser (10.6 μm). Details of the special applications and advantages of each are discussed in other chapters of this book. From a safety standpoint, it is worthwhile to remember that of these three types of lasers the $CO_2$ laser's far-infrared-wavelength radiation does not penetrate the ocular media of the eye and is therefore far less of a hazard to the eye than the other two types of lasers for the same power level.

Hazardous laser reflections are the primary safety concern from the standpoint of laser radiation safety. When endoscopic delivery systems (Auth et al., 1976) are used, the concern for reflections is less, but one must still be concerned with backflash. The best illustration of the reflective hazards associated with a surgical laser beam in the open is that of a reflection from a flat metal surface for a beam with the following characteristics. A beam radiant power $\Phi$ of 20 W in a beam of initial diameter $a$ of 5 mm is focused to a spot diameter $D_f$ of 0.1 mm by a lens with a focal length $f$ of 50 mm. We shall make use of the fact that the divergence of a reflected beam from a focal spot on a flat specular surface is the same as the convergence of the initial beam. Beam divergence $\phi$ is defined as the change in beam diameter (i.e., $\Delta D$) divided by the path length, which in this case is $f$ for a change of diameter from 5 mm to 0.1 mm:

$$\phi = \Delta D/f = 4.9 \text{ mm}/50 \text{ mm} = 0.098 \text{ rad} \quad (1)$$

Obviously the divergence is enormous compared to a normal, collimated laser beam. However, despite this large divergence of 98 mrad, the large radiant power of 20 W requires calculating the laser-beam irradiance E at a distance $r_1$ from the reflecting surface. We shall assume a worst case of 100% reflectance, which may be approached for 10.6-μm radiation incident upon stainless steel or aluminum. The applicable formula is as follows:

$$E = 1.27\Phi/(a + r_1 \cdot \phi)^2 \quad (2)$$

At a distance of 30 cm, the irradiance would be as follows:

$$\begin{aligned} E &= 1.27(20)/[0.1 + (30)(0.098)]^2 \\ &= 2.9 \text{ W/cm}^2 \end{aligned}$$

At a viewing distance $r_1$ of 100 cm, the irradiance would be much lower:

$$\begin{aligned} E &= 1.27\ (20)/\ [0.1 + (100)(0.098)]^2 \\ &= 0.26 \text{ W/cm}^2 \end{aligned}$$

## Protective Measures

By the present ANSI Z-136.1 limits given in Table 3.2, the maximum permissible exposure duration for an irradiance of 2.9 $W/cm^2$ is 0.11 s and for an irradiance of 0.26 $W/cm^2$ is 2.8 s for the 10.6-$\mu$m wavelength. For the argon and neodymium wavelengths, these irradiances would be hazardous for extremely short durations, and eye protection would be absolutely essential. Even for the $CO_2$ laser wavelength, the use of clear plastic eye protectors would be advisable. The aforementioned irradiances would not present a very serious risk of skin injury although they would exceed ELs for the skin for durations almost the same as for the $CO_2$ laser. A considerable experience with laser surgical equipment has demonstrated that eye protection is essential and skin protection is often not called for. Certainly face shields and heavy protective clothing are unnecessary when one is using CW lasers.

Reflections of argon and neodymium laser radiation back through a fiber-optic endoscope (backflash) must be attenuated with protective filters built into the endoscopic viewer. Studies by Gulacsik et al. (1979) showed that the reflections back through the laser catheter were of the order of 2 mW for a specular reflection backflash returning through the endoscope per watt of power at the distal end of the fiber-optic delivery system used for Nd-YAG systems, and less than 1 mW/W for the argon systems. They used a quartz glass target to represent the worst-case specular reflection from the mucosal membrane of the intestine. Thus, minimal filtration would be required to protect the surgeon's eye from injury during momentary viewing. Eye protection having an optical density of 3 or 4 would be required at the argon wavelengths to provide protection as well as comfortable viewing during extended exposures. An optical density of 1.5–2 would be required at the neodymium-YAG wavelength. The operator's exposure when viewing a diffuse reflection was always far less, and added eye protection would not be required purely for such viewing.

The BRH requires that medical laser products (like all laser products marketed in the United States) have a protective housing that prevents human access to hazardous laser radiation at all points except the designated exit port of a beam. Laser emission should not be present at connections of beam guides and at fiber-optic connectors. The connectors of fiber-optic cables to the laser output should therefore be designed so that if the cable is removed, a spring-loaded shutter or similar device terminates any laser emission.

Laser surgical instruments are often operated by a footswitch to allow the surgeon freedom for his or her hands. The footswitch should be operable only after a master control switch is thrown. An emergency shutdown switch should also be located at a point of ready access.

Quite often surgeons have available a fire-resistant target such as alumina or silicon-carbide firebrick to focus a hand-held laser "scalpel." This inanimate target aids the surgeon in developing a feel for the instrument and provides a visible indication of the size and location of the focal spot. Metallic surfaces are not acceptable for this practice.

Eye protection for all personnel within the operating room is almost always required for laser surgical operations. Surgeons using $CO_2$ laser instruments should be reminded that materials that do not appear specular (mirrorlike) to the eye may be specular at the 10.6-$\mu$m wavelength (e.g., enamel metal and brushed metal surfaces). The beam should not be directed near any such surface, particularly if the surface is flat. Fortunately, most surgical instruments have convex metal surfaces that produce highly divergent reflections, and these instruments should be used in preference to any with flat surfaces. If instruments having concave surfaces must be used, such instruments should first be tested by directing a laser beam at the surface under controlled conditions to determine the extent of any recollimation of the beam upon reflection.

As a summary, the following standard precautions may significantly reduce the chance of personnel injury from laser radiation in a setting where laser surgery is employed:

1. Drape the area of surgical incision with wet towels or gauze, usually sterile saline solution, rather than dry towels to avoid towel or gauze combustion.
2. Use focusing guides that not only assist the surgeon in keeping the focal spot on the tissue but also reduce the chance of hazardous specular reflection because of their geometry.
3. Exclude combustible anesthetic gases from laser surgical procedures (see Snow et al., 1974).
4. Employ a positive-action (dead-man) switch. This may be either a hand-operated switch or footswitch to ensure rapid shutoff in case of emergency.
5. Prohibit operation and potential misuse of the laser by unauthorized personnel. This may best be accomplished by the use of a key-switch master control. This device is required in the United States by the BRH regulation for all surgical lasers manufactured since August 1976.

## LASER RETINAL PHOTOCOAGULATORS

Far more common than other surgical lasers, the funduscopic laser photocoagulators used in treating retinal diseases require many of the precautions previously discussed. Although the ophthalmic lasers emit less optical power than the aforementioned surgical lasers, they are still class IV. Almost all ophthalmic photocoagulators employ an argon laser, although ruby lasers were at one time developed for treating detached retinas. The optical delivery systems in common commercial instruments differ, but the majority now use a slit-lamp biomicroscope which can be adjusted to deliver a variable cone of radiation to the retina. The beam generally is of a small divergence, and the optical power entering the eye normally exceeds 0.2 W and may range upward to 1.5 W. Although the power normally delivered to the eye is less than 0.5 W (the upper limit of class III), this beam power still represents a serious eye hazard if misdirected. Unfortunately, because of the low divergence of the beams now used with contact lenses, the beam irradiance does not decrease rapidly with distance. The ophthalmologist views the fundus under treatment through the viewing optics (Fig. 3.2).

The reflection of the treatment beam from the cornea is a very small fraction of the initial beam power but may be of concern. A collimated beam striking the

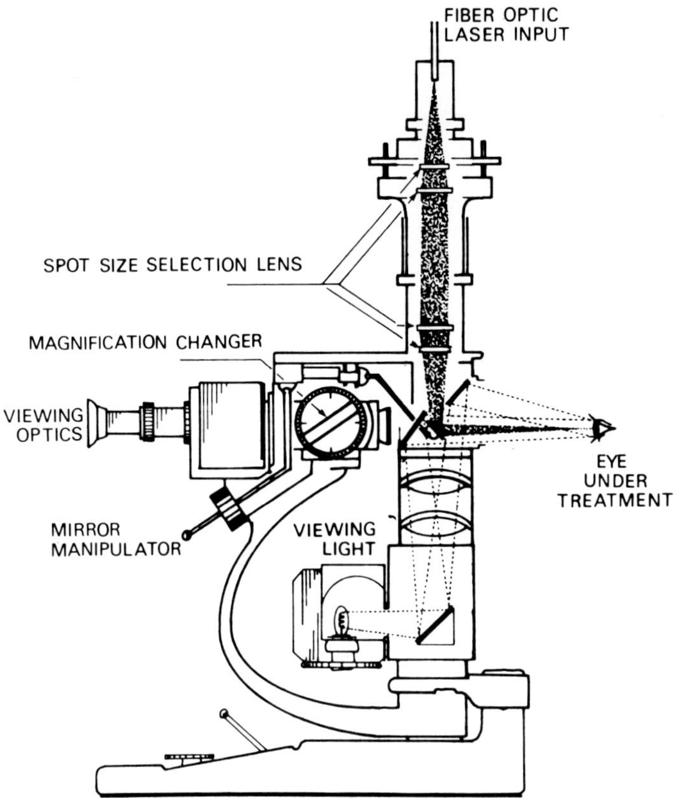


**Fig. 3.2.** Cross-sectional view of laser retinal photocoagulator illustrates laser-beam path for a slit-lamp delivery system using fiber-optic beam input from the laser. (Adapted from Sliney DH, Wolbarsht ML, Safety with Lasers and Other Optical Sources. Plenum Publishing Corp., New York, 1980.)

clear cornea would provide the sharpest cone of back-reflection. As the beam strikes the exposed corneal surface, only a 2% normal reflection is encountered. This value is calculated by the classic Fresnel equation (Sliney and Wolbarsht, 1980), using a refractive index of 1.33 for the cornea. A reflection at a distance $r_1$ of 30 cm from the cornea may be of the order of 10m W/cm$^2$ for 1 W incident upon a 3-mm corneal spot. Because of the design of most delivery systems, a reflected beam from the bare cornea is terminated by the instrument itself. However, when a gonial contact lens is used (the common practice), a hazardous reflected beam can be deflected at angles that pass through openings in some instruments or to the side of the instrument (Jenkins, 1979). Reflections from a low-power alignment beam less than 1 mW initially are not hazardous for any reasonable exposure duration. All specular reflections from the contact lens should be considered hazardous, even if the contact lens is anti-reflection-coated. In the latter case, the hazard still extends to 1.6 m from the lens. All personnel except the ophthalmologist viewing the fundus should wear appropriate eye protection. The

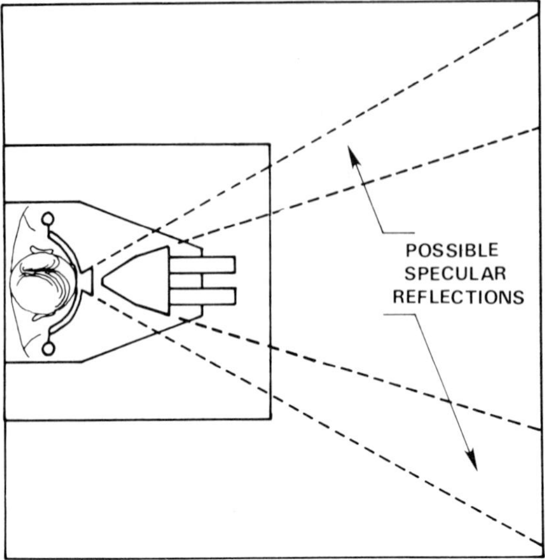


**Fig. 3.3.** Secondary beams from a retinal photocoagulator. Reflected from flat surfaces on corneal contact lens, these beams represent a potential hazard to the eyes of adjacent, unprotected personnel. (Adapted from Jenkins DL, Non-Ionizing Radiation Protection Special Study No. 25-42-0310-79. Hazard Evaluation of the Coherent Model 900 Photocoagulator Laser System, Jan.-Feb. 1979. US Army Environmental Hygiene Agency. Aberdeen Proving Ground, MD, [NTIS No. ADA 068713].)

ophthalmologist is protected by a filter in the viewing optics, which is always in place during the use of the therapy beam.

The ophthalmologist adjusts the low-power beam on the retina prior to using the treatment beam. As he or she must see the beam on the retina, there is no filter in place in the sighting optics. The specular reflections from a contact lens that is not anti-reflection-coated would be of the order of a few microwatts, which may appear dazzling to the ophthalmologist but are not hazardous even in the context of the number of possible exposures in 1 day.

The only serious safety problem encountered with the argon laser photocoagulators has been the reflected secondary beam from a contact lens (Fig. 3.3).

## LASER DIAGNOSTIC EQUIPMENT

Although the laser's unique characteristics suggest that it could be useful in medical diagnosis, it is not as yet widely used for this purpose. One of the most interesting applications has been the utilization of the speckle characteristics of coherent laser light for direct measurement of refractive errors of the human eye. The laser power used in these applications is very low. A 1-mW HeNe laser is adequate if the ambient illumination is low, and special precautions for such a low-power laser are minimal. In another application, HeNe-laser interference fringes can be produced at the retina despite serious loss of transparency in the anterior structures of the eye (Green, 1970). In these cases, the retinal irradiances are very safe (Wolbarsht and Landers, 1979). Holographic studies of the retina and laser Doppler measurement of eye movement (Riva et al., 1979) are still other nontherapeutic laser applications in ophthalmology that do not require exposure levels exceeding current ELs. For all the diagnostic techniques other than holography, the retina is always exposed to a very low irradiance, well within the comfort range and therefore well below hazardous levels. It is only when the output of the laser system is focused on the retina that there should be any concern for hazard.

Laser microprobes used in cell studies or for chemical analysis require enclosure or baffling of the target spot. Such pulsed laser systems are also sometimes used in controlled areas where eye protection is worn. One problem reported with such instruments has been the spread of potentially toxic materials (Marich et al., 1972). This problem may be unique to pulsed laser microprobes.

Many of the ophthalmic laboratories in the United States now use automatic lens refractometers which make use of a class II HeNe laser. The lens to be measured is placed over a lens cone on a lens holder, and the laser beam is directed up through the lens. The operator of the instrument is normally unable to place his or her eye within the beam, and scattered radiation is perfectly safe to view. Only if a mirror is placed at the location where the lens is positioned can the beam be deflected out into the room, and then the power is within the class II range which is safe to view momentarily.

Still other laser applications such as cell sorting (Mullaney et al., 1974) and ultrasonic imaging (Harding and Baker, 1968) in which lasers play a role in the instrument present no hazard for the user. With product performance requirements of the federal government applied to these devices, potentially hazardous exposures could occur only to servicing technicians. A very comprehensive laser safety training program should be mandatory for technicians who service laser equipment containing class III or class IV lasers.

Alignment lasers that emit class II levels—typically ranging from 0.04 to 0.1 mW per beam—are used for patient positioning in radiation teletherapy. In this application the laser beam should not be directed at the patient's eyes even though the levels would almost always be safe. This policy would avoid unwarranted concerns on the part of the patient.

## SUMMARY

With the ever-increasing use of lasers in medicine and surgery, it is essential that the designers of such equipment be knowledgeable regarding the adverse effects of laser radiation and the need for appropriate hazard-control measures. It is also essential to remember that ELs were developed for the normal person and may not always apply to a photosensitive patient or to a patient receiving certain medications or under anesthesia.

## REFERENCES

American Conference of Governmental Industrial Hygienists (ACGIH) (1976) A Guide for Control of Laser Hazards, ACGIH. PO Box 1937, Cincinnati, Ohio.

American National Standards Institute (ANSI) (1976) Safe Use of Lasers, Standard Z-136.1-1976. ANSI, 1430 Broadway, New York.

Auth DC, Lam VTY, Mohr RW, Silverstein FE, Rubin CE (1976) A high-power gastric photocoagulator for fiberoptic endoscopy. IEEE Trans BME 23(2): 129–135.

Burch JM, Gates JWC (1967) Lasers: Practical control and protection in experimental laboratories. Ann Occup Hyg 10(Laser Safety Suppl.): 65–73.

Gamaleya NF (1977) Laser biomedical research in the USSR. In Wolbarsht ML (ed) Laser Applications in Medicine and Biology. Plenum Publishing Corp., New York, vol. 3, pp. 1–173.

Goldman L (1967) Laser laboratory design. In: CRC Handbook of Laboratory Safety. Chemical Rubber Co., Cleveland, Ohio, pp. 294–301.

Goldman L, Hornby P (1965) The design of a medical laser laboratory. Arch Environ Health 10: 493–497.

Goldman L, Rockwell RJ (1971) Lasers in Medicine. Gordon and Breach, New York.

Green DG (1970) Testing the vision of cataract patients by means of laser-generated interference fringes. Science 168: 1240–1242.

Gulacsik C, Auth DC, Silverstein FE (1979) Ophthalmic hazards associated with laser endoscopy. Appl Opt 18(11): 1816–1823.

Harding DC, Baker DW (1968) Laser Schlieren optical system for analyzing ultrasonic fields. Biomed Sci Instrum 4: 223–230.

Jenkins DL (1979) Non-Ionizing Radiation Protection Special Study No. 25-42-0310-79, Hazard Evaluation of the Coherent Model 900 Photocoagulator Laser System, Jan.–Feb. 1979. US Army Environmental Hygiene Agency. Aberdeen Proving Ground, Maryland (NTIS No. ADA068713).

Marich KW, Orenberg JB, Treytl WJ, Glick D (1972) Health hazards in the use of the laser microprobe for toxic and infective samples. Am Ind Hyg Assoc J 33(7): 488–491.

Mullaney PG, Steinkamp JA, Crissman HA, Cram LS, Holm DM (1974) Laser flow microspectrophotometers for rapid analysis and sorting of individual mammalian cells. In: Wolbarsht ML (ed) Laser Applications in Medicine and Biology.Plenum Publishing Corp., New York, vol. 2, pp. 151–204.

Riggle GC, Hoyle RC, Ketcham AS (1971) Laser effects on normal and tumor tissue. In: Wolbarsht ML (ed) Laser Applications in Medicine and Biology. Plenum Publishing Corp., New York, vol. 1, pp. 35–65.

Riva CE, Timberlake GT, Feke GT (1979) Laser Doppler technique for measurement of eye movement. Appl Opt 18(14): 2486–2490.

Rockwell RJ Jr, Goldman L (1974) Research on Human Skin Laser Damage Thresholds. Final Report, Contract F41609-72-C-0007. USAF School of Aerospace Medicine, Brooks AFB, TX, prepared by Department of Dermatology and Laser Lab., Medical Center, University of Cincinnati.

Sliney DH, Wolbarsht ML (1980) Safety with Lasers and Other Optical Sources. Plenum Publishing Corp., New York.

Snow JC, Kripke BJ, Strong MS, Jako GJ, Meyer MR, Vaughan CW (1974) Anesthesia for carbon-dioxide laser microsurgery on the larynx and trachea. Anesth Analg (Cleve) 53: 507–512.

US Department of Health Education and Welfare (USDHEW) (1979) Title 21, Code of Federal Regulations, Part 1040, Light Emitting Products, Govt. Printing Office, Washington, D.C.

Wolbarsht ML (ed) (1972) Laser Applications in Medicine and Biology, vol. 1. Plenum Publishing Corp., New York.

Wolbarsht ML, Landers MB III (1979) Lasers in ophthalmology: The path from theory to application. Appl Opt 18: 1518–1526.

World Health Organization (1981) Optical radiation, with particular reference to lasers. In: Manual for Non-Ionizing Radiation. WHO European Office, Copenhagen.

# 4

# Instrumentation for Laser Biology and Laser Diagnostic Medicine

*Leon Goldman*

Prior to the development of laser technology, Bessis had developed techniques for microirradiation with ultraviolet light. He was also one of the early pioneers in using laser microirradiation. This technique has continued to develop through studies on the impact of microirradiation on red blood cells and the continuing drama of the phagocytosis of these cells by white blood cells. With the developments by Rounds et al. and Berns et al., microirradiation was extended into operations on various types of tissues and eventually to work on chromosomes. Laser microirradiation is reviewed in detail in Chapter 6.

The development of the laser microscope continued with the use of this microscope for microemission spectroscopy. From the early laser microprobe, the laser microprobe mass analyzer (LAMMA) was developed by Kaufmann et al. This new laser microprobe has had an extraordinary range of use, whether the specimen be biologic, technical, organic, or even inorganic. The lasers in this new microprobe are both the HeNe and the Nd-YAG, Q-switched. The pulse duration is 20–30 ns. This is combined with the mass spectrometer. For biomedical applications, the specimen is freeze-dried and embedded in plastic. On the basis of the determination of trace metals K, Na, Ca, and Fe in the various states, and of the numbers of tissues examined, the use of the laser microprobe mass analyzer on soft biologic tissues would appear to be the next step in the progress in the use of this instrument and may possibly be a means of overcoming the limitations of cryotechniques.

## OTHER ADVANCES IN LASER BIOLOGY AND DIAGNOSIS

To introduce the next phases of the new laser biology, it is well to review the various topics of the Europhysics Conference of September of 1979. These were as follows:

1. Laser spectroscopy of biomolecules
2. Laser flash photolysis of biomolecules
3. Physics and chemistry of laser-induced processes in biomolecules
4. Biologic processes induced by the laser
   a. Photodynamic therapy
   b. Biostimulation effects
   c. Photodermatology

The biologic processes included the following:

1. Photodynamic therapy
2. Biostimulation effects
3. Photodermatology
4. Photophysiology
5. Photopharmacology

The instrumentation for laser biology should emphasize, in general, these themes.

## Laser Spectroscopy

Further developments of laser spectroscopy will have a tremendous importance in both biology and medicine. In brief, the laser spectroscopy includes the following types:

1. Raman
2. Acoustical—substituting laser for xenon
3. Infrared of Kaiser (1979), with attenuated total reflection (ATR) prism and simple mouth probe plus analyses of blood serum, sugar, urea, alcohol, and lipids
4. Resonance fluorescence with a continuous-wave dye laser
5. Resonance ionization—pulsed laser for photoionization of the atom (Nayfeh, 1979)

Work with the amorphous polymers (Aviram) indicates that in the field of so-called mechanophotochemistry, the use of the laser should be considered in the conversion of light energy to mechanical motion. In biology and medicine, this would be helpful in the design of test models of devices for such purposes as protection from the sun and relief for those suffering from skin disorders or light sensitivity. Ultraviolet lasers in this field might offer great potential.

These techniques will all be adapted to uses for biologic purposes and not limited to the chemical laboratory for strictly analytic techniques.

## The Laser in Acoustic Microscopy

The relationship of the laser to acoustic microscopy also has potentially great significance in biology and medicine. An acoustic microscope with sonic lenses may be focused on fresh, unfixed tissue. The imagery is made visible on a television screen by laser so that changes in the morphology of the living tissue may be observed through the sonic microscope. An example of this is the use of the acoustic microscope to study the dynamics of the heart of the chick embryo after exposure to various cardiac drugs.

It is possible also to develop techniques for observing the effect of cellular structure in response to dynamic changes such as radiation, either ionizing or nonionizing, and to observe the dynamics of the cells during these periods. More extensive experience with these types of scopes and further developments to improve imagery are needed. Here, too, is another area of challenge in the ever-expanding field of optoelectronics.

## Laser Doppler Techniques

Laser Doppler techniques have shown great promise in studies of blood flow, including microtechniques. The latter could be used for studies of microcirculation in the skin, nail bed, lips, tongue, deep-muscle tissue, and even over the surface of the brain. In-vivo blood-flow mapping can also be done with the transmitting fiber optic inserted inside the blood vessel.

Other studies are also possible, especially in the field of peripheral circulation, including aggregation of platelets, thrombogenesis and thrombolysis, cellular fluorescence, and endothelial cell dynamics. Rounds et al. (1979) and Berns et al. (1976) have studied tissue cultures of cardiac muscle cells exposed to laser microirradiation. This material is serving as a test model for the action of cardiac drugs on arrhythmias. Laser vascular dynamics can be used for the study of stroke (laser Doppler velocimetry and laser canalization of occluded vessels) and for aortocoronary bypass surgical techniques.

## Laser-induced X-Ray Diffraction

Laser-induced x-ray diffraction is one of the spin-offs of laser-induced nuclear fusion studies. With glass lasers, 200 billion watts, and nanosecond exposures, it is possible now through the work of the laboratory of laser energetics of the University of Rochester to carry out kinetic studies of such fascinating biologic processes as photosynthesis. This will have great potential for the future in the study of many types of biologic processes in nanosecond time, thus helping to reveal the dynamics of some of the essential processes of physiology, immunology, respiration, etc.

## Laser Nephelometry

A practical instrument today in the immunology laboratory is the laser computer nephelometer. This instrument not only provides quantitative data on IgG, IgA, IgM, $C_3c$, $C_4$, albumin, and immune complexes, but also on transferrin and the rheumatoid factor. The instrument may be used also for cerebrospinal-fluid analyses. This extraordinary instrument can be developed further to facilitate other studies of other immunoglobulins as well as other materials to aid laboratory research and development in the field of immunology.

In immunology, with the new cell-sorter technology by the laser, specific monoclonal antibodies in hybridoma technology can be developed for immunotherapeutics. This will make it possible to analyze the inflammatory infiltrate in relation to the immunologic response of the patient.

Also, in immunology, the significant experiments of Waidelich and Mester et al. suggest that the laser (HeNe) and also the lasers HeCd and Kr may be used as immunosuppressive and immunostimulating agents. Clinically, this has been of some value in the healing of chronic ulcers and in delaying graft rejection. It is hoped that this delay in graft rejection will eventually have value in organ transplants.

## Transillumination

Another laser diagnostic technique that requires further investigation is laser transillumination of tissue (Fig. 4.1). The present goal is the early recognition of cancer of the breast with the 2-mm mass (Figs. 4.2 and 4.3). With the present concern about the exposure of the younger woman to x rays during mammography and xerography, it is essential to determine whether laser transillumination is superior to these procedures of breast examination and to thermography. Two laser systems are being presently considered: the dye laser and the infrared laser. In the past, HeNe and HeCd lasers have also been used in an attempt to provide imagery of the different masses in the breast without extensive dispersion of the incident beams. With the infrared sources, special photographic techniques are necessary, with special sensitized films in the use of sensitive image converters to obtain photographs for the patient's record. This, too, is a fertile field for cooperative research and endeavor to provide an effective, safe, sensitive diagnostic method. The background for this is reviewed in detail by Greenberg and Tribbe in Chapter 22.

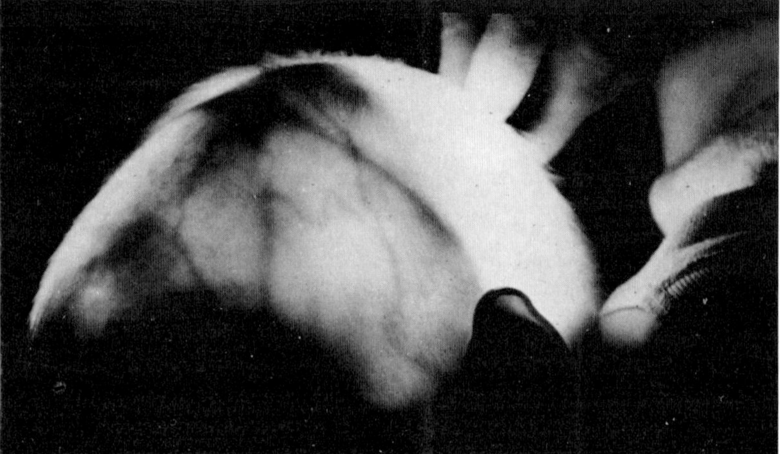

**Fig. 4.1.** Deep krypton laser transillumination of a progressive, inoperable, vascular birthmark of scalp and oral cavity to locate major feeder vessels for possible surgery. Infant died before surgery could be initiated.

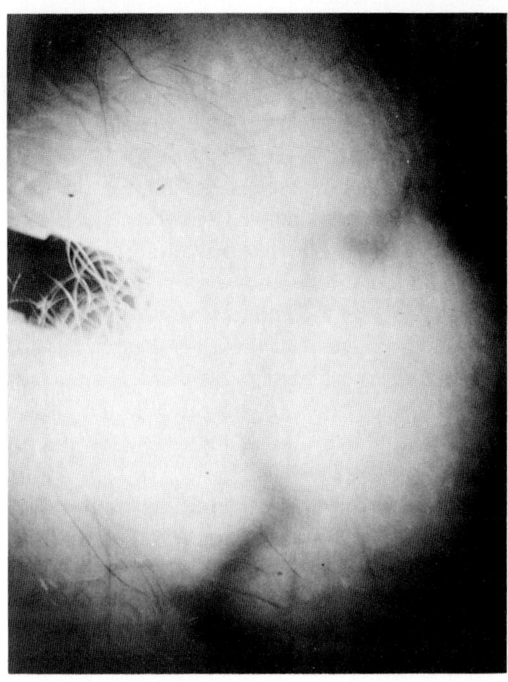

**Fig. 4.2.** Helium-neon laser transillumination of normal breast, showing only blood vessels.

**Fig. 4.3.** Helium-neon laser transillumination of breast, showing diffuse densities of birthmark of the skin surface.

## THE LASER IN COMMUNICATIONS AND INFORMATION HANDLING

Finally, in the field of laser diagnosis, there is the current development in the field of communications and information handling for the better deliverance of health care. This can be accomplished by the medical center that provides expertise for the examination of the patient, and detailed laboratory studies of all types that are transmitted to the central medical facility. Some trial project models have been used for community clinics and even distant villages, but these are a substitute for additional expertise when highly trained and experienced personnel are not available. Laser systems available for such communications systems include the HeNe, high outputs, Nd, and $CO_2$. The controls with closed-circuit television and microwave systems must be evaluated also in this connection.

Before long, the extraordinary developments in transmission of laser systems by fiber optics will be applied to patient care, teaching and training at all levels of patient care, and educational programs for medical and paramedical personnel.

Information handling of in-house record material for data image processing for medical records offers another of the innumerable challenges to the communication systems and information-handling engineers. The video disks with lasers offer possibilities for medical education and training in all fields of medicine and nursing, as well as in fields of art and culture. These advances demand detailed evaluation by educators and sociologists, together with experts in many areas of laser technology.

For laser diagnostic medicine, there are challenges in the clinical laboratory, even in addition to laser biochemistry for its analytical techniques. There is also an opportunity for detailed expansion in the field of transillumination, even to microtransillumination, in many facets of heart disease diagnosis by various types of profilometer surveys—even intravascular examinations by catheters and inspection of atheromas—and holography of cardiovascular dynamics. There is obvious need for continued development in acoustic holography, and the great potential that this has for early cancer diagnosis is also obvious. This can improve the imagery of echocardiography.

A new field of laser diagnostic medicine which promises much for the future is laser-induced fluorescence. This has been shown to be of value for the localization of early cancer of the lung and, in preliminary studies in China, for ulcerations of the cervix—whether benign or malignant. Moreover, laser-induced fluorescence has been used in investigative studies for the photodynamic therapy of tumors. As Sacchi indicates, fluorescence, long important in basic and applied biomedical research, is now at an early stage for clinical application.

For the marketplace, the diagnostic instrumentation field will have much greater potential than the surgical treatment area.

## SUMMARY

In the new field of laser diagnostic medicine, there will be much in the future to interest the biomedical engineer, especially at the graduate level (Tokuda et al.,

1979). The importance of the engineer will again be demonstrated in the health program for humankind.

## REFERENCES

Aviram A (1979) Personal communication.

Berns M, Rattner JB, Meredith S, Witter M (1976) Current laser microirradiation studies. Ann NY Acad Sci 26:160.

Bessis M., Ter-Pogassian (1965) Micropuncture of cells by means of a laser beam. Ann NY Acad Sci 122:659.

Kaiser N (1979) Laser absorption spectroscopy with ATR prism. J Fahrenfort Spectrochem Acta 17: 689.

Kaufmann R, Hillenkamp F, Wechsung R (1979) The new laser microscope mass analyzer (LAMMA). A new instrument for biomedical microprobe analysis. Med Progr Technol 6:106.

Mester E, Nagylucskay T, Tisza S, Mester A (1977) Personal communication.

Nayfreh MH (1979) Laser detection of single atoms. Am Scientist 67:204.

Rounds DE, Olsen RS, Bouher J (1979) Measurements of the cell migration index with a HeNe laser. Ann NY Acad Sci 26:152.

Tokuda AR, Auth DC, Bruckad AP (1979) Holograph of the human eye. Laser + Elektro-optik 2:38.

Waidelich W (1979) Personal communication.

# 5

# Flow Cytometry: The Use of Lasers for Rapid Analysis and Separation of Single Biological Cells

*Gary C. Salzman*

The term *flow cytometry* describes a relatively new technique for making rapid measurements on individual biological cells as they pass in single file through a laser beam. The early history of this rapidly expanding technology has been reviewed by Mullaney et al. (1976). The development of the argon-ion laser enabled precise measurement of cellular DNA content, using fluorescent stains which bind stoichiometrically to DNA. The technology has since expanded to include flow cytometer instruments for (1) studies of doubly stained cells by means of multiple lasers and fluorescence detectors, (2) single chromosome analysis, (3) measurements of scattered light with multiple detectors, (4) studies of polarized fluorescence emission from single cells, and (5) scanning and imaging of cells as they pass through a laser beam. The present review surveys some of the laser-related instrumentation developments in this subfield of automated cytology and indicates some new directions for growth in this research area.

## ELEMENTS OF FLOW CYTOMETRY

### Fluid-filled Flow Chamber

In the fluid-filled flow chamber developed by Steinkamp et al. (1973, 1979) at the Los Alamos Scientific Laboratory (Fig. 5.1), a cell suspension is injected into the center of a rapidly moving sheath fluid stream under conditions of laminar flow.

This work was supported by the U.S. Department of Energy under contract No. W-7405-ENG36 and by the National Institute of General Medical Sciences under grant No. GM 26857.

The author expresses appreciation to J. C. Martin and M. E. Wilder and to Dr. M. R. Raju for critically reviewing the manuscript. Also, thanks to J. Brown for patiently typing and retyping the manuscript.

The cells are accelerated by hydrodynamic forces to a velocity of approximately 10 m/s as the combined fluid stream passes through the 100-$\mu$m-diameter volume-sensing orifice (Coulter, 1956). The cell sample stream may be only 20 $\mu$m in diameter at this point. The approximately 10- to 20-$\mu$m-diameter cells are spaced about 1 cm apart. Cell sample concentration is typically $10^6$ cells/ml at a cell analysis rate of 1000 cells/s. Another sheath fluid enters the flow chamber near the intersection of cell and laser beam and guides the cell sample stream out of the chamber through a 100-$\mu$m-diameter exit orifice.

The cell nucleus is typically stained with a fluorochrome which binds stoichiometrically to DNA and which can be excited by one of the available laser wavelengths. As the stained cell passes through the focused laser beam, the fluorochrome is excited and emits a pulse of fluorescent light (Fig. 5.2).

A cell emitting fluorescence within a specified intensity range can be separated physically from the cell sample by means of the cell-sorting technique developed by Fulwyler (1965). The flow chamber is vibrated at approximately 40 kHz with a piezoelectric transducer so that the fluid jet containing the cells is broken into a uniform stream of droplets (Sweet, 1964). When the cell with the desired properties is about to separate from the stream into a droplet, a pulse of charge is applied to the stream. A droplet breaking off during this charging pulse carries away some of the charge. A short distance below the chamber, the droplet stream passes

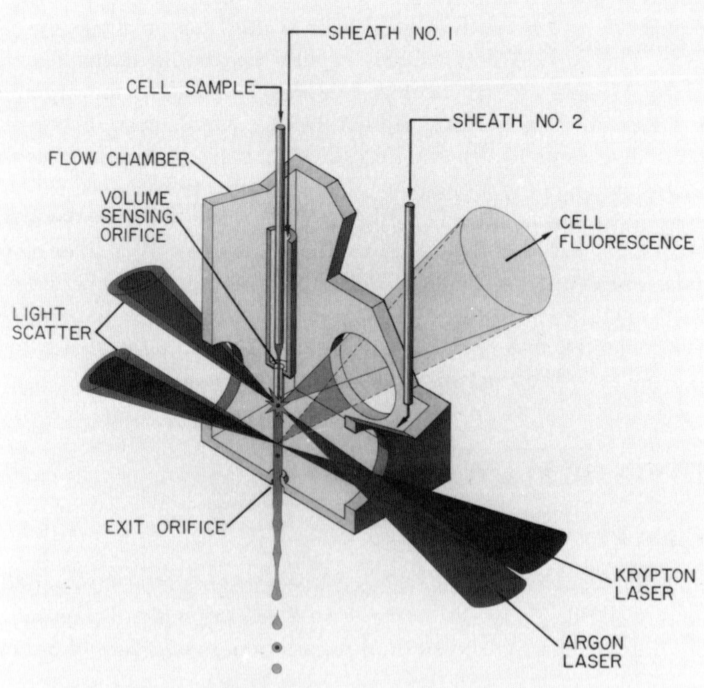


**Fig. 5.1.** Cut-away view of fluid-filled flow chamber for a cell-sorting flow cytometer. This chamber incorporates a volume-sensing orifice and dual laser beams for multiple fluorochrome studies. (Steinkamp et al., J Histochem Cytochem 27:273, 1979.)

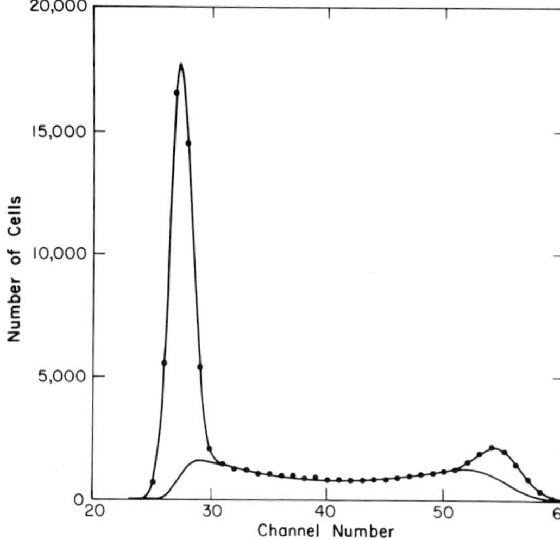


**Fig. 5.2.** Frequency histogram for sample of propidium-iodide–stained Chinese hamster tissue-culture cells excited at 488 nm with argon laser. Curves indicate computer fit to data, according to a program developed by Dean and Jett (1974) and Jett (1978). *Lower curve,* DNA synthesis (S) phase cells. (Crissman et al., Methods in Cell Biology, vol 9. Academic Press, New York, 1975.)

through an electrostatic deflection field of approximately 10 kV/cm where the charged droplet containing the cell of interest is separated from the uncharged droplet stream and subsequently captured in a test tube or on a microscope slide for later analysis.

### Stream-in-Air Flow Chamber

The other major approach to flow chamber design has been the stream-in-air concept [Bonner et al. (1972) and Arndt-Jovin and Jovin (1974)] in which the sample stream is injected into the center of a sheath flow and the two concentric streams jet out of a 50- to 75-$\mu$m-diameter nozzle into the air. The focused laser beam intersects the stream in the air about 1 mm below the nozzle. This flow chamber design is simpler than the enclosed chamber of Steinkamp et al. (1973) and is the basis for two commercial cell sorters. In the future we may see a return to enclosed flow chambers as resolution requirements become more stringent.

## DUAL LASER STUDIES

Investigators interested in simultaneous measurements of nuclear DNA content as well as other cellular parameters, such as cytoplasmic protein content, have been limited to stains that can be excited by the same laser line but that have well-separated emission spectra. Propidium iodide has been used as a nuclear DNA stain in combination with fluorescein isothiocyanate as a cytoplasmic protein stain (Steinkamp and Crissman, 1974). Both of these stains can be excited at the argon laser wavelength of 488 nm. Their emission spectra do overlap to some extent; so narrow band filters and/or signal subtraction schemes are used to correct the fluorescence data.

The range of choices for stains has been greatly expanded by the addition of a second laser to flow cytometers in a number of laboratories (Stohr, 1976; Stohr et al., 1977; Shapiro et al., 1977; Dean and Pinkel, 1978; Steinkamp et al., 1979). In the dual laser flow cytometer developed by Dean and Pinkel (1978) (Fig. 5.3), the two laser beams are separated by 200 $\mu$m so that the stains in a cell are excited sequentially by the two different laser wavelengths and produce two spatially separated beams of fluorescent light. These separated beams are appropriately filtered and detected by photomultiplier tubes.

The fluorescence absorption spectra of mithramycin bound to DNA and rhodamine 640 bound to bovine serum albumin (Fig. 5.4A) are well-separated. The fact that their fluorescence emission spectra (Fig. 5.4B) overlap significantly is not a problem since fluorescence signals are separated both spatially and in time. Dual laser instruments have been constructed only in a few laboratories because of the large capital costs of the high-powered argon and krypton lasers. Also, since relatively few experimental results have been published, it is not yet clear whether this approach will be cost-effective.

## LIGHT SCATTERING

Light scattering is an attractive parameter for flow cytometry because it requires neither fixation nor staining of the cells. Viable cells can be separated physically using light-scattering measurements with a cell sorter. Cell sizing has been the major use for flow cytometric light-scattering measurements, although efforts are being made with multiple-detector systems to extract additional morphologic information from cells.

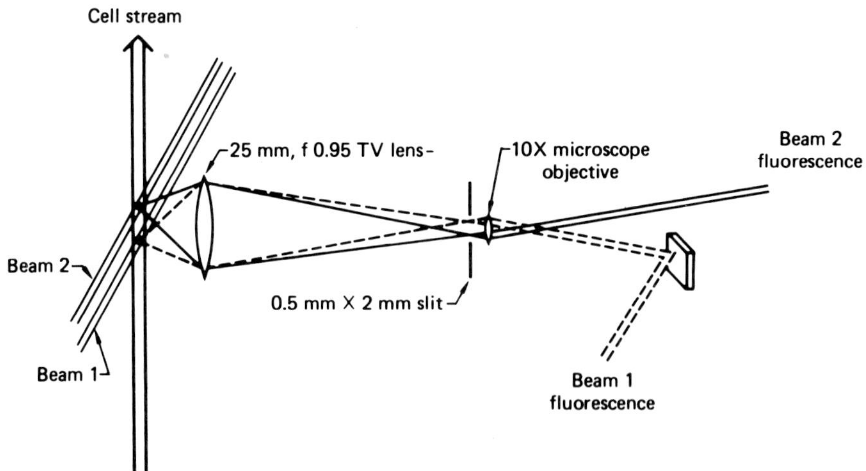


**Fig. 5.3.** Schematic drawing of light collection optics for the dual laser flow cytometer developed by Dean and Pinkel. The two fluorescence beams are detected by separate photomultiplier tubes. (Dean and Pinkel, J Histochem Cytochem 26:622, 1978.)

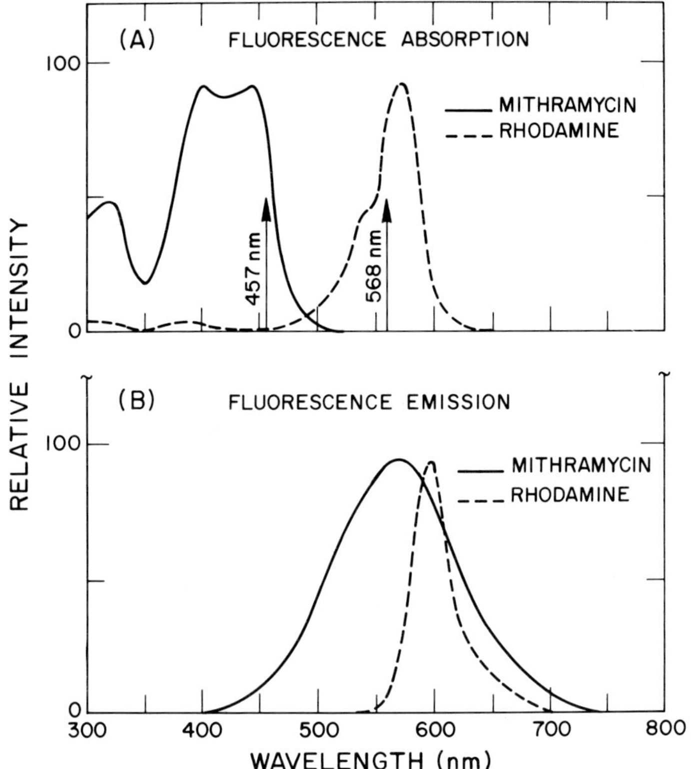


**Fig. 5.4. A.** Fluorescence excitation spectra for DNA stained with mithramycin and for bovine serum albumin stained with rhodamine 640. Mithramycin is excited by the 457-nm argon laser line, and rhodamine by the 568-nm krypton laser line. **B.** Fluorescence emission spectra for mithramycin and rhodamine. (Steinkamp et al., J Histochem Cytochem 27:273, 1979.)

In a flow cytometer developed by Mullaney et al. (1969) the argon laser light scattered by each cell is detected in an annular region between 0.5° and 2° with respect to the laser-beam direction. They showed that the photodiode detector signal increased linearly with spherical particle volume over a diameter range between 6 and 14 $\mu$m.

Loken et al. (1976) have developed a sweep scatter-flow cytometer in which an argon laser beam is expanded parallel to the cell stream. A photomultiplier detector is positioned so that light scattered at small angles with respect to the laser-beam direction enters the detector just as the cell enters the laser beam. As the cell moves downward through the beam, the detector views increasingly larger scattering angles. The continuous signal from the detector is stored in a waveform recorder and later transferred to a computer. Scattered light is detected over an angular range between 1° and 49° with an angular resolution of 1°.

Salzman et al. (1975) have developed a flow cytometer (Fig. 5.5) with which the light scattered from a single cell can be sampled at up to 32 angles in the forward

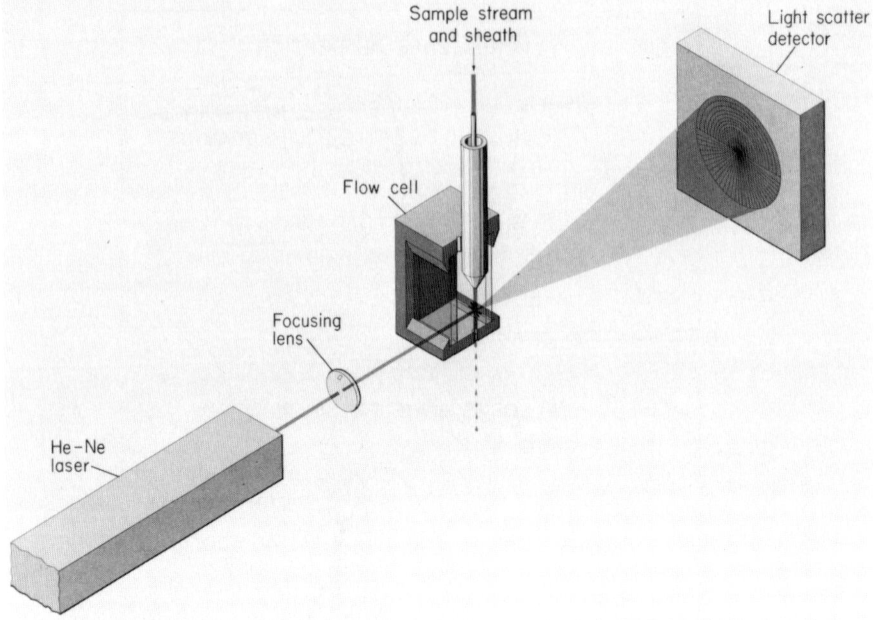


**Fig. 5.5.** Schematic drawing of multiangle light scatter flow cytometer, showing 5-mW HeNe laser beam focused into a flow chamber similar to that shown in Figure 5.1. Forward-scattered light is sampled simultaneously at 32 angles between 0° and 21°. (Mullaney et al., Ann NY Acad Sci 267:176, 1976.)

direction. Two detector arrays are used with this system (Figs. 5.6 and 5.7). The first array integrates over 180° in azimuthal angle and has higher polar angular resolution at small angles than at larger angles. It spans an angular range from 0° to about 21°. The second detector is a cross array constructed from individual photodiodes (Fig. 5.7). It is intended for use in studying cell asymmetry and orientation. Hybrid integrated-circuit preamplifiers are mounted on the back of the array.

Recent theoretical studies by Kerker et al. (1979) and Meyer (1979) indicate that backscattering from cells may be more sensitive to internal morphological changes than forward scattering. Bartholdi (1979) and Bartholdi et al. (1980) recently developed a 360° light-scattering flow cytometer (Fig. 5.8). In this system the cells intersect the focused argon laser beam at the primary focus of an ellipsoidal reflector. Light scattered from a cell at polar angles between 2.5° and 177.5° above and below the laser beam is reflected toward the secondary focus of the elliptical mirror. A special detector array (Fig. 5.9) intercepts this cone of scattered light. The 60 detector elements, each subtending a polar angle of 3°, are located on 6° centers around a 2-cm-diameter circle. Signals from a subset of 32 of the detectors can be transferred to the computer on a cell-by-cell basis for later analysis.

Experiments carried out to date have not led to widespread use of light scattering for precise measurement of changes in cell morphology. Reasons for this

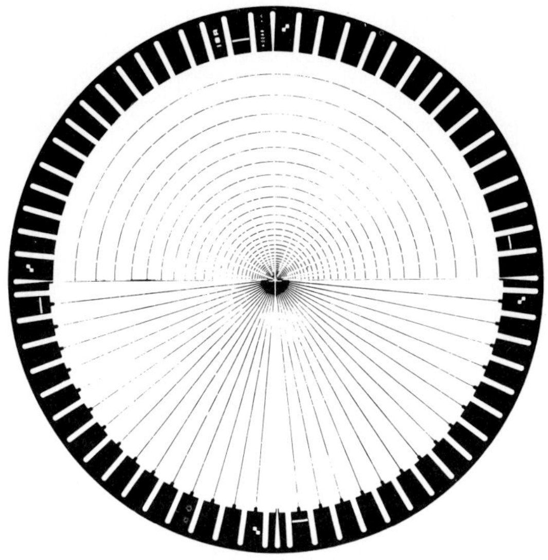

**Fig. 5.6.** A detector used with multiangle scatter flow cytometer. The 64-element photodiode array consists of 32 concentric rings spanning an azimuthal angle of 180° and 32 wedges. (The detector is a commercial product of Recognition Systems, Inc., Van Nuys, California.)

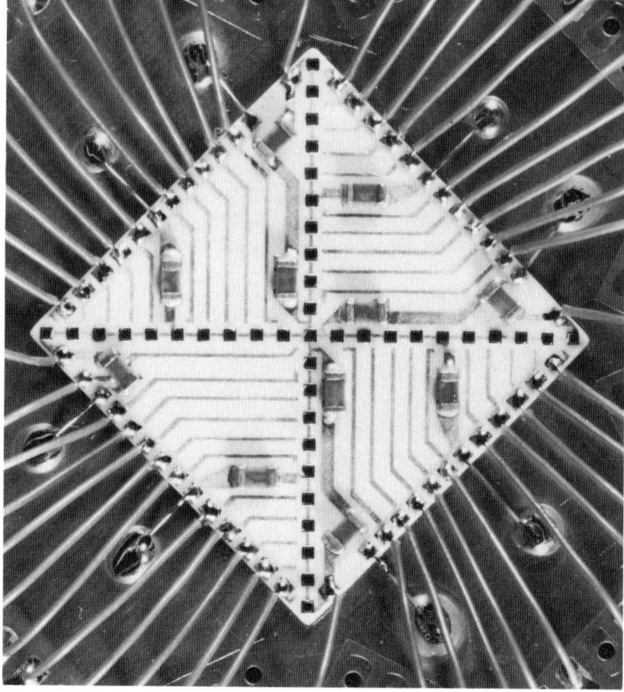

**Fig. 5.7.** Cross-array detector used with multiangle scatter flow cytometer. The 40 individual photodiodes are each 0.76 $mm^2$ with active areas of 0.25 $mm^2$. The 11 rectangular objects are decoupling capacitors. Leads from the photodiodes are attached to hybrid circuit preamplifiers on the back of the array. (Constructed in the hybrid circuit facility at the Los Alamos Scientific Laboratory.)

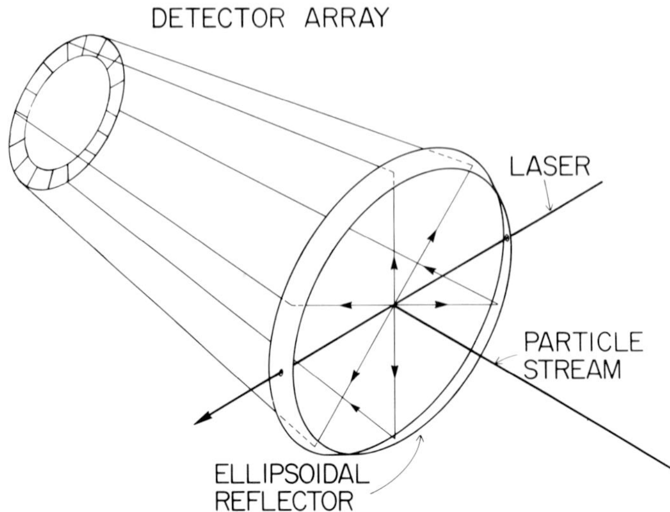


**Fig. 5.8.** Schematic drawing of 360° flow cytometer, showing the relationship between the ellipsoidal reflector and the photodiode detector array. Forward-scattered light from a cell at the intersection of the particle stream and laser beam is reflected toward the left side of the detector array. Backscattered light is reflected toward the right side of the array. (Bartholdi, PhD thesis, Clarkson College of Technology, 1979.)

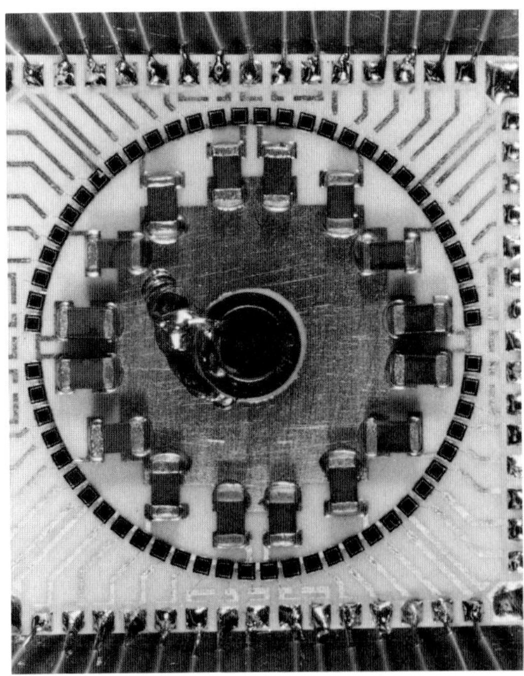

**Fig. 5.9.** Photodiode array with 60 elements, used with 360° light-scattering flow cytometer. Photodiodes (0.5 $mm^2$) are on a 2-cm diameter circle. Individual hybrid preamplifiers are on back of the substrate. (Constructed in the hybrid circuit facility at the Los Alamos Scientific Laboratory. Bartholdi, PhD thesis, Clarkson College of Technology, 1979.)

include the inability to control the many variables present in a light-scattering experiment. Among these are cell shape, orientation, and refractive index. Modeling studies coupled with carefully controlled experiments are required before the full potential of light scattering is realized in flow cytometry.

## HIGH-EFFICIENCY FLUORESCENT LIGHT COLLECTION

Two problems in flow cytometry instrumentation are the collection of light from weakly fluorescent cells and the artifacts caused by orientation effects in asymmetric cells. In most flow cytometers, a lens is the first element for light collection, and less than 10% of the available light is captured. Spherical mirrors have been used by Arndt-Jovin and Jovin (1974) to increase the collection efficiency to about 30%.

A paraboloid flow cytometer developed by Skogen-Hagenson (1980) has a fluid-filled chamber in which the cell stream intersects the laser beam at the focal point of the paraboloid mirror (Fig. 5.10). Scattered and fluorescent light are reflected

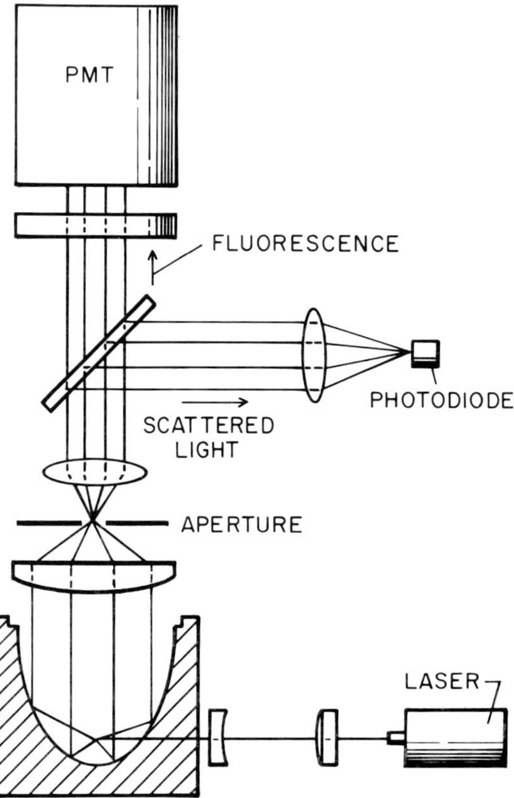


**Fig. 5.10.** Schematic drawing of a cross-sectional view of the paraboloid flow cytometer. An argon laser is used to excite fluorochromes bound to stained cells as they pass through the paraboloid focus. The cell sample stream is perpendicular to the plane of the page. A dichroic filter separates the scattered and fluorescent light. *PMT*, photomultiplier tube. (Skogen-Hagenson, PhD thesis, Iowa State University, 1980.)

from the gold-plated surface and focused by a lens onto a 0.5-mm-diameter aperture so that light from only a small volume surrounding the paraboloid focus is passed into the rest of the optical system. A dichroic beam splitter is used to direct scattered and fluorescent light to different photodetectors.

This flow cytometer collects approximately 80% of the available fluorescent light. It has been used in several immunofluorescence experiments and in detecting the fluorescence from adriamycin in tissue-culture cells at chemotherapeutic dose levels. The predecessor of this instrument, an ellipsoid of revolution, was used to study bacterial nucleotide fluorescence (Skogen-Hagenson et al., 1977).

The flow cytometric fluorescence distribution from stained mature sperm cells should exhibit a single symmetric peak, indicating haploid DNA content. Most flow cytometers, however, produce fluorescence-intensity distributions that are skewed to higher fluorescence values (Gledhill et al., 1976). This is caused by the random orientation of the flat sperm cells with respect to laser-beam direction and fluorescence detector. More fluorescent light is emitted from the edge of a cell than from the flat sides (Van Dilla et al., 1977). The paraboloid flow cytometer produces symmetric fluorescence-intensity frequency histograms because it collects fluorescent light over a large solid angle and is, therefore, less sensitive to cell orientation. Another approach to the cell orientation problem has been to taper the sample inlet tube so that hydrodynamic shear forces cause the flat cells to rotate into a fixed plane (Stovel et al., 1978; Dean et al., 1978; Pinkel et al., 1979). This technique apparently works only with relatively low flow rates (Stovel et al., 1978).

The high efficiency of this instrument in light collection may lead to its use in a commercial instrument using a small laser, although such an application may be hindered because the flow chamber is unsuitable for cell sorting or fluorescence polarization studies.

## CHROMOSOME ANALYSIS INSTRUMENTATION

As flow cytometers and preparative techniques improved, investigators were able to contemplate DNA measurements on individual chromosomes. Gray et al. (1975a, 1975b) first demonstrated that individual chromosomes of the Chinese hamster cell line could be sorted on the basis of DNA measurements. Other investigators [Stubblefield et al. (1975); Carrano et al. (1976); Cram et al. (1979a)] have expanded this work to other cell lines and to human chromosomes. The 23 types of human chromosomes were resolved into 12 groups using the DNA stain Hoechst 33258 excited by an argon laser operating in the ultraviolet (351- + 364-nm lines) at a power of 0.8 W (Gray et al., 1979a).

The dual laser flow cytometer described earlier (Dean et al., 1978) was used recently to resolve the human karyotype in 20 groups (Gray et al., 1979a). The chromosomes were stained with Hoechst 33258 and with chromomycin A3. The two argon lasers were operated in the UV range (351 + 364 nm) and at 458 nm, respectively. This improvement in resolution occurred because the Hoechst stain binds preferentially to adenine-thymine–rich regions in the DNA (Latt and Wohlleb, 1975), and the chromomycin A3 binds preferentially to guanine-cytosine–rich

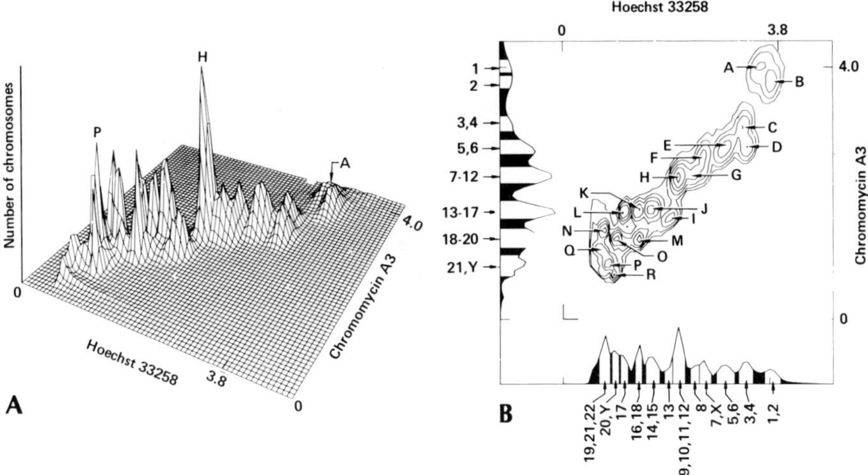


**Fig. 5.11. A.** Two-parameter-frequency histogram, showing number of human chromosomes as a function of Hoechst 33258 and chromomycin A3 fluorescence. **B.** Contour plot of same data. Chromosome numbers are identified on marginal-frequency histograms. (Gray et al., 1979a.)

regions (Latt, 1977). An isometric display of the two-parameter frequency histogram was obtained in this experiment (Fig. 5.11).

Although the karyotyping of human chromosomes has been the major thrust of the work in this area, another important use of this technique may be in the study of subtle changes in tissue-culture-cell karyotypes under the influence of suspected mutagenic and carcinogenic chemicals.

## PULSE SHAPE ANALYSIS METHODS

The measurement of cell nuclear and cytoplasmic diameters has been shown to be a useful tool in pathology. Wheeless and Patten (1973), and Wheeless et al. (1975) have developed a flow system in which the one-dimensional fluorescence contour of a cell can be measured as it passes through a slit-focused argon laser beam. This waveform is then analyzed to extract nuclear and cytoplasmic diameters.

Steinkamp and Crissman (1974) and Steinkamp et al. (1976) have developed a similar technique in which the time duration of the fluresecence signal above a fixed threshold from a stained nucleus is used to determine nuclear diameter, and the time duration for a scattered light signal is used to measure cytoplasmic diameter. Sharpless et al. (1975), and Sharpless and Melamed (1976) have shown that these fixed-threshold time-of-flight measurements depend on signal amplitude as well as signal duration. Leary et al. (1979) have developed a variation of this method in which the rise time over a constant fraction of a fluorescent or scattered light pulse is used for nuclear or cytoplasmic diameter measurement, respectively.

Cambier et al. (1979) and Wheeless et al. (1979) have developed a flow cytometer specifically directed toward automated prescreening for cervical cancer. The acridine-orange–stained flat epithelial cells pass through a slit-focused 488-nm argon laser beam inside a fluid-filled chamber. The photomultiplier-tube signal from the detected fluorescence is digitized as each cell passes through the slit of laser light. Since the nuclear fluorescence is brighter than the cytoplasmic fluorescence, the nuclear and cytoplasmic diameters and the nuclear fluorescence can be calculated from the waveform. The two parameters, nuclear fluorescence and nuclear-to-cytoplasmic diameter ratio, are used to discriminate between normal and abnormal cells. Since the orientation cannot be controlled for every cell, fluorescence scans are made along three mutually orthogonal axes (Fig. 5.12). This flow cytometer has also been modified so that a fluorescent image of the cell can be captured along with the slit-scan waveforms (Kay et al., 1979).

To further improve chromosome resolution, Gray et al. (1979c) adapted the slit-scan technique of Wheeless and Patten (1973) to a flow chamber similar to that of Eisert et al. (1975). The argon laser beam is focused to a slit whose smallest dimension is approximately 1 $\mu$m at the $1/e^2$ intensity points. Servo-controlled hydrodynamic focusing is used to constrain the chromosome sample stream to a 3-$\mu$m diameter. The slit-scanned fluorescent chromosome waveforms are digitized at 10-ns intervals with a flow velocity of 4 m/s. The centromere of a chromosome is usually somewhat less fluorescent than the chromosome arms, so the fluorescent waveform has a dip at the centromere. Various algorithms are used to compute the centromeric index (i.e., the ratio of the longest arm lengths to the total chromosome length). It is hoped that this additional parameter will allow all human chromosome types to be resolved.

Cram et al. (1979b) have modified the flow cytometer of Arndt-Jovin and Jovin (1974) so that the fluorescent images of chromosomes can be scanned in the image plane rather than in the object plane, as is done by Gray et al. (1979c). The primary advantage of this approach is that the width of the scanning slit is no longer determined by the spot size of the focused laser beam but is defined by an adjustable slit in front of the photomultiplier-tube detector. They have used this flow cytometer configuration to detect what they believe to be cells in anaphase and telophase. Gray et al. (1979b) have since modified their system to incorporate image plane scanning as well as object plane scanning..

Pulse shape analysis may prove to be particularly useful for the detection of abnormal chromosomes such as dicentrics. It may also be useful for increased cell size resolution in cases where the plasma membrane is severely perforated, as occurs in ethanol fixation.

## FLUORESCENCE POLARIZATION

The fluorescent light emitted by a fluorophore bound to some cell moiety is partially polarized. This occurs because some fluorescent molecules are rigidly bound to structures within the cell or on the cell surface and cannot rotate between the time they are preferentially excited by polarized laser light and the time of flu-

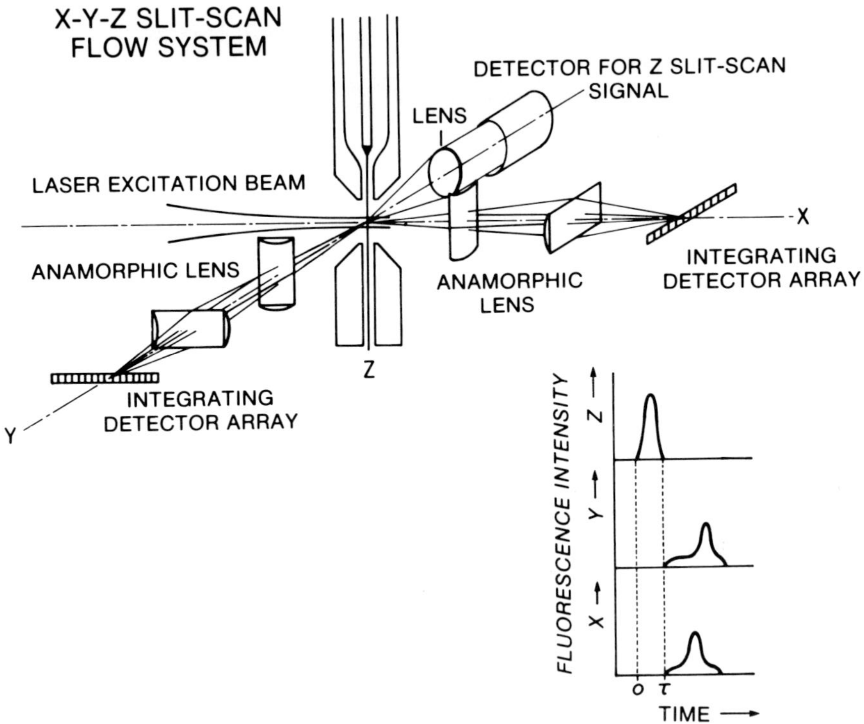


**Fig. 5.12.** Schematic drawing of *X-Y-Z* slit-scan flow cytometer designed for prescreening for cervical cancer. Velocity of cell controls Z-slit scan through slit-focused beam. Detectors *X* and *Y* integrate photodiode arrays with microchannel plate intensifiers in front of them. *At bottom,* three scans from a typical cell, needed to reduce cell misclassification rate to an acceptable level. (Cambier et al., 1979.)

orescent emission. This area of research has been extensively reviewed by Jovin (1979). This polarization of fluorescence has been used for several purposes: (1) to examine cytoplasmic microviscosity (Price et al., 1977), (2) to study the kinetics of fluorescein accumulation in the cytoplasm (Epstein et al., 1977; Pinkel et al., 1978; Udkoff and Norman, 1979), (3) to estimate membrane fluidity (Arndt-Jovin and Jovin, 1976), (4) to study energy transfer between fluorophores bound to surface components so as to measure distances between binding sites (Chan et al., 1979), and (5) to study the dye-binding characteristics of individual chromosomes (Cram et al., 1979a).

In the flow cytometer fluorescence polarimeter (Fig. 5.13) developed by Pinkel et al. (1978), the gains of the two photomultipliers are adjusted for equal signal strength when the half-wave retarder is rotated so that the beam polarization is horizontal, and the detected fluorescence polarization should be zero. The argon laser beam polarization is normally perpendicular to the horizontal plane. Specially designed diffusers are placed in front of each photomultiplier to depolarize the

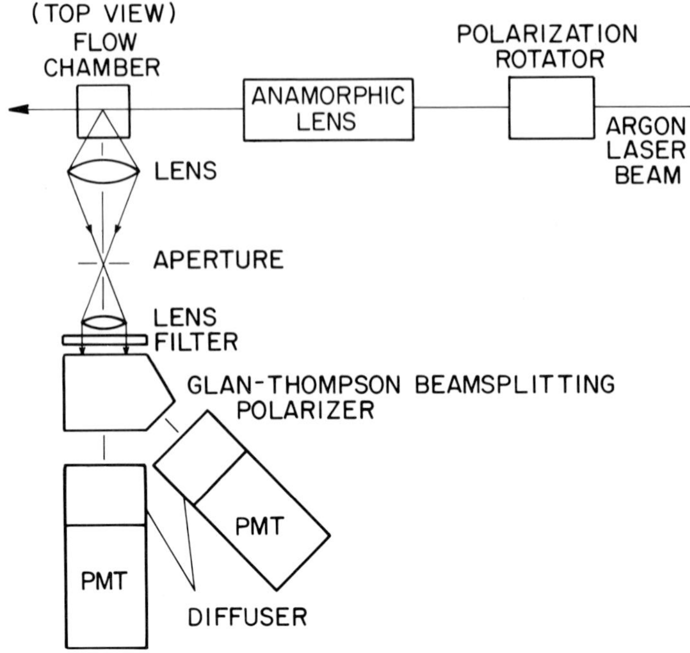


**Fig. 5.13.** Flow cytometer fluorescence polarimeter. In normal operation, the polarization rotator is set so that the laser beam is polarized perpendicular to the plane of the paper. Polarization of the fluorescent light pulse from a cell passing through the laser beam is analyzed by the Glan-Thompson prism, which directs vertical and horizontal components of the fluorescence polarization to different photomultiplier tubes (PMT). Diffusers are placed in front of PMTs to eliminate photocathode polarization effects. (Redrawn from Pinkel et al., 1978.)

detected light so that effects due to polarization sensitivity of the photocathode are eliminated.

This application of flow cytometry may lead to significant contributions to molecular biology and to better understanding of events within the cell and on the cell surface.

## DATA ACQUISITION AND COMPUTER-CONTROLLED SORTING

Most of the flow cytometers in operation today use commercially available one- and two-parameter pulse-height analyzers. This limits the user's ability to study the correlations among the many pieces of information available about each cell as it passes through the flow chamber. Arndt-Jovin and Jovin (1974) have developed a computer-controlled cell sorter that can acquire up to 10 parameters from each cell, generate on-line frequency histograms of each parameter or ratios of two parameters, and make sorting decisions based on windows set on each parameter or ratio of two parameters.

Salzman et al. (1978) have developed a four-parameter data acquisition and processing system in which the four signals from each cell are saved as correlated events on a mass storage device, in addition to on-line frequency histogram generation and computer-controlled sorting. The storage of each correlated event in this list mode enables the user to study the relationships among the parameters in great detail (Fig. 5.14). When a window is set around the second peak in the DNA histogram and the 40,000 correlated events are reprocessed to generate new gated frequency histograms, one obtains the cross-hatched histograms. Others have since developed similar data acquisition systems (Miller et al., 1978).

The recently developed Los Alamos Cell Analysis (LACEL) data acquisition and sorting system (Fig. 5.15) has two pertinent features: (1) A correlated raw event can contain parameters with mixed resolutions of 1024, 512, and 256 channels; and (2) sorting windows are established under computer control, but the actual sorting decision is made in hardware. This second feature is necessary for high-speed sorting, particularly with stream-in-air geometry flow chambers where the time between laser-beam interrogation of a cell and droplet breakoff is approximately 150 $\mu$s.

Time has recently been added as a new parameter in flow cytometry (Martin

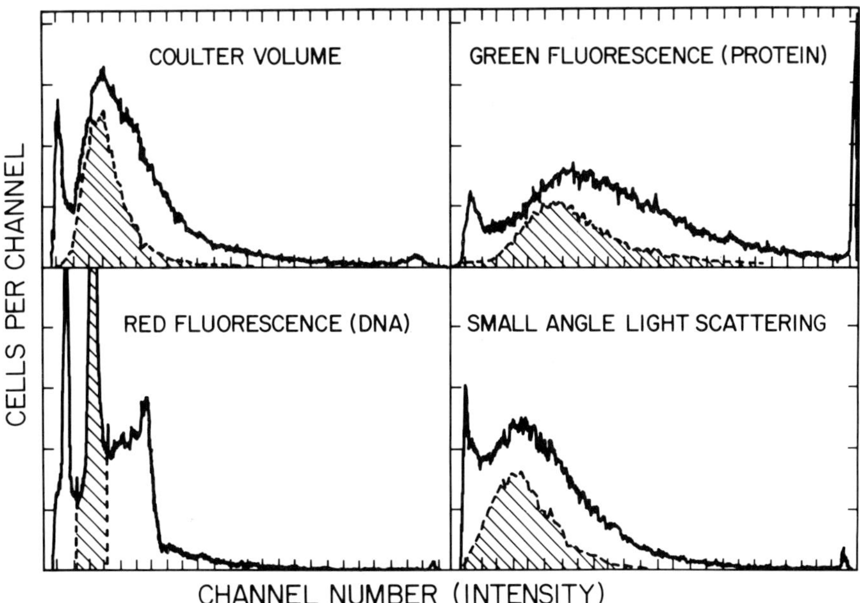


**Fig. 5.14.** Four single-parameter frequency histograms from a sample of primary Lewis lung carcinoma containing aneuploid tumor cells. *Full scale* on *ordinate* is 1024 cells per channel. *Solid curves*, approximately 40,000 cells. *Cross-hatched curves*, results of regenerating-frequency histograms from stored correlated events based on a window set in the DNA histogram. (Salzman et al., 1978.)

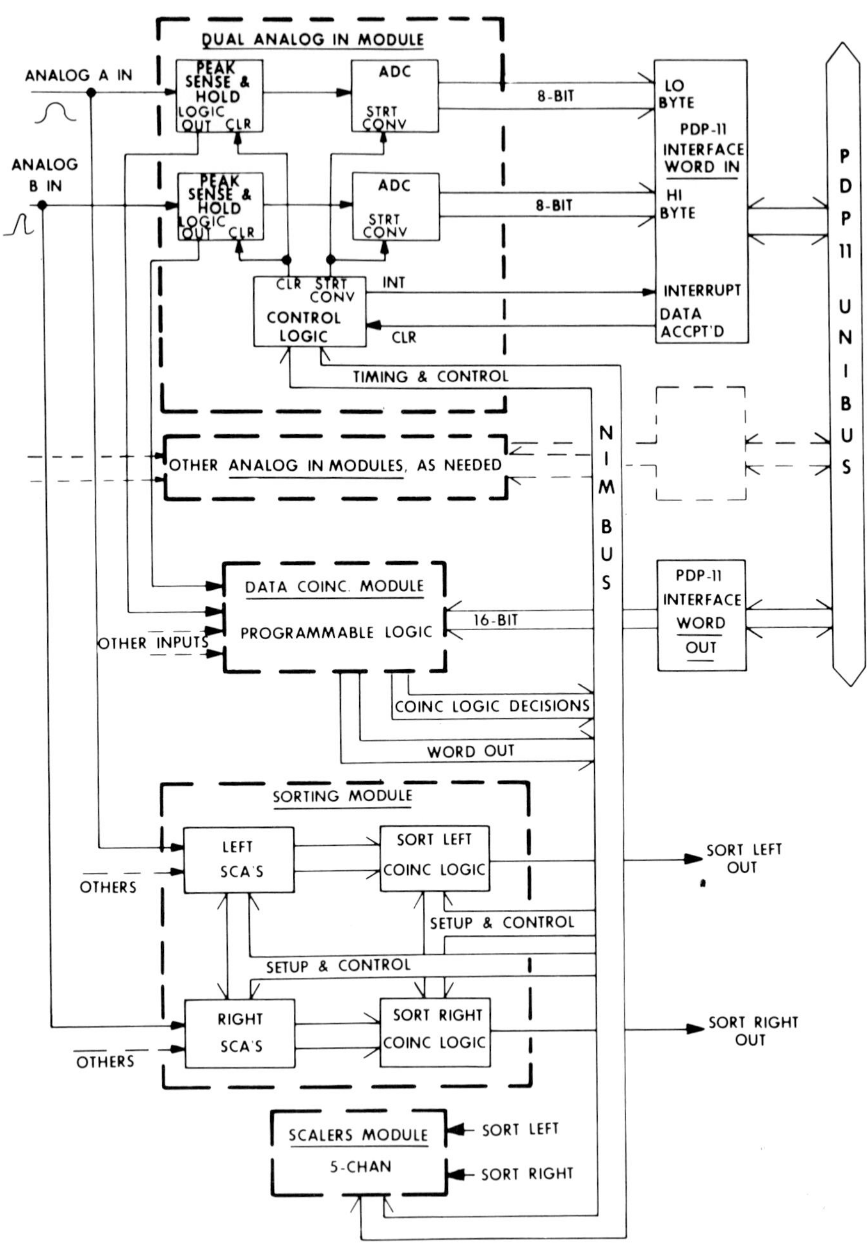


**Fig. 5.15.** Block diagram of LACEL data acquisition and sorting system. Each parameter has its own analog-to-digital converter (*ADC*) which can have a resolution of 1024, 512, or 256 channels. Sorting windows are established under computer control; actual sorting decisions are made under hardware control.

and Swartzendruber, 1979). In this technique, one of the analog-input signals to the data acquisition system of Salzman et al. (1978) is replaced by a signal whose level increases linearly with time. The method has been used to study the enzyme kinetics of esterase activity in several cell lines as well as the kinetics of dye leaching from ethanol fixed mouse spleen cells stained with mithramycin.

A considerable amount of attention has been given to the analysis of the single-parameter frequency histograms from flow cytometric measurements of DNA content (Dean and Jett, 1974; Baisch et al., 1975; Fried, 1976; Jett, 1978). The major goal in this work has been the extraction of the number of cells in each phase of the cell cycle. Statistical methods have only recently been applied to the quantitation of subtle changes in single-parameter frequency histograms of data from flow cytometers (Young, 1977; Bartels, 1979; Bagwell et al., 1979). Little effort has been given to the use of statistical methods for the analysis of multiparameter flow cytometric data. A wealth of information may be going to waste in many of the multiparameter experiments now being carried out. There is also a need for better display techniques for this multiparameter data.

## COMMERCIAL FLOW CYTOMETERS

The Becton Dickinson Fluorescence Activated Cell Sorter (FACS) is based on the stream-in-air design of Bonner et al. (1972). With this flow cytometer one can measure light scattered from cells in the forward direction as well as several colors of fluorescence in a direction orthogonal to both the sample stream and the laser beam. The latest model, the FACS IV, incorporates a user-programmable microprocessor and the capability for correlated event or list mode data acquisition. Light-scattering measurements with this flow cytometer have been analyzed by Salzman et al. (1979).

The Coulter Electronics cell sorter based on the design of Bonner et al. (1972) incorporates two-color fluorescence and forward-angle scattered light measurements. It uses several microprocessors to control multiparameter data acquisition and list mode data storage.

The Ortho Instruments Cytofluorograf System 50 is based on the pioneering work of Kamentsky et al. (1965). It incorporates an enclosed flow chamber with flat windows and argon and HeNe lasers as standard equipment. The HeNe laser is used for extinction, and small- and large-angle scattering measurements. Detectors are provided for multicolor fluorescence measurements. A computer interface is provided so that list mode data acquisition is possible. As in the other instruments, sorting is by the electrostatic technique described earlier. A modular flow cytometer originally developed by Dittrich and Gohde (1969) can be added to the System 50. It uses an epiillumination system to achieve the highest resolution fluorescence measurements now available from commercial flow cytometers. This epiillumination also avoids the sperm orientation artifact encountered by Gledhill et al. (1976).

The early commercial flow cytometers used pulse-height analyzers and offered little data analysis capability. Most recent versions offer some type of computer-based data acquisition and processing. Biologists planning to purchase flow cytometers should examine the data-handling options carefully so that they can make optimal use of the data produced by the instrument.

## SUMMARY

Flow cytometry began with the need for rapid quantitation of the volume and DNA content of individual biological cells. Development of the argon laser as a light source for these instruments led to rapid growth in the field. The introduction of electrostatic sorting hardware allowed the physical separation of cells based on DNA content and other measurements. Fluorochromes were introduced as stains for DNA, protein, and cell-surface properties. Since the excitation spectra of the fluorochromes frequently did not overlap, flow cytometers incorporating multiple lasers were developed. Small-angle light scattering was initially used for cell sizing. Flow cytometers have now been developed to sample the scattered light pattern over a larger angular range to quantitate changes in cell morphology. Pulse-shape analysis techniques have been developed to measure fluorescent profiles of cells as they pass through the laser beam. Fluorescence polarization measurements in flow cytometers have opened new areas for biological investigation. Analysis of subcellular components has been extended to chromosomes, a development that may lead to automated karyotyping. New data analysis methods have been developed to handle multiparameter flow cytometric data.

The increasing dependence of the technique of flow cytometry on ever more sophisticated instrumentation and on data analysis methods has created a need for multidisciplinary teams of biologists, chemists, physicists, engineers, and statisticians.

## REFERENCES

Arndt-Jovin DJ, Jovin TM (1974) Computer controlled multiparameter analysis of cells and particles. J Histochem Cytochem 22:622–625.

Arndt-Jovin DJ, Jovin TM (1976) Cell separation using fluorescence emission anisotropy. In: Marchesi VT (ed) Membranes and Neoplasia: New Approaches and Strategies, vol. 9. Progress in Clinical and Biological Research. Alan Liss, New York, pp. 123–136.

Bagwell CB, Hudson JL, Irvin GL III (1979) Nonparametric flow cytometry analysis. J Histochem Cytochem 27:293–296.

Baisch H, Gohde W, Linden WA (1975) Analysis of pulse cytophotometric data to determine the fraction of cells in various phases of the cell cycle. Radiat Environ Biophysics 12:31–40.

Bartels PH (1979) Numerical evaluation of cytologic data. I. Description of profiles. Anal Quant Cytol 1:20–29.

Bartholdi M (1979) 360 degree light scattering photometer for single particle analysis. PhD thesis, Clarkson College of Technology, Potsdam, New York.

Bartholdi M, Salzman GC, Hiebert RD, Kerker M (1980) Differential light scattering photometer for rapid analysis of single particles in flow. Appl Optics 19:1573–1581.

Bonner WA, Hulett HR, Sweet RG, Herzenberg LA (1972) Fluorescence activated cell sorting. Rev Sci Instrum 43:404–409.

Cambier JL, Kay DB, Wheeless LL Jr (1979) A multidimensional slit scan flow system. J Histochem Cytochem 27:321–324.

Carrano AV, Gray JW, Moore DH II, Minkler JL, Mayall BH, Van Dilla MA, Mendelsohn ML (1976) Purification of the chromosomes of the Indian muntjac by flow sorting. J Histochem Cytochem 24:348–354.

Chan SS, Arndt-Jovin DJ, Jovin TM (1979) Proximity of lectin receptors on the cell surface measured by fluorescence energy transfer in a flow system. J Histochem Cytochem 27:56–64.

Coulter WH (1956) High speed automatic blood cell counter and cell size analyzer. National Electronics Conference Proceedings 12:1034–1042.

Cram LS, Arndt-Jovin DJ, Grimwade BG, Jovin TM (1979a) Fluorescence polarization and pulse width analysis of chromosomes by a flow system. J Histochem Cytochem 27:445–453.

Cram LS, Arndt-Jovin DJ, Grimwade BG, Jovin TM (1979b) One dimensional image analysis of microspheres and Chinese hamster cells in a flow cytometer/flow sorter. In: Proceedings of the Fourth International Symposium on Flow Cytometry, Voss, Norway, June 4–8, 1979.

Crissman HA, Mullaney PF, Steinkamp JA (1975) Methods and applications of flow systems for analysis and sorting of mammalian cells. In: Methods in Cell Biology, vol 9. Academic Press, New York, pp. 179–246.

Dean PN, Jett JH (1974) Mathematical analysis of DNA distributions derived from flow microfluorometry. J Cell Biol 60:523–527.

Dean PN, Pinkel D (1978) High resolution dual laser flow cytometry. J Histochem Cytochem 26:622–627.

Dean PN, Pinkel D, Mendelsohn ML (1978) Hydrodynamic orientation of sperm heads for flow cytometry. Biophys J 23:7–14.

Dittrich W, Gohde W (1969) Impulsfluorometrie bei Einzelzellen in Suspensionen. Z Naturforsch 24B (Part 3): 360–361.

Eisert W, Ostertag R, Niemann EG (1975) Simple flow microphotometer for rapid cell population analysis. Rev Sci Instrum 46:1021–1024.

Epstein M, Norman A, Pinkel D, Udkoff R (1977) Flow system fluorescence polarization measurements on fluorescein diacetate stained EL-4 cells. J Histochem Cytochem 25:821–826.

Fried J (1976) Method for the quantitative evaluation of data from flow microfluorometry. Comput Biomed Res 9:263–276.

Fulwyler MJ (1965) Electronic separation of biological cells by volume. Science 150:910–911.

Gledhill BL, Lake S, Steinmetz LL, Gray JW, Crawford JR, Dean PN, Van Dilla MA (1976) Flow microfluorometric analysis of sperm DNA content. Effect of cell shape on the fluorescence distribution. J Cell Physiol 87:367–375.

Gray JW, Carrano AV, Moore DH II, Mendelsohn ML, Van Dilla MA (1975a) High speed quantitative karyotyping by flow microfluorometry. Clin Chem 21:1258–1262.

Gray JW, Carrano AV, Steinmetz LL, Van Dilla MA, Moore DH II, Mayall BH, Mendelsohn ML (1975b) Chromosome measurement and sorting by flow systems. Proc Nat Acad Sci (USA) 72:1231–1234.

Gray JW, Langlois RG, Carrano AV, Burkhart-Schulte K, VanDilla MA (1979a) High resolution chromosome analysis: One and two parameter flow cytometry. Chromosoma 73:9–27.

Gray JW, Lucas J, Pinkel D, Peters D, Ashworth L, Van Dilla MA (1979b) Slit-scan flow cytometry: Analysis of Chinese hamster M3-1 chromosomes. In: Proceedings of the Fourth International Symposium on Flow Cytometry, Voss, Norway, June 4–8, 1979.

Gray JW, Peters D, Merrill JT, Martin R, Van Dilla MA (1979c) Slit scan flow cytometry of mammalian chromosomes. J Histochem Cytochem 27:441–444.

Jett JH (1978) Mathematical analysis of DNA histograms from asynchronous and synchronous cell populations. In: Lutz D (ed) Pulse Cytophotometry. European Press, Ghent, Belgium, pp. 93–102.

Jovin TM (1979) Fluorescence polarization and energy transfer. In: Melamed MR, Mullaney PF, Mendelsohn ML (eds) Flow Cytometry and Sorting. John Wiley & Sons, New York, pp. 137–165.

Kamentsky LA, Melamed MR, Herman D (1965) Spectrophotometer: New instrument for ultrarapid cell analysis. Science 150:630–631.

Kay DB, Cambier JL, Wheeless LL Jr (1979) Imaging in flow. J Histochem Cytochem 27:329–334.

Kerker M, Chew H, McNulty PJ, Kratohvil JP, Cooke DD, Sculley M, Lee MP (1979) Light scattering and fluorescence by small particles having internal structure. J Histochem Cytochem 27:250–263.

Latt SA (1977) Fluorescence probes of chromosome structure and replication. Can J Genet Cytol 19:603–623.

Latt SA, Wohlleb J (1975) Optical studies of the interaction of 33258 Hoechst with DNA, chromatin and metaphase chromosomes. Chromosoma 52:297–316.

Leary JF, Todd P, Wood JCS, Jett JH (1979) Laser flow cytometric light scatter and fluorescence pulse width and pulse rise time sizing of mammalian cells. J Histochem Cytochem 27:315–320.

Loken MR, Sweet RG, Herzenberg LA (1976) Cell discrimination by multiangle light scattering. J Histochem Cytochem 24:284–291.

Martin JC, Swartzendruber DE (1979) Time: A new parameter for kinetic measurements in flow cytometry. Science 207:199–200.

Meyer RA (1979) Light scattering from biological cells: Dependence of back scatter radiation on membrane thickness and refractive index. Appl Opt 18:585–588.

Miller MH, Powell JI, Sharrow SO, Schultz AR (1978) Rapid data collection, analysis, and graphics for flow microfluorometry instrumentation. Rev Sci Instrum 49:1137–1142.

Mullaney PF, Steinkamp JA, Crissman HA, Cram LS, Crowell JM, Salzman GC, Martin JC (1976) Laser flow microphotometry for rapid analysis and sorting of mammalian cells. Ann NY Acad Sci 267:176–190.

Mullaney PF, Van Dilla MA, Coulter JR, Dean PN (1969) Cell sizing: A light scattering photometer for rapid volume determination. Rev Sci Instrum 40:1029–1032.

Pinkel D, Dean PN, Lake S, Peters D, Mendelsohn ML, Gray JW, VanDilla MA, Gledhill B (1979) Flow cytometry of mammalian sperm: Progress in DNA and morphology measurement. J Histochem Cytochem 27:353–358.

Pinkel D, Epstein M, Udkoff R, Norman A (1978) Fluorescence polarimeter for flow cytometry. Rev Sci Instrum 49:905–912.

Price GB, McCutcheon MJ, Taylor WB, Miller RG (1977) Measurement of cytoplasmic fluorescence depolarization of single cells in a flow system. J Histochem Cytochem 25:597–600.

Salzman GC, Crowell JM, Goad CA, Hansen KM, Hiebert RD, LaBauve PM, Martin JC, Ingram M, Mullaney PF (1975) A flow system multiangle light scattering instrument for cell characterization. Clin Chem 21:1297–1304.

Salzman GC, Hiebert RD, Crowell JM (1978) Data acquisition and display for a high speed cell sorter. Comput Biomed Res 11:77–88.

Salzman GC, Wilder ME, Jett JH (1979) Light scattering with stream in air flow systems. J Histochem Cytochem 27:264–267.

Shapiro H, Schildkraut R, Curbelo R, Brough-Turner R, Webb R, Brown D, Block M (1977) Cytomat-R: A computer-controlled multiple laser source, multiparameter flow cytophotometer system. J Histochem Cytochem 25:836–844.

Sharpless T, Melamed MR (1976) Estimation of cell size from pulse shape in flow cytofluorometry. J Histochem Cytochem 24:257–264.

Sharpless T, Traganos F, Darzynkiewicz Z, Melamed MR (1975) Flow cytofluorometry discrimination between single cells and cell aggregates by direct size measurements. Acta Cytol 19:577–581.

Skogen-Hagenson MJ, Salzman GC, Mullaney PF, Brockman WH (1977) A high efficiency flow cytometer. J Histochem Cytochem 25:784–789.

Skogen-Hagenson MJ (1980) A high efficiency flow cytometer. PhD thesis, Iowa State University, Ames, Iowa.

Steinkamp JA, Crissman HA (1974) Automated analysis of DNA, protein and nuclear to cytoplasmic relationships in tumor cells and gynecologic specimens. J Histochem Cytochem 22:616–621.

Steinkamp JA, Fulwyler MJ, Coulter JR, Hiebert RD, Horne JL, Mullaney PF (1973) A new multiparameter separator for microscopic particles and biological cells. Rev Sci Instrum 44:1301–1310.

Steinkamp JA, Hansen KM, Crissman HA (1976) Flow microfluorometric and light scatter measurement of nuclear and cytoplasmic size in mammalian cells. J Histochem Cytochem 24:292–297.

Steinkamp JA, Orlicky DA, Crissman HA (1979) Dual laser flow cytometry of single mammalian cells. J Histochem Cytochem 27:273–276.

Stöhr M (1976) Double beam application in flow techniques and recent results. In: Gohde W, Schumann J, Buchner T (eds) Second International Symposium on Pulse-cytophotometry. European Press, Ghent, Belgium, pp. 39–45.

Stöhr M, Eipel H, Goerttler K, Vogt-Schaden M (1977) Extended application of flow microfluorometry by means of dual laser excitation. Histochemistry 51:305–313.

Stovel RT, Sweet RG, Herzenberg LA (1978) A means for orienting flat cells in flow systems. Biophys J 23:1–6.

Stubblefield E, Deaven L, Cram LS (1975) Flow microfluorometric analysis of isolated Chinese hamster chromosomes. Exp Cell Res 94:464–468.

Sweet RG (1964) High frequency oscillography with electrostatically deflected ink jets. Stanford Electronics Laboratory Report No. SU-SEL-64-004, Technical Report No. 1722-1, Stanford University, Stanford, California.

Udkoff R, Norman A (1979) Polarization of fluorescein fluorescence in single cells. J Histochem Cytochem 27:49–55.

Van Dilla MA, Gledhill BL, Lake S, Dean PN, Gray JW, Kachel V, Barlogie B, Gohde W (1977) Measurement of mammalian sperm DNA by flow cytometry: Problems and approaches. J Histochem Cytochem 25:763–773.

Wheeless LL, Cambier JL, Cambier MA, Kay DB, Wightman LL, Patten SF (1979) False alarms in a slit scan flow system: Causes and occurrence rates: Implications and potential solutions. J Histochem Cytochem 27:596–599.

Wheeless LL, Hardy JA, Balasurbramanian N (1975) Slit scan flow system for automated cytopathology. Acta Cytol 19:45–52.

Wheeless LL, Patten SF (1973) Slit scan cytofluorometry. Acta Cytol 17:333–339.

Young IT (1977) Proof without prejudice: Use of the Kolmogorov-Smirnov test for the analysis of histograms from flow systems and other sources. J Histochem Cytochem 25:935–941.

# 6

# Current Developments in Laser Microirradiation

*M. W. Berns, M. Kitzes, P. A. McNeill*
*S. P. Peterson, K. Strahs, J. B. Rattner*
*J. Burt, S. Brenner, L. K. Chong*
*L. -H. Liaw, M. Hammer-Wilson, A. Siemens*

Laser microirradiation was introduced in experimental cytology in 1962 by Bessis and his colleagues in Paris (Bessis et al., 1962). Since that time, numerous studies have been conducted using various laser sources to produce alterations at the subcellular level. These studies have been extensively reviewed over the past 10 years (see reviews by Berns and Salet, 1972; Moreno et al., 1969; Berns, 1974a, 1974b, 1975, 1978; Berns et al., 1976). The present review will briefly describe the studies discussed in the previous reviews and will concentrate on work conducted in our laboratory since that time. Because of space constraints, we will not review the important UV laser microbeam studies conducted on tissue culture nuclei by Cremer et al. (1976) and the laser microbeam studies conducted by Salet (1972) and Salet et al. (1979) on myocardial cell mitochondria.

## LASER MICROBEAM

The microbeam employs a laser system that may be operated in several different configurations, depending upon the particular wavelength that is needed. The basic source is a pulsed Nd-YAG laser that employs intracavity frequency doubling to produce 532 nm. The power of this beam is between 2 and 5 kW/180 ns pulse. The beam is either directed into a microscope which focuses it to a submicron spot, or used to stimulate a dye laser. The 532-nm beam can also be further frequency-shifted to 265 nm by an external, temperature-modulated potassium dihydrogen phosphate (KDP) crystal. If used to stimulate a dye laser, the 532-nm beam is

This research was supported by NIH grants HL 15740, GM 23445 RR01192, and U.S. Air Force grant AFOSR-80-0062.

passed into a dye laser (Chromatix #1050) that has one of several dyes circulating from an external 1-liter reservoir (dye used: rhodamine 6G, fluorescein, Kiton red S, or coumarin). Using these dyes makes it possible to produce a series of laser wavelengths between 450 and 700 nm. By employing another intracavity frequency-doubling crystal, one-half of each of these wavelengths can be attained. The entire laser system provides a wide range of wavelengths spanning the spectrum between 250 and 700 nm.

The laser is used in conjunction with a Zeiss photomicroscope III that has been equipped with quartz UV-transmitting optics (Fig. 6.1). Both the tube head and the objectives permit efficient transmission of wavelengths down to 200 nm. The laser beam is deflected into the microscope by a dichroic filter that is coated to reflect > 90% of the laser energy and to transmit wavelengths significantly different from those of the laser light. The image of the target cell that is viewed through the microscope is projected through the filter into a high-light-sensitivity television camera (RCA #TC1000) and subsequently through a videotape machine (GYYR #DAS-300) to a television monitor (Sony #CMV115). A crosshair on the monitor screen denotes the point of laser focus. Careful movement of the microscope mechanical stage locates the target region of the cell under the crosshair, and the laser is fired. The laser is attenuated with different combinations of neutral-density filters, depending upon the wavelength employed and whether or not an external photosensitizing agent is added to the cells prior to laser irradiation. The size of the focused spot is controlled by using microscope objectives of different magnification: Zeiss Neofluar 40×, spot diameter 1–2 μm; Zeiss Neofluar 100×, spot diameter 0.25–1 μm; Zeiss Ultrafluar 32×, spot diameter 1.5–3 μm; Zeiss Ultrafluar 100×, spot diameter 0.25–0.75 μm.

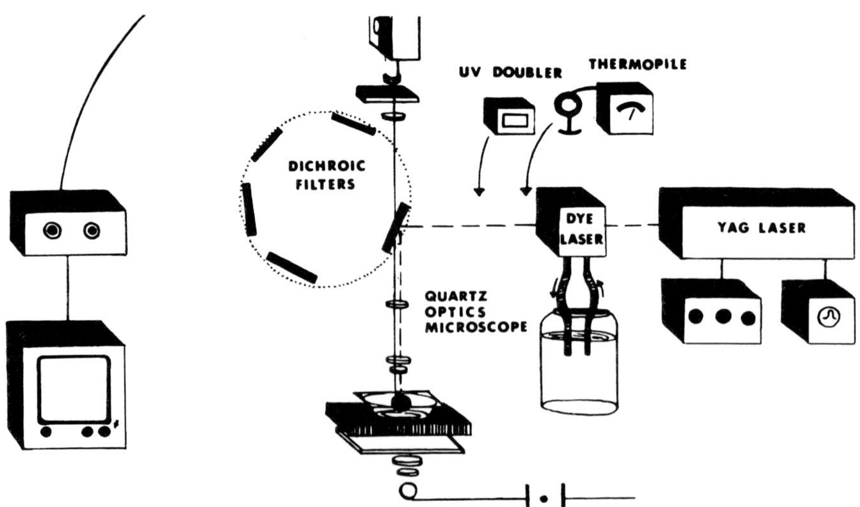


**Fig. 6.1.** Diagram of microbeam apparatus.

## CELL CULTURE

Most of the experiments described in this review employed either the established cell line $PtK_2$ from the rat kangaroo, *Potorous tridactylis*, or primary cultures of neonatal rat heart muscle cells. The *Potorous* cells are characterized by the fact that they remain flat during cell division, thus permitting clear visualization of their internal organelles, especially the chromosomes. The $PtK_2$ cells are epithelial and near diploid in karyology. They are grown in $T_{35}$ plastic flasks prior to seeding into standard culture chambers for irradiation. If visible laser wavelengths are to be employed, the cells are injected into Rose chambers with standard no. 1 thickness coverglasses. However, if ultraviolet laser light is to be used (wavelength below 325 nm), the Rose chamber coverglass upon which the cells are growing is made of quartz, with a thickness of less than 0.37 mm. When photosensitizing agents are employed in the experiments, the agent is injected directly into the Rose chamber at an appropriate period of time prior to irradiation.

Following irradiation, the cells are either observed by means of time-lapse photography for several days or fixed for electron microscopy. The follow-up may continue for several days by simply leaving the cells in the Rose chamber under the time-lapse videotape system. The cells are videotaped continually, and by means of the playback feature of the video system, they can be tracked easily. In some experiments, the Rose chambers are opened in a sterile laminar flow hood, and with the use of a pneumatic micromanipulator, the nonirradiated cells are cleared away from the irradiated cells (Berns, 1974c). The chamber is reassembled, and the cells are observed for additional time periods under the video system.

The rat myocardial cells are established according to the technique of Mark and Strasser (1966) and modified by us in later studies (Kitzes et al., 1977). Individual mitochondria in the contracting myocardial cells are microirradiated, and cytoplasmic stress fibers in the nonmuscle endothelial cells are irradiated (Strahs and Berns, 1979).

## ELECTRON MICROSCOPY

A main feature of our work involves precise ultrastructural analyses of the target organelle at varying time periods following irradiation. To accomplish this, the cells are fixed for electron microscopy, relocated, and serially sectioned with a diamond knife. The sections are then examined with the transmission electron microscope and correlated with light microscope photographs that were taken before and after irradiation. These procedures have been described in detail elsewhere (Brinkley et al., 1967; Rattner and Berns, 1974; Berns and Richardson, 1977).

## CHROMOSOME STRUCTURE AND FUNCTION

One of the earliest applications of the laser microbeam was the alteration of a submicron-sized area of an individual chromosome in dividing tissue culture cells

(Berns et al., 1969). In those studies, the blue-green beam of a low-power, pulsed argon laser (peak power of 2–3 W) was focused onto chromosomes that had been sensitized with the dye acridine orange. In low concentrations this dye was nontoxic to the cells, and it permitted selective sensitization of nucleic acids to the visible laser light. The combined approach of vital staining and laser microbeam irradiation permitted the disruption of a highly localized area of chromatin. In later studies, the low-power argon laser was replaced with a 35-W pulsed argon laser, and the optical system was redesigned to maximize the amount of laser energy passing through the microscope (Berns et al., 1971). With this system, energy densities in the 0.5-μm focused spot were between 50 and 1000 μJ. The result on individual chromosomes was the production of highly localized, discrete lesions without the need for presensitization with a vital dye, such as acridine orange (Berns et al., 1971). When these laser lesions were analyzed cytochemically and compared to the laser lesions produced with the acridine orange pretreatment, a differential molecular effect was observed (Berns and Floyd, 1971). These results are presented in Table 6.1. The net result of these studies was the demonstration that by varying the laser energy and/or the use of a nucleic-acid–specific photosensitizing agent, different molecular components of the chromosome could be affected, e.g., either DNA or histone. More recent studies (Peterson and Berns, 1978a, 1978b) employing light-activated, nucleic-acid–binding molecules—the psoralens—in combination with 365-nm argon laser light have demonstrated the capacity to selectively alter DNA and/or RNA in chromatin and organelles containing nucleic acid. These studies will be discussed in detail later.

Following the cytochemical analysis of laser microirradiated chromosomes, studies were undertaken to define the structural alterations at the electron microscope level (Rattner and Berns, 1974). These studies were necessary to define both the nature and the extent of the damage. For example, it was important to determine if the limitation of the lesions as observed with the light microscope correlated with the area of damage observed with the electron microscope. The results of these studies clearly demonstrated that electron-dense lesion material was confined to a portion of the chromosome correlating exactly with the "pale" lesion area observed with the light microscope. Unirradiated chromatin, as well as the cytoplasm and nucleoplasm in close proximity to the irradiation site, appeared to be unaffected. Furthermore, the nature of the ultrastructural damage appeared to be of two major classes, depending upon whether DNA-damaging or protein-damaging irradiation conditions were employed (Table 6.1). The ultrastructural dam-

**Table 6.1.** Alteration of Chromosomal Components

| | Acridine orange (μg/ml) | Laser energy ($\mu J/\mu^2$) | Feulgen reaction | Alkaline-fast green | Nucleolar organizer functions |
|---|---|---|---|---|---|
| DNA | 1–0.001 | 50 | − | + | − |
| Histone | 0 | 300 | + | − | + |
| DNA + histone | 1 | 300 | − | − | − |
| DNA + histone | 0 | 1000 | − | − | − |

age in the case of protein lesions appeared to comprise electron-dense, interconnected aggregates of material, and the DNA-altered chromatin comprised much smaller, spherical, electron-dense material.

## CHROMOSOME ELIMINATION

After the development of the capability for selective alteration of subchromosomal regions, the method was employed to study a specific problem of chromosome stability. By focusing the green laser beam [from any of the following lasers: second harmonic of the yttrium aluminum garnet (YAG) laser, an organic dye laser, or a 35 W argon laser] into the centromere region of a chromosome in metaphase $PtK_2$ cells, it was possible to damage that region sufficiently so that the chromosome became detached from the mitotic spindle. The cells usually continued through division with the irradiated chromatids either being lost from the cell or being incorporated into a micronucleus (Berns, 1974c). The cells were subsequently isolated by micromanipulation and cloned. The use of this method for selected removal of entire chromosomes, made it possible to generate daughter cells deficient in a particular chromosome. Of particular interest was the discovery that the subsequent clonal population of cells contained the normal number of the removed chromosome. This experiment was repeated numerous times with the same result. It appeared that some mechanism existed to replace the lost chromosome. It was hypothesized that either a nondisjunction event or selective endoreduplication of the unirradiated homologue was occurring.

## NUCLEOLAR ORGANIZER

One of the fundamental questions with regard to the potential usefulness of the laser microbeam in genetic studies was whether it could be used to inactivate specific genetic regions of the chromosome. In the early laser microbeam experiments, it was demonstrated that focusing the green laser beam into the secondary constriction region of the chromosomes was effective in inactivating the nucleolar organizer genes (Berns et al., 1970a; Ohnuki et al., 1972). In these studies, the chromosomes were sensitized with acridine orange prior to laser microirradiation of the secondary constriction region in metaphase or anaphase. The daughters of such an irradiated cell were deficient in the number of nucleoli corresponding to the number of irradiated secondary constrictions. This fine level of microsurgery was extended even further to include microirradiation of either the secondary constriction directly or of the chromosome region immediately proximal to the secondary constriction (Berns and Cheng, 1971). The results of these studies suggested that the region proximal to the secondary constriction in some way regulates secondary constriction activity.

More recent experiments have employed the 265-nm wavelength of the frequency quadrupled, neodymium-YAG laser. In these studies, the nucleolar organizer region was irradiated either by focusing the laser into the secondary constriction in anaphase or focusing it into the nucleolus just as it was disappearing in midprophase (Berns et al., 1979). In 23% of the cases (14/59), irradiation of one prophase nucleolus resulted in the formation of daughter cells that were deficient in one nucleolus. Furthermore, when these cells were isolated and cloned by micromanipulation, a deficiency of one nucleolus occurred in all the cells in the clonal population. The cells used in this study were from a stable tetraploid $PtK_2$ line that normally had two nucleoli per cell. The ribosomal genes have been shown to be located just below the centromere on the X chromosome. Both X chromosomes have a clear secondary constriction (Branch and Berns, 1976) in this region. In the clonal cells that descended from an irradiated cell, each nucleus had one nucleolus instead of two. Giemsa-trypsin banding of the clonal cells revealed that each cell still had two X chromosomes but that one of the X chromosomes was deficient in a light-staining region just below the centromere. These results demonstrate that one group of nucleolar genes was either deleted or inactivated by laser microirradiation. Furthermore, the genetic deficiency can be correlated with an altered chromosome-banding pattern.

## MITOSIS AND MITOTIC ORGANELLES

The process of mitosis has been studied extensively with the laser microbeam. Experiments have involved irradiation of centriolar regions or centromeres and the subsequent analysis of cell behavior and ultrastructure.

These types of experiments have been possible because the flat nature of the rat kangaroo cells permits clear visualization of the centriolar regions and the centromeres during mitosis (Rattner and Berns, 1976a, 1976b). The centriolar duplexes first appear as phase-dark dots in an otherwise "clear" zone adjacent to the nucleus in prophase. As mitosis progresses, the duplexes are observed separating from each other as they migrate to opposite poles of the cell.

### Microbeam Studies

Microbeam studies have been undertaken to selectively damage the centriolar region in order to ascertain the roles of its components in the mitotic process. For example, it has been possible to selectively damage the pericentriolar cloud material by green laser microirradiation following treatment with acridine orange (Berns et al., 1977). In these studies, it appeared that the damage was localized to the material surrounding the centriole rather than to the centriole itself. When the irradiation was performed in prophase, the cells were able to organize opposite poles and even enter a metaphase configuration. However, there was no chromatid separation or anaphase movement of chromosomes, though the cells did undergo cytokinesis. These results strongly suggest that the pericentriolar material plays a critical role in regulating chromosome movement. Furthermore, the apparent binding of acridine orange to this region suggests the presence of a nucleic acid.

## Experiments With Psoralens

Subsequent studies employing light-activated, nucleic-acid–binding components (psoralens) further confirmed that a nucleic acid component is present in the centriolar region (Peterson and Berns, 1978b). In these studies, four different psoralen compounds were tested with respect to their ability to inhibit mitosis following exposure of the centriolar region to 365-nm laser light. Of the four psoralen compounds tested, only one [4′-aminomethyl-4,5′, 8-trimethyl (AMT) psoralen] was efficient in blocking mitosis. This was the only psoralen compound that had been shown to have a high affinity for RNA as well as DNA. The other three psoralen compounds had high affinities for DNA only, and mitotic blockage did not result when cells treated with these compounds were exposed to 365-nm laser light in their centriolar zones. These experiments suggest further that the nucleic acid found in the centriolar region is RNA. When the ultrastructure of the mitotically blocked irradiated cells was examined, both control and irradiated centriolar zones showed no structural damage. However, there was a marked lack of microtubules in or around the irradiated centriolar regions. Numerous mitochondria and other cytoplasmic organelles had moved in between the centriolar region and the chromosomes. Normally, these organelles are excluded from this region of the mitotic cell by the spindle.

The fact that the irradiated centrioles and pericentriolar material appeared normal structurally yet were still unable to organize a spindle suggests that the laser plus AMT-psoralen was affecting the spindle-organizing capacity of this region at the molecular level.

## Spindle Organization

Another experiment that suggested a spindle-organizing function for the pericentriolar region as opposed to the centriole itself was an experiment in which the 473-nm wavelength of the YAG laser was used to irradiate nonphotosensitized centriolar regions (Berns and Richardson, 1977). The result of this type of irradiation was the destruction of the centriole without the production of apparent damage in the pericentriolar material. The cells were able to continue through mitosis even though the centrioles had been destroyed in prophase. Electron micrographs clearly demonstrated normal numbers of microtubules associated with the pericentriolar material. The apparent role of the pericentriolar material in spindle organization and function has been corroborated by in-vitro biochemical polymerization studies (Gould and Borisy, 1977) and by studies in $PtK_2$ cells demonstrating centriole-deficient poles in somatic cells undergoing a meiotic-like reduction division (Brenner et al., 1977).

## Chromosome Movement

The other major aspect of mitosis that has been studied with the laser microbeam involves chromosome movement and distribution. As discussed earlier in this review, irradiation of the centromere region damages the kinetochore and results in the chromosome's becoming detached from the spindle. Of particular interest was the observation that if both kinetochores on one chromosome are irradiated in metaphase, the chromosome drifts off the metaphase plate, but the two chromatids remain attached to each other. However,when the nonirradiated chromosomes undergo initial chromatid separation immediately prior to the beginning of anaphase movements, the irradiated chromatids also separate from each other. The irradiated chromatids do not have kinetochores or spindle attachment sites, and they simply drift about in the cell, often becoming incorporated into a micronucleus. These results demonstrate that the event of chromatid separation is distinct from chromatid movement toward the poles. Furthermore, the initial separation of chromatids from each other does not involve microtubules creating a pulling force at the centromere region (Brenner et al., in press).

If cells with micronuclei created by kinetochore irradiation are observed until they enter the subsequent mitosis, the chromosomes are seen to condense in the micronucleus. The chromosomes contain two chromatids each, thus demonstrating that irradiation in the centromere region (and its subsequent inactivation) does not prevent chromosome replication during interphase. However, these chromosomes do not attach to the spindle during either the first or second mitosis following the one in which irradiation occurred. The descendant cells continued to have micronuclei produced around the chromosomes that were descendants of the original irradiated ones. This finding thus suggests that the ability to synthesize or repair a kinetochore was permanently affected by the irradiation one or two cell divisions earlier. Since very little is known about kinetochore structure, function, or synthesis, these microbeam studies are some of the first experimental results on these very small structures.

**Chromosome Movement on the Mitotic Spindle.** Other studies have been directed more specifically toward chromosome movement on the mitotic spindle. One series of experiments was designed to investigate the function of the kinetochore in chromosome movement. A single kinetochore of a double chromatid chromosome was irradiated at prometaphase of mitosis in $PtK_2$ cells. It was of interest to see what effect the irradiation of the single kinetochore would have on the orientation of the remaining kinetochore and on the subsequent movement of the chromosome and chromatids. It was thought possible that such irradiation would produce behavior similar to that of a univalent in meiosis (Nicklas, 1961), in which one or more reorientations are induced followed by nondisjunction.

In most cases, the chromosome immediately moves toward the pole to which the nonirradiated kinetochore is oriented while the remaining chromosomes congress on the metaphase plate (McNeill and Berns, 1979a). In some instances, however, the chromosome reorients and moves back across the spindle to the opposite pole, thus exhibiting the same behavior as a univalent (McNeill and Berns, in press). In either situation, at anaphase, the chromatids of the irradiated chromosome separate, but the damaged chromatid does not move toward the opposite pole. It remains parallel to, and slightly separated from, the undamaged chromatid, resulting in nondisjunction of the irradiated chromosome.

Electron microscopy of such a chromosome shows a normal kinetochore on the nonirradiated chromatid. The irradiated chromatid exhibits either no recognizable kinetochore structure or a typical "inactive" kinetochore appearance in which the trilayer structure is present but has no microtubules associated with it.

**Chromatid Separation.** The separation of the chromatids, which occurs at the beginning of anaphase in the absence of the bipolar tension associated with two functional kinetochores, suggests that the initial separation and hence the "anaphase trigger" are not dependent on the kinetochore region and are not due to microtubule-mediated forces. In an attempt to shed more light on this problem, the region between the sister kinetochores of a single chromosome has been irradiated (McNeill and Berns, 1979b). Preliminary results show an induced separation of the kinetochores that is not followed by premature separation of the chromatids. This indicates that the chromosome is held together by some interaction of the chromosome arms until anaphase initiation.

## NUCLEOLUS

The nucleolus is an organelle that has been a target for classic ultraviolet microbeamists for years (Moreno, 1971; Sakharov and Voronkova, 1966). In fact, the first major demonstration that the function of the nucleolus was in cellular RNA synthesis was made by Perry et al. (1961) employing UV inactivation of nucleoli followed by $^{3}$H-cytidine autoradiography.

The green argon laser was first applied to study nucleolar function in 1969 (Berns et al., 1969). In this study, the drug quinacrine hydrochloride was used as a photosensitizing agent. This compound appeared to bind selectively to the nucleolus. Since it had some absorption between 490 and 540 nm, enough of the 488 wavelength of the argon laser was efficiently absorbed to result in selective damage to this organelle. These experiments demonstrated that a chromophore can be used in conjunction with the laser even if there is only a weak absorption in the region of the laser wavelength used. Very effective nucleolar lesions were produced, even though the relative amount of light absorbed at 488 nm was low. These studies also demonstrated that the drug itself (without laser treatment) had only a temporary effect on the cells' RNA synthesis.

The previous studies indicated that combining laser microirradiation with quinacrine treatment could be a useful approach to the study of nucleolus function. A subsequent study was undertaken in which the drug actinomycin D was used to induce segregation of the two major nucleolar subcomponents—the pars granulosa from the pars fibrillar. Cells with the segregated nucleoli were next treated with quinacrine hydrochloride, and then one of the two segregated components was irradiated with the laser microbeam (Brinkley and Berns, 1974). After differential destruction of either the pars granulosa or pars fibrillar, the cells were incubated in $^{3}$H-uridine and examined autoradiographically. With this rather complex experimental approach, it was possible to ascribe differential functions to the two main nucleolar subcomponents.

In a succeeding study (Meredith and Berns, 1976), a precise electron microscope analysis of cells treated under the various drug and irradiation conditions demonstrated that the laser lesions were confined to the regions irradiated. However, these experiments also revealed that in the control sequence where laser microirradiation of the nucleoplasm without drug treatment occurred, small ultrastructural lesions were detected even though no alteration was observed with the light microscope. These results demonstrated that light microscope analysis alone was not sufficient to assay for laser damage.

Numerous other studies involving nucleolus organization and function have already been described earlier in this review, in the section Nucleolar Organizer.

## THE NUCLEAR ENVELOPE

The nuclear envelope is a cell structure that has been very difficult to study by traditional methods. Most of what is known about this structure is based upon descriptive light and electron microscopy.

In recent studies, we have been investigating the role of the chromatin in nuclear envelope formation at the end of mitosis (Peterson and Berns, 1978a). The 365-nm wavelength of an argon laser was focused onto varying amounts of chromatin in mitosis. The cells were irradiated in the presence of various psoralen derivatives to create monoadducts and diadducts in the DNA. The cells were followed through mitosis, and the reformation of the nuclear envelope was assayed by light and electron microscopy. When all the chromatin was irradiated, no new nuclear envelope was formed. However, partial nuclear envelopes were formed when either the total laser dosage was reduced or one-fourth to one-half of the chromatin was irradiated. The studies also revealed that numerous nuclear pore complexes were present, either free in the cell or as part of the nuclear envelope, regardless of the irradiation conditions. This result suggests that the formation of the nuclear pore complexes is separate from the actual synthesis of the nuclear membrane. The psoralen effect on the reduction of the amount of nuclear envelope strongly implicates DNA in nuclear envelope formation.

## MYOCARDIAL CELL CONTRACTILITY

Extensive studies have been conducted in which the laser has been focused into individual mitochondria of contracting heart ventricle cells (Berns et al., 1970b, 1972a, 1972b; Adkisson et al., 1973; Berns and Cheng, 1973; Rattner et al., 1976; Waymire et al., 1976; Kitzes et al., 1977; Strahs et al., 1978; Burt et al., 1979). These studies have permitted the investigation of cardiac muscle cell contractility and cell-to-cell interactions in vitro. By selective alteration of a single mitochondrion or a single myofibril (Strahs et al., 1978), it was possible to alter precisely the contractile pattern of a single cell and cells electrically coupled to the irradiated cell (Kitzes et al., 1977). In addition, by recording the membrane action potentials by microelectrode impalement of the irradiated cell, it was possible to demonstrate that the laser-induced, altered contractile pattern was characterized by a change in the action potential. Furthermore, the recovery of the cell to a rhythmic contractile pattern was accompanied by a recovery of the action potential (Kitzes et al., 1977). It was also demonstrated that the ability to induce an altered contractile pattern depended upon the cell's exhibiting a typical pacemaker action potential rather than a nonpacemaker action potential (Kitzes et al., 1977). Scanning electron microscopy of laser-irradiated myocardial cells revealed a slight bulge in the cell membrane directly above the irradiated mitochondrion (Burt et al., 1979). These observations support the electrophysiological implication of the cell membrane in the aberrant contractile pattern.

## STRESS FIBER AND INTERMEDIATE FILAMENT IRRADIATION

The laser microbeam has been used selectively to alter stress fibers and bands of intermediate filaments (100 Å) in cultured nonmuscle cells (Strahs and Berns, 1979). Wavelengths of 532, 537, and 280 nm were used, and no artificial chromophores were employed. Lesions were assayed by a combination of phase contrast, polarizing, and transmission electron microscopy (TEM).

Stress fibers 1–2 μm in diameter were narrowed or completely severed by irradiation at 532, 537, and 280 nm. Stress fibers could be grouped into two classes: (1) those whose severed ends separated during the first few seconds following laser irradiation (46% of fibers irradiated) and (2) those fibers that showed no movements (54%). Microtubules that paralleled stress fibers persisted in the presence of colcemid for up to 5 h, and alignment of the severed stress fiber ends was maintained even in their absence. Injured stress fibers appear to be repaired within 1 h of irradiation. Bands of 100-Å filaments were induced in nonmuscle cells in secondary cultures of neonatal rat heart by exposure to colcemid. Lesions that appeared as phase-dense spots were induced in these bands by irradiation at 532, 537, and 280 nm. The positions of the lesions in the band, relative to one another, did not change over several hours despite movements of the entire band.

These studies demonstrate that (1) stress fibers may be an excellent system in which to study subcellular repair, (2) induced bands of 100-Å filaments probably move passively in the cell containing them, and (3) laser irradiation of cytoplasmic filaments in nonmuscle cells does not require the introduction of an artificial chromophore.

## SUMMARY

In this review, we have attempted to demonstrate how the laser microbeam can be used to study a variety of cellular components. The ability to produce defined molecular alterations in submicron areas of specific target structures permits a rather precise manipulation of cell structure and function. This approach is being used to study rather basic problems in chromosome organization and function, cell mitosis, nucleolus function, nuclear envelope synthesis, cell contractility, and cytoskeletal elements. Any structure that can be visualized with the light microscope is within the resolution of laser microbeam irradiation.

## REFERENCES

Adkisson KP, Baic D, Burgott S, Cheng WK, Berns MW (1973) Argon laser microirradiation of mitochondria in rat myocardial cells in tissue culture. IV. Ultrastructural and cytochemical analysis of minimal lesions. J Mol Cell Cardiol 5:559–564.

Berns MW (1974a) Recent progress in laser microbeams. Int Rev Cytol 39:383–411.

Berns MW (1974b) Microbeams. In: Wolbarsht ML (ed) Laser Applications in Medicine and Biology, vol. 2. Plenum Press, New York, pp. 1–40.

Berns MW (1974c) Directed chromosome loss by laser microirradiation. Science 186:700–705.

Berns MW (1975) Dissecting the cell with a laser microbeam. In: Joussot-Dubien J (ed) Lasers in Physical Chemistry and Biophysics. Elsevier Publishing Company, Amsterdam, pp. 389–401.

Berns MW (1978) The laser microbeam as a probe for chromatin structure and function. In: Stein G, Stein J, and Kleinsmith L (eds) Methods in Cell Biology, vol. 18. Academic Press, New York, pp. 277–294.

Berns MW, Cheng WK (1971) Are chromosome secondary constructions nucleolar organizers: A re-evaluation using a laser microbeam. Exp Cell Res 69:185–192.

Berns MW, Cheng WK (1973) Argon laser microirradiation of mitochondria in rat myocardial cells in tissue culture. Pacemaker versus non-pacemaker cells. Life Sci 12:469–474.

Berns MW, Floyd AD (1971) Chromosome microdissection by laser: A functional cytochemical analysis. Exp Cell Res 67:305–310.

Berns MW, Richardson SM (1977) Continuation of mitosis after selective laser microbeam destruction of the centriolar region. J Cell Biol 75:977–982.

Berns MW, Salet C (1972) Laser microbeams for partial cell irradiation. Int Rev Cytol 33:131–154.

Berns MW, Olson RS, Rounds DE (1969) *In vitro* production of chromosomal lesions. Nature (Lond) 221:74–75.

Berns MW, Ohnuki Y, Rounds DE, Olson RS (1970a) Modification of nucleolar expression following laser microirradiation of chromosomes. Exp Cell Res 60:133–138.

Berns MW, Gamaleja N, Duffy C, Olson R, Rounds DE (1970b) Argon laser microirradiation of mitochondria in rat myocardial cells in tissue culture. J Cell Physiol 76:207–214.

Berns MW, Cheng WK, Floyd AD, Ohnuki Y (1971) Chromosome lesions produced with an argon laser microbeam without dye sensitization. Science 171:903–905.

Berns MW, Gross DCL, Cheng WK, Woodring D (1972a) Argon laser microirradiation of mitochondria in rat myocardial cells in tissue culture. II. Correlation of morphology and function in single irradiated cells. J Mol Cell Cardiol 4:71–83.

Berns MW, Gross DCL, Cheng WK (1972b) Argon laser microirradiation of mitochondria in rat myocardial cells in tissue culture. III. Irradiation of multicellular networks. J Mol Cell Cardiol 4:427–434.

Berns MW, Rattner JB, Meredith S, Witter M (1976) Current laser microirradiation studies. Ann NY Acad Sci 267:160–175.

Berns MW, Rattner JB, Brenner S, Meredith S (1977) The role of the centriolar region in animal cell mitosis: A laser microbeam study. J Cell Biol 72:351–367.

Berns MW, Chong LK, Hammer-Wilson M, Miller K, Siemens A (1979) Genetic microsurgery by laser: Establishment of a clonal population of rat kangaroo cells ($PTK_2$) with a directed deficiency in a chromosomal nucleolar organizer. Chromosoma 73:1–8.

Bessis M, Gires F, Mayer G, Nomarski G (1962) Irradiation des organites cellulaires á l'aide d'un laser á rubis. C R Acad Sci [*D*] 225:1010–1012.

Branch AB, Berns MW (1976) Nucleoli and ploidy in *Potorous* cells ($PTK_2$) *in vitro*. Chromosoma 56:33–40.

Brenner S, Branch A, Meredith S, Berns MW (1977) The absence of centrioles from spindle poles of $PTK_2$ undergoing meiotic-like reduction division *in vitro*. J Cell Biol 72:368–379.

Brenner SL, Liaw L-H, Berns MW (in press) Laser microirradiation of kinetochores in mitotic $PtK_2$ cells: Chromatid separation and micronucleus formation. Cell Biophysics.

Brinkley L, Berns MW (1974) Laser microdissection of actinomycin D segregated nucleoli. Exp Cell Res 87:417–422.

Brinkley BR, Murphy P, Richardson LC (1967) Procedure for embedding in situ selected cells cultured *in vitro*. J Cell Biol 35:279–283.

Burt JM, Strahs KR, Berns MW (1979) Correlation of cell surface alterations with contractile response in laser microbeam irradiated myocardial cells: A scanning electron microscope study. Exp Cell Res 118:341–351.

Cremer C, Cremer T, Zorn C, Schoeller L (1976) Effects of laser UV-microirradiation ($\lambda$ = 2573A) on proliferation of Chinese hamster cells. Radiat Res 66:106–121.

Gould RR, Borisy GG (1977) The pericentriolar material in Chinese hamster ovary cells nucleates microtubule formation. J Cell Biol 73:601–615.

Kitzes M, Twiggs G, Berns MW (1977) Alteration of membrane electrical activity in ray myocardial cells following selective laser microbeam irradiation. J Cell Physiol 93:99–104.

Mark GE, Strasser FF (1966) Pacemaker activity and mitosis in cultures of newborn rat heart ventricle cells. Exp Cell Res 44:217–233.

McNeill PA, Berns MW (1979a) Laser microirradiation of a single kinetochore in mitotic $PTK_2$ cells. In vitro 15:206.

McNeill PA, Berns MW (1979b) The role of the kinetochore in the initiation of anaphase movement, studied by laser microirradiation. J Cell Biol 83:374a.

McNeill PA, Berns MW (in press) Chromosome behavior following laser microirradiation of a single kinetochore in mitotic $PtK_2$ cells. J Cell Biol.

Meredith S, Berns MW (1976) Light and electron microscopy of laser microirradiated nucleoli and nucleoplasm in tissue culure cells. J Morphol 150:785–804.

Moreno G (1971) Effects of UV microirradiation on different parts of the cell. II. Cytological observation and unscheduled DNA synthesis after partial nuclear irradiation. Exp Cell Res 65:129–139.

Moreno G, Lutz M, Bessis M (1969) Partial cell irradiation by ultraviolet and visible light: Convention and laser sources. Int Rev Exp Pathol 7:99–137.

Nicklas RB (1961) Recurrent pole to pole movements of the sex chromosome during prometaphase I in Melanoplus differentialis spermatocytes. Chromosoma 12:97–115.

Ohnuki Y, Olson RS, Rounds DE, Berns MW (1972) Laser microbeam irradiation of the juxtanucleolar region of prophase nucleolar chromosomes. Exp Cell Res 71:132–144.

Perry RP, Hell A, Errera M (1961) The role of the nucleolus in ribonucleic acid and protein synthesis. I. Incorporation of cytidine into normal and nucleolar inactivated HeLa cells. Biochim Biophys Acta 49:47–57.

Peterson SP, Berns MW (1978a) Chromatin influence on the function and formation of the nuclear envelope shown by laser-induced psoralen photoreaction. J Cell Sci 32:197–213.

Peterson SP, Berns MW (1978b) Evidence for centriolar region RNA functioning in spindle formation in dividing $PTK_2$ cells. J Cell Sci 34:289–301.

Rattner JB, Berns MW (1974) Light and electron microscopy of laser microirradiated chromosomes. J Cell Biol 62:526–533.

Rattner JB, Berns MW (1976a) Centriole behavior in early mitosis of rat kangaroo cells ($PTK_2$). Chromosoma 54:387–395.

Rattner JB, Berns MW (1976b) Distribution of microtubules during centriole separation in rat kangaroo *(Potorous)* cells. Cytobios 15:37–43.

Rattner JB, Lifsics M, Meredith S, Berns MW (1976) Argon laser microirradiation of mitochondria in rat myocardial cells. VI. Correlation of contractility and ultrastructure. J Mol Cell Cardiol 8:239–248.

Sakharov VN, Voronkova LN (1966) Consequences of UV-microbeam irradiation of the nucleoli of living cell. Genetika 6:144–148.

Salet C (1972) A study of beating frequency of a single myocardial cell. I. Q-switched laser microirradiation of mitochondria. Exp Cell Res 73:360–366.

Salet C, Moreno G, Vinzens FA (1979) A study of beating frequency of a single myocardial cell. III. Laser microirradiation of mitochondria in the presence of KCN or ATP. Exp Cell Res 120:25–29.

Strahs KR, Berns MW (1979) Laser microirradiation of stress fibers and intermediate filaments in non-muscle cells from cultured rat heart. Exp Cell Res 119:31–45.

Strahs KR, Burt JM, Berns MW (1978) Contractility changes in cultured cardiac cells following laser microirradiation of myofibrils and the cell surface. Exp Cell Res 113:75–83.

Waymire K, Kitzes M, Meredith S, Twiggs G, Berns MW (1976) Argon laser microirradiation of mitochondria in rat myocardial cells in tissue culture. VII. Fibrillation in ventricle and auricle cells. J Cell Physiol 89:345–354.

# 7

# Laser Fluorescent Microirradiation: A New Technique

*A. Andreoni, A. Longoni*
*C. A. Sacchi, O. Svelto*

The technique of fluorescence microscopy has been increasingly used for structural studies of biologic molecules (Konev, 1967; Udenfried, 1969; Duchesne, 1973). This technique is particularly valuable and sensitive for the investigation of biophysical and biochemical processes in single cells or organelles, even in the living state. Current trends in this field are, for example: (1) the biophysical study of the secondary structure of nucleic acids, (2) the biochemical study of enzymatic reactions that either produce fluorescent emission or occur on a fluorogenic substrate (Prenna et al., 1977; Kohen et al., 1978), and (3) the study of membrane properties related either to the potential-dependent release and uptake of fluorescent dyes or to the fluorescence recovery after photobleaching (Jacobson,1979).

The fluorescence emission may be due either to the biomolecule itself (primary fluorescence) or to a suitable dye bound to a specific position of the biomolecule (secondary fluorescence). In primary fluorescence, which in general requires UV excitation, information on isolated biomolecules can readily be obtained. On the other hand, when the UV absorption overlap of many cellular constituents makes it difficult to study a given biomolecule interacting with others, secondary fluorescence allows the study of biomolecules in their natural environment (i.e., in situ), provided that suitable stains are chosen that bind selectively to the given biomolecule (Andreoni, 1979).

Furthermore, in the latter situation, the fluorescence properties of the staining agent depend, in general, on its mechanism of interaction with the biomolecule. In both examples, however, the fluorescence parameters of interest are the polarization, the emission and the excitation spectrums, the decay time, and the quan-

This work was supported by the Italian National Research Council through the Special Program "Tecnologie Biomediche."

tum yield. In particular, the measurement of the decay time is an especially valuable technique in the investigation of a large variety of biophysical processes (Brand and Gohlke, 1972). In fact, fluorescence time behavior is, in general, strongly dependent on the paths along which the energy of the excited molecule is released to the surroundings.

In our laboratory, we applied ourselves to the study of the complexes that are formed when a dye belonging to the acridine family is bound both to synthetic polynucleotides and to native DNA. As described in the section on biologic applications later in this chapter, study of these complexes has implications in several fields—in particular, it can be useful for understanding the origin of the fluorescence patterns of chromosomes when they are stained with some of the acridine dyes.

In studies on time-resolved fluorescence, decay-time constants in the nanosecond or subnanosecond range often must be measured. In addition, the fluorescence must be excited selectively in small portions of single cells or cellular organelles. That is why we built up a laser microfluorometer with $\sim$ 0.2 ns temporal resolution and $\sim$ 0.3 $\mu$m spatial resolution. Since two basic techniques are currently used for the measurement of fluorescence decay-time constants, a short outline and a comparison of these techniques are presented in the next section.

## THE MEASUREMENT TECHNIQUES FOR FAST FLUORESCENCE DECAYS

The fluorescence signals excited by laser microirradiation are expected to be very weak, mainly because of the smallness of the irradiated volume. Typically, a few tens of photons are emitted per excitation pulse. Thus, only photodetectors with internal gain, usually photomultiplier tubes (PMT), can be used.

A detected photon releases at the photocathode of the PMT one electron which, after internal multiplication, gives a current pulse [single electron response (SER)] at the output. Depending on the PMT types, the SER pulses have durations ranging from somewhat less than 1 ns to a few nanoseconds and an average charge ranging from $10^4$ to $10^8$ electrons. The PMT current waveform resulting from a detected fluorescence pulse is a superposition of SER pulses.[1]

In general, two techniques for the measurement of fast fluorescence decays may be adopted: the so-called single photon (SP) detection technique, and one that we call the light flux (LF) technique. The SP technique is applicable when the light intensity is low (detected photon rate $\ll$ reciprocal of the width of the SER pulses): In this case, SER pulses can be individually resolved. The probability distribution of the arrival time of the SER pulses in relation to a synchronism signal (usually obtained from the excitation pulse) is proportional to the fluorescence pulse. However, when the SER pulses cannot be resolved, the LF technique may be applied.

[1]In this regard see, for instance, the RCA photomultiplier manual (1970).

In this case, the fluorescence pulse is considered as a continuous light flux. The PMT current waveform is correspondingly treated as an analog variable whose average shape is proportional to the fluorescence decay.

The SP technique offers a number of advantages over the LF technique. In fact, the requirements of high linearity of the PMT and of high stability of its gain, typical of the LF technique, are not necessary in the SP techniques. Furthermore, dark-current contributions can be reduced in SP techniques by means of circuits for pulse discrimination, as a result of their different statistical distribution compared with that of the SER pulses. Finally, the overall time resolution of the SP technique is, in general, better than that of the LF technique because of the irrelevance of the statistical spread of the SER pulse width in the SP technique.

However, a problem associated with SP techniques is that to avoid distortions in the probability distribution of the arrival time, the probability of detecting more than one photon per fluorescence pulse must be kept very low, possibly by attenuating the light intensity. Thus, if the repetition rate of the excitation source is low (as is often the case with pulsed laser excitation), the total measurement time, with the SP technique, may become impractically long. In such a case, if a light level higher than the maximum limit of the SP techniques is available, LF techniques would be more convenient.

The apparatus for SP measurement can be readily assembled with commercial instruments. It is based on a time-interval–to-pulse-height converter (TPHC) circuit and on a multichannel analyzer (MCA) set in a pulse-height analyzer (PHA) working mode. Descriptions of the operation of this kind of apparatus are available (Cova et al., 1973).

The LF technique may be implemented in different ways. A widely adopted, completely analog approach is based on the so-called boxcar detector (Cova and Longoni, 1979; Malmstadt et al., 1974). The detector retrieves a repetitive signal by filtering the uncorrelated noise. This approach may suffer from some limitations typical of the analog instrumentation, such as impracticability of large filtering time-constants, gain and zero-level drifts, microphonisms, etc. Furthermore, distortions of the averaged waveform may result when appreciable photodecomposition takes place in the time required by the detector to scan the whole waveform.

Some of these drawbacks can be overcome by sampling and digitizing the PMT output and then performing a digital averaging on the digitized data (Amsel and Bosshard, 1970; Cohn, 1969; Steingraber and Berlman, 1963). We recall here that the signal-to-noise (S/N) ratio enhancement obtained in this way is of the order of $\sqrt{N_A}$, where $N_A$ is the number of samples averaged at each point of the waveform (Cova and Longoni, 1979; Hewlett-Packard Journal, April 1968). Usually, in the case of short fluorescence pulses, only one sample per light pulse can be taken. Depending on the sampler type, the rise time of the instrument can be as low as a few tens of picoseconds. This technique was applied in our experiments with a conventional sampling oscilloscope. So far, only one commercial instrument is capable of taking a high number of samples in each short fluorescence pulse (up to 512 samples in a 10-ns time interval). However, its rise time of 0.5 ns sets a limit to its capability of measuring subnanosecond decay times.

## THE LASER MICROFLUOROMETER

### Technology

The experimental apparatus (Fig. 7.1) developed in our laboratory (Sacchi et al., 1974; Sacchi and Andreoni, 1975) is based on (1) a subnanosecond-pulsed tunable dye laser, (2) a microscope system for fluorescence microscopy (Leitz MPV) with a PMT, and (3) a digital signal-averager. The averager is provided with on-line monitoring capability, mass storage for the data acquired, and an interface with a host computer for off-line data handling.

**The Dye Laser.** Described in detail by Andreoni et al. (1975), the dye laser is pumped by a nitrogen laser that generates pulses with peak power up to 500 kW, duration of 2.5 ns, and a repetition rate of up to 50 Hz. The special design of the dye cell enables this laser to generate pulses with a duration of ~ 0.4 ns and peak power up to 10 kW. The laser beam is diffraction-limited and can be focused down to the resolving spot of the microscope, i.e., to ~ 0.3 $\mu$m. With a suitable choice of the laser dye, the wavelength can be tuned over the whole visible and near-UV spectrum. As indicated in Figure 7.1, the laser beam enters the fluorescence microscope after passing two lenses and two diaphragms which select the central part of the beam. Both the lenses and the diaphragms, together with the microscope optics, determine the spot size on the plane of the sample. A beam splitter sends a small fraction of the laser power on a fast photodiode (Hadron TRG 105 C, rise time 0.3 ns). Its output enables the laser power to be monitored and the digital averager to be triggered externally.

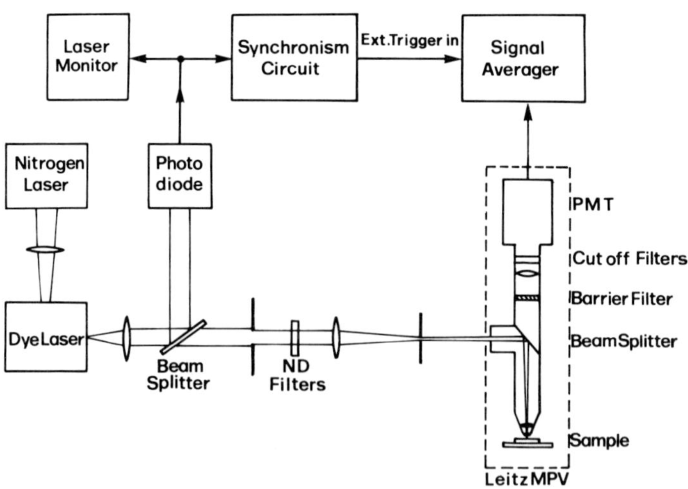


**Fig. 7.1.** Block diagram of laser microfluorometer. *PMT*, photomultiplier tube; *ND*, neutral density filters; *MPV*, microscope system for fluorescence microscopy.

**Fluorescence Microscopy.** The MPV apparatus is a commercial instrument for fluorescence microscopy. It includes a microscope with side windows both for the entrance of the laser beam and for the illumination of the sample by a conventional lamp. The microscope objective itself collects the fluorescence light, which is then focused on the photocathode of a photomultiplier mounted at the top of the microscope. The desired band of the fluorescence spectrum is selected by suitable barrier filters. In our experiments, the photomultiplier RCA 70045D with $\sim$ 0.7 ns rise time was used.

When the measurements are performed in situ—i.e., on smears prepared by histochemical techniques—the irradiated volume may be as small as a few cubic microns. For this reason, and because of fluorescence and detection efficiencies, the fluorescence signal may be very weak—typically, a few photons per nanosecond. Since this light level is higher than the limit for the single-photon (SP) technique and the laser repetition rate is rather low, the LF technique is more convenient. The PMT output must be averaged since, at such low emission rates, the emission statistics introduce fluctuations of the order of the signal itself.

**The Averager.** The averager is based on general-purpose laboratory instrumentation such as a conventional sampling oscilloscope and a multichannel analyzer. The PMT output is first sampled by the sampling oscilloscope. An analog-to-digital conversion (ADC) of the sampled signals is then performed, and finally a digital averaging of the signals is done by means of the multichannel analyzer. Note that the overall rise time of the averager (Fig. 7.2) is of the order of that of the sampling oscilloscope (i.e., as short as a few tens of picoseconds).

*Sampling of the Fluorescence Signal.* A conventional fast sampling oscilloscope (Tektronix 564, with S1 plug-in sampling head, rise time of $\sim$ 350 ps) takes one sample of the PMT output at each repetition of the light pulse. The waveform reconstruction on the oscilloscope display is obtained by sampling the input at different times (House, 1971). In our case, the delay of these times in relation to the triggering signal is increased by a constant step at each repetition (sequential scanning mode). At each sampling, the oscilloscope provides a voltage-output signal (vertical output, Y) (Fig. 7.2) whose height is proportional to the sampled amplitude and remains practically constant until the next sampling operation. This output, therefore, gives a slowed-down replica of the input repetitive fast waveform. An analog-to-digital conversion of this slow waveform can now be easily performed.

*Analog-to-Digital Conversion of Sampled Data.* The slow output Y of the oscilloscope is fed, after suitable amplification, to a voltage-to-frequency converter. The free-running voltage-controlled oscillator performs a highly linear conversion of the input signal to an output frequency $f$ (nonlinearity $< 0.01\%$ of full scale, in our case). At each sample, a strobe signal from the oscilloscope triggers the measurement of the frequency: the voltage-controlled oscillator (VCO) pulses are counted during a time interval with a precisely controlled duration ($T_m$). Thus, a number ($T_m \times f$) proportional to the value of Y, is obtained.

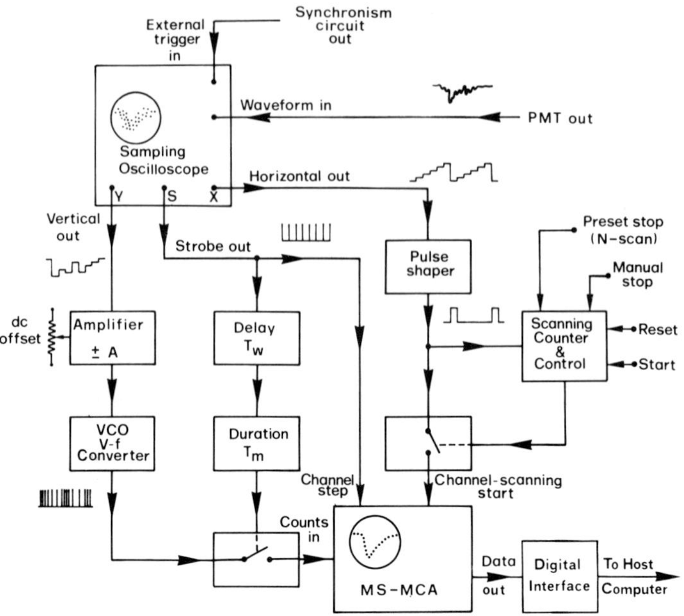


**Fig. 7.2.** Block diagram of digital averager. *PMT*, photomultiplier tube; *Y*, vertical voltage output signal; *S*, strobe signal; *X*, horizontal output signal; *N-scan*, number of preset scans; *A*, amplifier; $T_w$, "waiting" time; *VCO*, voltage-controlled oscillator; *V-f*, voltage-to-frequency converter; $T_m$, controlled time interval; *MS*, multiscaler; *MCA*, multichannel analyzer.

*Scanning the Fluorescence Waveform.* The frequency measurement and the digital averaging operations are performed by a multichannel analyzer (MCA), operating in the multiscaler (MS) mode. Thus, the MCA behaves like a scaler associated with a multicell digital memory: In the *n*th cell (channel) it stores the number of pulses counted by the scaler in the *n*th time interval ($T_m$). In our case, a Silena System 27 MCA was used. The start of the channel scan is synchronized with the start of the sampling oscilloscope scan, by using suitable control logic. A one-to-one correspondence is kept between sampling time-position and memory-cell address (*n*). At each sample, the scaler is enabled to operate and the address *n* is increased by one.

*Averaging the Digitized Signals.* Repeated scans of the signal can be automatically performed. To enhance the S/N ratio, the number of *V-f* pulses counted at the *n*th sampling of each scanning of the signal is added to the previous content of the *n*th memory cell. This averaging method, based on multiple fast scans, is less sensitive to slow spurious effects, such as photodecomposition processes or laser-intensity drifts, than are methods based on a single slow scan such as that performed by the boxcar detector. Moreover, in contrast to the usual ADC methods (e.g., successive approximation AD conversion), the adopted ADC procedure is free from systematic deviations in the average (DeLotto and Osnaghi, 1967).

*Other Features of the Apparatus.* To enhance the performances of the averager described, an additional simple circuit, which we called "base-line subtractor," was also employed. The aim of this circuit is to subtract automatically, from the measured signal, the light background not correlated with the laser pulse and any instrumental offset, with associated possible slow drift. To enhance the linearity of the $V$-$f$ conversion, it is normally useful to avoid the lower part of the VCO input dynamic range by offsetting the input signal with a constant voltage. The base-line subtractor circuit provides an echo-trigger pulse for the oscilloscope at a time instant intermediate between two laser pulses. In correspondence with the echo pulse, the sampling and the AD conversion are performed as usual, but the resulting number is subtracted from the content of the memory cell. The channel address is stopped only after the set of two sampling actions (true measurement and echo measurement). Moreover, the alternate samples that are displayed on the oscilloscope make it possible to check accurately the adjustment (dot-response control) of the oscilloscope itself. By using light choppers synchronized with the laser pulse, it would be possible also to subtract light background and electromagnetic interference correlated in time with the laser pulse, but at the expense of doubling the time required for a measurement.

Another feature of the apparatus that should not be overlooked is the continuous monitoring of the acquisition and averaging process by means of the oscilloscope and of the MCA displays, respectively.

A magnetic tape for the mass storage of the averaged waveform is provided by the MCA. A digital interface (Standard IEEE 488) to a host computer for further data handling (e.g., deconvolution of the apparatus response from the measured curves, resolution of multiexponential decays, etc.) was developed.

In a typical response curve (prompt response) of the overall apparatus to the excitation pulse (Fig 7.3), the time width of $\sim$ 1 ns is due to the convolution of the laser pulse with the response time of both the PMT and the signal averager.

## Properties of the Laser Microfluorometer

The advantages of using the laser instead of conventional lamps in connection with fast-detection electronics and averaging instrumentation can now be evidenced by summarizing the performances of our microfluorometer.

1. The laser light can be concentrated, thus giving high power-density excitation, over very small regions (with dimensions of the order of a wavelength) to excite the fluorescence selectively in single cellular organelles. In fact, we checked photographically that the laser beam can be focused down to a spot diameter equal to the resolving diameter of the microscope ($\sim$ 0.3 $\mu$m).
2. The short duration, the clean shape (free from low-level tails), and the high stability of the laser pulses, in connection with the response time of the detection electronics, make possible the measurement of fluorescence-decay times even in the subnanosecond

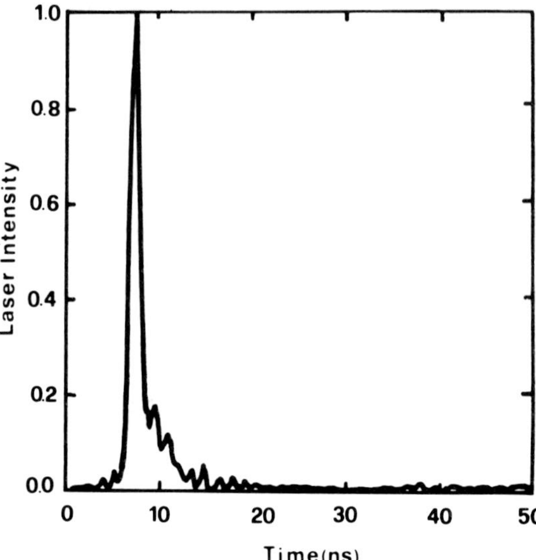


**Fig. 7.3.** Prompt response of the whole apparatus.

range. In our study, even if the prompt response of the system has a time width of ~ 1 ns, its shape and the overall residual fluctuations after the averaging process produce a precision of the lifetime measurement of ~ 0.2 ns (at least in the case of decays with a single time-constant).

3. The sample irradiation with laser pulses of high intensity and short duration turned out to be very important for greatly decreasing, if not practically suppressing, the photodecomposition of fluorescent dyes, during a typical measurement cycle (Sacchi et al., 1974; Andreoni et al., 1979a). This result, which has been commonly obtained in our experiments, is particularly relevant compared with the results obtained with UV lamps in ordinary fluorescence microscopy. In this case, a fading of the fluorescence due to the photodecomposition often occurs in a few seconds, thus making it difficult to perform reliable measurements. The absence of dye photodecomposition with pulsed laser excitation is probably due to the small amount of energy density normally used despite the high power-density (Andreoni, 1979).
4. The spectral properties of the laser can be very useful for optimizing the fluorescence excitation conditions. In fact, owing to its monochromaticity, laser light can selectively excite fluorescent substances with different excitation spectra. Furthermore, with tunable lasers, the wavelength can be tuned to the peak of the excitation spectrum of the fluorescent substance, thus yielding the most intense emission.
5. The extremely high power-density may greatly increase sensitivity. As a consequence, fluorescent materials, including important types of drugs, can be localized and measured in very low concentration. Furthermore, the available excitation intensity is usually high enough to saturate the fluorescence transition. Measurement of the saturation intensity leads to a straightforward evaluation of the absorption cross-section of the transition itself (Sacchi et al., 1974). This quantity is of great biologic relevance, since its magnitude is certainly affected by the interaction of the fluorescent probe with the substrate and the cellular ambient.
6. The polarization of the laser light makes possible polarization measurements of the fluorescent emission, thus giving information on the overall shape of the biologic macromolecules and on their orientational relaxation (Rigler, 1979).

7. Finally, it is worth noting that some performances of our microfluorometer have, quite recently, been improved. In fact, a new nitrogen-pumped dye laser, built in our laboratory (Cubeddu and De Silvestri, 1979) has been used. It generates pulses with a duration (full width half maximum: FWHM) of ~ 150 ps at a repetition rate of up to 150 Hz. The fluorescent waveform is now measured by a crossed-field photomultiplier (Varian 154 M, rise time ~ 100 ps, fall time ~ 150 ps). In this way, decay times of the order of ~ 100 ps or even shorter might be measured by appropriate deconvolution.

## EXAMPLES OF BIOLOGIC APPLICATIONS

The study of laser-induced fluorescence has already been applied to several cases that are of biologic interest (Andreoni et al., 1979a). Here, we consider examples of biologic molecules that can profitably be studied with laser techniques and that require, when investigated in situ (i.e., on histochemical preparations), the high spatial resolution given by the microfluorometer.

### Acridine Dyes

We have studied the fluorescence properties of the complexes formed when a dye of the acridine family is bound to DNA. These complexes present many interesting properties, with implications of relevance in several fields—from chemical physics to biophysics, and from pharmacology to medicine.

The acridines form a large family of fluorescent dyes, which absorb in the blue and emit in the green region of the spectrum. Most of them are specific stains for DNA (Albert, 1966). Among the dyes of interest, we mention acriflavine, proflavine, quinacrine, and quinacrine mustard (QM). When an acridine dye is added to a solution of DNA, acridine-DNA complexes are formed.

In suitable staining conditions, the complexes result from the intercalation of the acridine ring between two neighboring base-pairs of the DNA double helix (Peacocke, 1973). These complexes have been quite extensively studied, but the mechanism of their formation is still unclear. Experimentally, they present two main important properties. The first one is that their fluorescence quantum yield depends strongly on the binding site (Michelson et al., 1972; Schreiber and Daune, 1974; Latt and Brodie, 1976). Indeed, it increases when the dye molecule intercalates two adenine-thymine (AT) base-pairs (e.g., by a factor 4 for QM) and decreases (by a factor ~ 10 for QM) when the molecule intercalates either two guanine-cytosine (GC) base-pairs or a GC-AT sequence. The second important property of the acridines is that they give characteristic fluorescence patterns when used to stain the DNA of metaphase chromosomes of both mammalians and plants (Caspersson et al., 1970). These patterns, formed by regions (bands) ~ 1 $\mu$m wide and with a more intense fluorescence, are so reproducible that they are used for chromosome recognition and characterization (Modest and Sengupta, 1973). The bands, whose origin is still unclear, could be regions with a higher concentration of either AT-AT sequences or fluorescent dye, compared with the surrounding regions. Comparison of the fluorescence time decay excited by the laser in the bands and out of them could help to clarify their origin (Andreoni et al., 1979a). This would be of obvious relevance in genetics and in the study of diseases that alter the banding patterns (Manolov and Manolova, 1972; Rowley, 1973; Zankl and Kang, 1972).

## Fluorescent Drugs

Finally, it should be mentioned that important fluorescent drugs, such as actinomycin D (antibiotic drug) (Modest and Sengupta, 1973), daunomycin, and doxorubicin hydrochloride (antitumor agents) bind selectively to the DNA and present base-specific fluorescence properties and give fluorescent bands in chromosomes as the acridines.

## Acridine-DNA Complexes

An extensive study of the fluorescence properties of the acridine-DNA complexes has been made with our apparatus. Most of the experiments were performed with quinacrine mustard which gives the highest contrast and most stable fluorescence bands. The laser dye was a $1.5 \times 10^{-3}$ M solution of POPOP (l, 4-di-[2-(5-phenoxazolyl)]-benzene) in toluene that permitted tuning the wavelength to 419 nm, corresponding to the peak of the absorption spectrum of quinacrine mustard (QM) (Andreoni et al., 1979a).

In a first set of experiments, the decay curves of QM, either free in solution or bound to the synthetic polynucleotides polydA-polydT and polydG-polydC, were studied (Fig. 7.4). As expected from the quantum yield data, the decay time of QM bound to polydA-polydT is much longer ($\tau \simeq 18$ ns) than that of the free dye in solution ($\tau = 3.9 \pm 0.2$ ns) (Andreoni et al., 1979a). The decay curve of QM

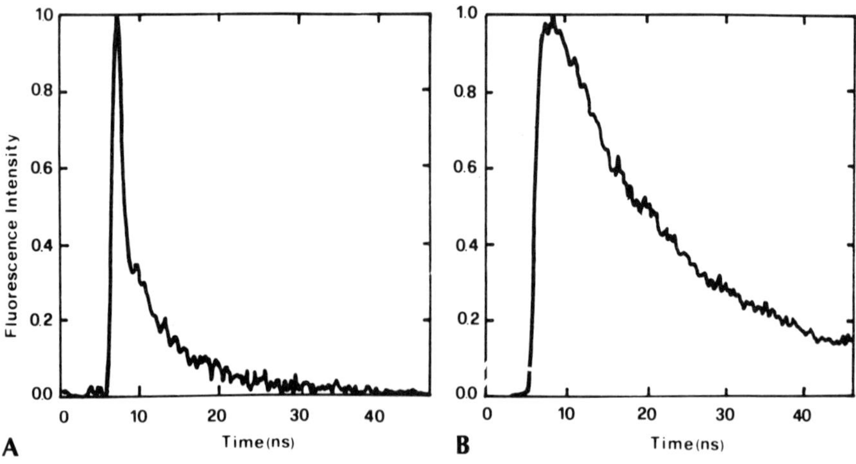


**Fig. 7.4.** Fluorescence-decay curve of quinacrine mustard bound to polydG-polydC **(A)** and polydA-polydT **(B)**.

bound to polydG-polydC is clearly not exponential but rather is formed by the superposition of a fast initial decay with time constant $\tau = 0.5 \pm 0.2$ ns and a slower tail with time constant $\tau \simeq 5$ ns. This behavior could be attributed to the formation of an excimer (i.e., an excited-state dimer) of the charge-transfer type between the excited QM molecule and the guanine residue (Andreoni et al., 1976). In a second set of experiments (Bottiroli et al., 1979), the fluorescence of several bacteria, with different known AT percentages and stained with QM, was studied, focusing the laser on a spot smaller than the bacteria themselves. To this end, preliminary measurements were made to compare the fluorescence responses of the cytologic preparations with those of the corresponding purified DNAs. It was found that the same fluorescence curve given by the bacterial smear was obtained from the DNA, provided that a suitable QM concentration was used (Bottiroli et al., 1979). This indicates that the fluorescence of the cytologic preparations is to be attributed to the dye bound to the DNA of the bacteria. After these preliminary measurements, a more extensive study of the stained bacteria was undertaken. All fluorescence-decay curves were interpreted in terms of nonradiative energy transfer in the Förster kinetics (Förster, 1948) between QM molecules bound to AT-AT (which behave as donors) and QM molecules bound to either AT-GC or GC-GC (considered as nonfluorescent acceptors) (Andreoni et al., 1979b; Bottiroli et al., 1979). In particular, results on the base-pair sequence distribution of in-situ DNAs were obtained (Andreoni et al., 1979b).

## Chromosomes

A preliminary study of the fluorescence patterns of chromosomes was also made. Two fluorescence curves of the *Vicia faba* M chromosome were obtained (Fig. 7.5), one by focusing the laser excitation outside and the other by focusing inside a fluorescent band. Apart from a scale factor (the in-band fluorescence was reduced by a factor 1.54), the two curves are almost identical. In our opinion, this fact indicates that the band considered was mainly due to a higher dye concentration (Andreoni et al., 1979a).

## Fluorescence Decay

A final example is the fluorescence decay of a $1.7 \times 10^{-3}$ M solution of the antitumor drug doxorubicin HCl physiologic solution, when excited at 476 nm, which corresponds to the peak of the absorption spectrum of doxorubicin HCl (Fig 7.6). We confirmed that this shape remains unchanged down to the minimum detectable concentration, i.e., $10^{-9}$ M (Andreoni et al., 1979a). This is two orders of magnitude less than the lowest concentration measurable by the best conventional fluorometers, i.e., 100 ng/cc. Preliminary experiments already carried out indicated the feasibility of in-situ measurements of drug distribution inside tissues and single cells in living conditions. The comparison between the decay curve obtained in situ with that shown in Figure 7.6 could also give information on the interaction of the drug with cellular constituents (Andreoni, 1979).

Although the examples described indicate that interesting results have already

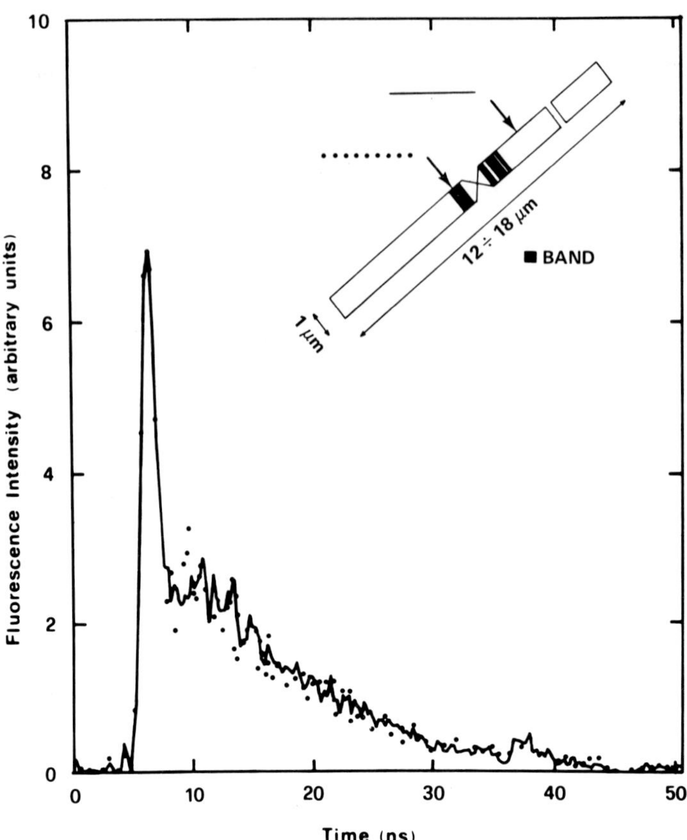


**Fig. 7.5.** Fluorescence-decay curves of *Vicia faba* M chromosome stained with quinacrine mustard. *Solid line,* laser excitation focused outside bands. *Dotted line,* laser excitation focused inside a band. *Arrows,* exact positions of excitation spot in schema of banding pattern.

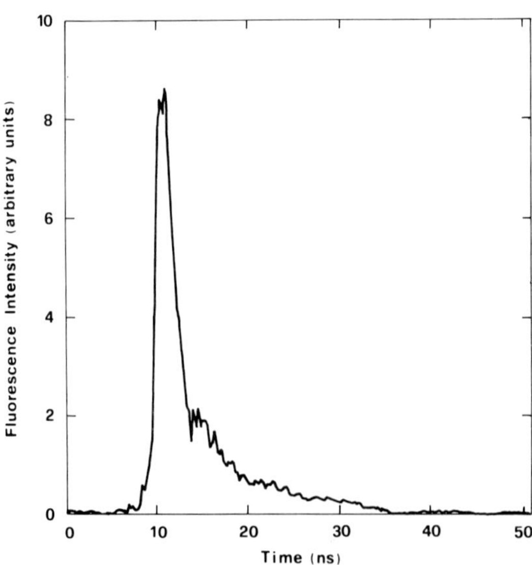


**Fig. 7.6.** Fluorescence-decay curve of $1.7 \times 10^{-3}$ M solution of doxorubicin HCl in physiologic solution.

been obtained, a good deal of work remains to be done: for example, (1) the nature of the interaction between fluorescent dye and DNA, (2) the systematic study of fluorescent-decay curves along a given chromosome, (3) the details of fast initial decays and energy-transfer processes in several kinds of samples, and (4) drug localization and interaction with cellular constituents. In all these instances, laser microirradiation promises to be a very useful investigative technique.

## SUMMARY

A laser microfluorometer particularly suitable for the measurement of fast fluorescence decays in microscopic biologic samples makes use of (1) a nitrogen-pumped dye laser as the source of excitation, (2) fluorescence microscopy, and (3) a signal averager. The main properties of the instrument include temporal resolution of $\sim$ 0.2 ns and spatial resolution of $\sim$ 0.3 $\mu$m. The instrument is now being used to study the fluorescence properties of the complexes formed by acridine dyes with DNA. Experiments are underway on synthetic polynucleotides, smears of bacteria with a known adenine-thymine percentage, metaphase chromosomes, and the antitumor agent doxorubicin HCl.

## REFERENCES

Albert A (1966) The Acridines. E Arnold, London.

Amsel G, Bosshard R (1970) Sampling and averging techniques in the analysis of fast random signals. Rev Sci Instrum 41:503–514.

Andreoni A (1979) In: Proceedings of the International School of Quantum Electronics: Lasers in Biology and Medicine. Camaiore, Italy, August 19–31, 1979. Plenum Press, New York, pp. 165–178.

Andreoni A, Benetti P, Sacchi CA (1975) Subnanosecond pulses from a single-cavity dye laser. Appl Physics 7:61–64.

Andreoni A, Cova S, Bottiroli G, Prenna G (1979) Fluorescence of complexes of quinacrine mustard with DNA. II. Dependence on the staining conditions. Photochem Photobiol 29:951–958.

Andreoni A, Longoni A, Sacchi CA, Svelto O, Bottiroli G (1976) In: Mooradian A, Jaeger T, Stokseth P (eds) Tunable Lasers and Applications. Springer-Verlag, Berlin, pp. 303–313.

Andreoni A, Sacchi CA, Svelto O (1979) In: Moore CB (ed) Chemical and Biochemical Applications of Lasers, vol. IV. Academic Press, New York, pp. 1–30.

Bottiroli G, Prenna G, Andreoni A, Sacchi CA, Svelto O (1979) Fluorescence of complexes of quinacrine mustard with DNA. I. Influences of the DNA base composition on the decay time in bacteria. Photochem Photobiol 29:23–28.

Brand L, Gohlke JR (1972) Fluorescence probes for structure. Ann Rev Biochem 41:843–868.

Caspersson T, Zech L, Johansson C, Modest EJ (1970) Identification of human chromosomes by DNA-binding fluorescent agents. Chromosoma 30:215–227.

Cohn CE (1969) Digital computer processing of sampling-oscilloscope data. Nucl Instrum Meth 71:349–352.

Cova S, Bertolaccini M, Bussolati C (1973) The measurement of luminescence waveforms by single-photon techniques. Phys Stat Sol (a) 18:11–62.
Cova S, Longoni A (1979) In: Omenetto N (ed) Analytical Laser Spectroscopy. Wiley-Interscience, New York, chap. 7, pp. 411–491.
Cubeddu R, De Silvestri S (1979) A simple and reliable atmospheric pressure nitrogen laser. Opt Quant Elect 11:276–277.
DeLotto I, Osnaghi S (1967) On random signal quantization and its effects in nuclear physics measurements. Nucl Instrum Meth 56:157–159.
Duchesne J (1973) Physicochemical Properties of Nucleic Acids, vol I. Academic Press, New York.
Förster T ( 1948) Intermolecular energy migration and fluorescence. An Physik 2:55–75.
House CH (1971) In: Oliver BM, Cage JM (eds) Electronic Measurements and Instrumentation. McGraw-Hill, New York, chap. 11, pp. 350–426.
Jacobson K (1979) In: Proceedings of the International School of Quantum Electronics: Lasers in Biology and Medicine. Camaiore, Italy, August 19–31, 1979. Plenum Press, New York, pp. 271–288.
Kohen E, Kohen C, Hirschberg JG, Wouters A, Thorell B (1978) Multisite topographic microfluorometry of intracellular and exogenous fluorochromes. Photochem Photobiol 27:259–268.
Konev SV (1967) Fluorescence and Phosphorescence of Nucleic Acids. Plenum Press, New York.
Latt SA, Brodie S (1976) In: Birks JB (ed) Excited States of Biological Molecules. Wiley-Interscience, New York, pp. 178–189.
Malmstadt HV, Enke CG, Crouch SR, Horlick G (1974) Electronic Measurements for Scientists. WA Benjamin, Reading, Pennsylvania.
Manolov G, Manolova Y (1972) Marker band in the chromosome 14 from Burkitt lymphomas. Nature (Lond) 237:33–34.
Michelson AM, Monny C, Kovoor A (1972) Action of quinacrine mustard on polynucleotide. Biochimie 54:1129–1136.
Modest EJ, Sengupta SK (1973) In: Thaer AA, Sernetz M (eds) Fluorescence Techniques in Cell Biology. Springer-Verlag, Berlin, pp. 125–134.
Peacocke HR (1973) In: Acheson RM (ed) Heterocyclic Compounds: Acridines, vol IX. Wiley-Interscience, New York, pp. 723–759.
Prenna G, Bottiroli G, Mazzini G (1977) Cytofluorometric quantification of the activity and reaction kinetics of acid phosphatase. Histochem J 9:15–30.
Rigler R, Grasselli, P (1979) In: Proceedings of the International School of Quantum Electronics: Lasers in Biology and Medicine. Camaiore, Italy, August 19–31, 1979. Plenum Press, New York, pp. 151–164.
Rowley JD (1973) A new consistent chromosomal abnormality in chronic myelogenous leukaemia identified by quinacrine fluorescence and Giemsa staining. Nature (Lond) 243:290–293.
Sacchi CA, Andreoni A (1975) In: Helion HA (ed) Proceedings of the Second European Electro-Optics Market and Technology Conference, Mack Brooks Exh. Ltd, London, pp. 67–73.
Sacchi CA, Svelto O, Prenna G (1974) Pulsed tunable lasers in cytofluorometry. Histochem J 6:251–258.
Schreiber JP, Daune MP (1974) Fluorescence of complexes of acridine dye wih synthetic polydeoxyribonucleotides: A physical model of frameshift mutation. J Mol Biol 83:487–501.

Steingraber OJ, Berlman IB (1963) Versatile technique for measuring fluorescence decay times in the nanosecond region. Rev Sci Instrum 34:525–529.

Udenfried S (1969) Fluorescence Assays in Biology and Medicine, vol. II. Academic Press, New York.

Zankl H, Zang KD (1972) Cytological and cytogenetical studies on brain tumors. 4. Identification of the missing G chromosome in human meningiomas as no. 22 by fluorescence techniques. Humangenetik 14:167–169.

# 8

# The Laser Operating Room

*Leon Goldman*
*Edward Perry*

In most surgical quarters at the present time, the laser is part of an operating room—especially if it is the flexible, self-contained type of laser instrument. However, to avoid disturbing the alignment of the laser beam, it is preferable to have all laser surgical units assigned to one operating room so that excessive movements of the instrument are not necessary. If there is an extensive program of laser surgery for investigative studies, especially with high-output systems, it is recommended that there be a special operating room only for laser surgery.

In the past, special operating rooms were constructed with safety door interlocks connected to the firing line of the laser, protective glass enclosures for visitors, attempts to prevent specular reflections from walls and equipment, and concealed high-output electricity lines (American National Standard for the Safe Use of Lasers, 1979). The laser must be considered as a high-voltage electronic product. Certification of the high voltage should be affixed to the equipment and be easily available.

The specific details of the principles and practice of laser safety have been discussed earlier in Chapter 3. The present review is concerned with some general aspects of design and safety in the clinical treatment area.

Detailed records should be made of the type of laser, its number, wavelength, output power, beam diameter, divergence, purpose, use, dates of inspection, and the laser safety card required for such equipment. The beam exit spot should be marked on the equipment. The laser must be kept locked so that its use is restricted to only those assigned.

## THE LASER SAFETY OFFICER

The laser safety officer for the operating room is the laser technician. This officer is experienced in the use of the equipment and in laser safety programs. In our experience, the laser technician should be available for each laser operation to start and to monitor the equipment. The technician checks the equipment prior to each operation to be sure it is ready before the patient is admitted. The laser technician also ascertains that all personnel have adequate eye protection and that proper safety signs are posted on the door of the operating room and on the equipment. In addition to attending to these details of monitoring of the laser-output controls, the technician is responsible for seeing that the operating arm and its probe are sterile.

It is expected, of course, that the surgeon who will be performing the operation with the laser is experienced in and familiar with the principles of laser safety and surgical technology and will be using adequate eye protection.

## THE OPERATING ENVIRONMENT

The general setup of the laser operating room should be reviewed critically from time to time by the personnel, including the surgeon, technicians, anesthetist, and nurses, so that any necessary improvements may be made. All personnel should be aware also of the hazards of laser surgery.

### The Flammability of Surgical Drapes

At the present time, the use of disposable sterile paper drapes presents a great risk of fire hazards. Various types of protective cloths have been developed in an attempt to reduce the hazards of flammability with $CO_2$ lasers. However, these cloths made of various types of asbestos or charcoal-like materials should be thoroughly examined so that no particles from them will act as foreign bodies in tissue during the course of surgery. For practical purposes, sponges soaked in saline are adequate.

### Danger from Reflections and Other Hazards

Specular reflection from instrumentation should be avoided by operating surgeons and the assistants, for accidents may occur from impacts of reflection on the eyes and directly on the hands. Accidents may also occur as a result of electrical hazards (Ascher, personal communication). Volatilization of tissue fragments may cause air pollution. Suction should be used when necessary, and proper air flows should be maintained in the operating room.

### Operating Room Personnel

**Nurses.** The nurses who are assigned for laser surgery should have thorough instruction on the laser and the safety programs before assignment.

**The Anesthetist.** The anesthetist, especially for major operations, maxillofacial surgery, and operations in the oral cavity and larynx, must be experienced in laser surgical anesthesia. Basically, nonexplosive anesthesia is used, as for electrosurgery. In endotracheal anesthesia, special endotracheal tubes covered with saline-wet cloths and special flexible steel tubes have been used for $CO_2$ laser surgery.

Eye protection for the anesthetist is also important. Occasionally the anesthetist will work behind screens, but protective glasses are still necessary despite the fact that special protective glasses for argon, Nd-YAG, UV, and ruby lasers may reduce his or her visual acuity. The anesthetist should note that the $CO_2$ laser is an enclosed system and does not affect the closed system of anesthesia of the patient for $CO_2$ levels of the patient's air flow.

## THE PATIENT

Adequate eye protection for the patient is provided by the use of sterile, heavy cloths. For laser surgery about the face, special protective eye shields, such as plastic covered with silver, may be inserted over the eyeball. When local anesthesia is used for laser surgery on the face, the eye shields may be inserted with tetracaine hydrochloride (Pantocaine) eyedrops. After the eye shields have been removed, sterile oil drops or ophthalmic polymyxin B-bacitracin (Polysporin) may be used in the eye.

In the operation record, detailed laser output in standard terms should be recorded. In this manner, subsequent reviews of the records can be used to evaluate the effect of the laser surgery. Morever, for medical liability insurance in the United States, it is considered preferable to include a special rider in the malpractice insurance policy.

## LASER SURGERY OUTSIDE THE HOSPITAL

Another aspect of laser surgery is the outpatient come-and-go surgery, such as colposcopy, treatment of tattoos, port-wine marks, and similar defects. In outpatient centers, which are more economical, the same design and safety programs should prevail. When general anesthesia is to be used, the same safety measures and restrictions as those used for inpatients' laser surgery should be observed and followed.

In private office practice, the practitioner must assume responsibility for performance standards of the laser, for its maintenance and safety, and for the meticulous recording of case details.

## THE FUTURE OF LASER SURGERY

It is not known as yet whether the Medical Instruments Division of the U.S. Bureau of Radiological Health will adopt performance standards for the laser operator. At present, the medical laser industry, the various laser professional medical societies, and medical-center laser committees will all have to develop adequate teaching programs, rules, and regulations for operating the laser. If these prove satisfactory for protection of the patient and for the critical evaluation of laser therapy, then state and federal controls will not be necessary.

Therefore, the catalog of laser medical instrumentation is not the place to learn how to use the laser. Adequate educational programs for medical, paramedical, and nursing personnel are necessary. Ascher has often said that there are no bad laser systems, only bad, inexperienced operators (Goldman et al., 1969).

## REFERENCES

American National Standard For the Safe Use of Lasers (1979) Z 136.1.

Ascher P Personal communication.

Goldman L, Rockwell RJ Jr, Fidler JP, Altemeier WA, Siler VE (1969) Investigative laser surgery safety aspects. Biomed Eng 4(9):13.

# 9

# The Sharplan Carbon Dioxide Laser in Clinical Surgery: 7 Years' Experience

*Isaac Kaplan*
*Joshua Raif*

With the development of suitable instrumentation, human-engineered to fulfill the requirements of the clinical surgeon and designed to fit in with the physical conditions prevailing in the operating theater, laser surgery has advanced rapidly in the past few years. There are signs of even more rapid progress and general acceptance as its application and advantages in more and more fields of surgery are demonstrated.

The basic advantages are as follows:

1. Noncontact surgery
2. Dry-field, almost bloodless surgery
3. Highly sterile surgery
4. Highly localized and precise microsurgery
5. Clear field of view and easy access in confined areas
6. Prompt healing with minimal postoperative swelling and scarring
7. Apparent reduction in postoperative pain
8. No electromagnetic interference on monitoring instrumentation

A laser surgical system consists basically of the laser—a source of intense visible or infrared radiation that can be focused to submillimeter spot sizes—and a delivery system that conveys this radiation to either a handpiece or a microscope attachment.

## THE CARBON DIOXIDE LASER

Among the various systems currently used in medical practice, the carbon dioxide laser has proved itself as the most efficient laser "scalpel" as a result of its infrared wavelength of 10.6 μm which, contrary to visible wavelengths, is highly absorbed in water. When the focused beam of this laser is incident upon living tissue (75%–95% water), the resulting effect is that of highly localized tissue removal through evaporation.

The tissue-vaporized zone is surrounded by a thin layer of heat-coagulated tissue in which blood vessels smaller than 0.5 mm are cauterized, resulting in a dry, almost bloodless, procedure.

During laser surgery, both beam position and the tissue undergoing surgery are under the continuous vision of the surgeon. The progress of tissue incision is continuously monitored. Small tissue volumes are removed with single- or multiple-exposure pulses, whereas larger incisions are performed through progressive scans of the beam in the continuous mode.

## The Sharplan Systems

The apparatus employed by us and others engaged in clinical surgery with this modality are the Sharplan 791 and Sharplan 733 systems, of 50 W and 25 W, respectively. These are the only systems available for both free-hand surgery and microsurgery. Both systems employ flowing gas and water-cooled laser heads (Fig. 9.1). The lasing medium is a mixture of $CO_2$, $N_2$, and He, pumped through a water-cooled discharge tube at a pressure of 25 mmHg.

The discharge tube is terminated by two mirrors, one fully reflective and one partially reflective, which constitute the optical resonator. The discharge energy is transferred via the $N_2$ molecules to the $CO_2$ molecules, which emit infrared radiation at a wavelength of 10.6 μm. This radiation is amplified in the optical resonator to produce the high-intensity collimated laser beam. The optical resonator is specially designed to assure the best optical-beam shape, designated $TEM_{00}$. This lowest beam mode is essential for the best surgical results because it is the only beam pattern with the following characteristics:

1. Gaussian power distribution across the beam—no "hot spots" and peak power at beam center
2. Maxium focusing capability—to "diffraction-limited" spots
3. Minimal beam divergence—assuring highest efficiency in passage through delivery systems and attachments such as endoscopes

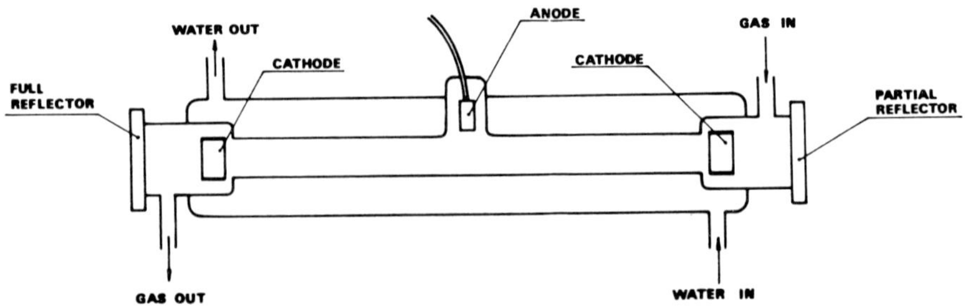


**Fig. 9.1.** Diagram of Sharplan 791 and 733 laser systems.

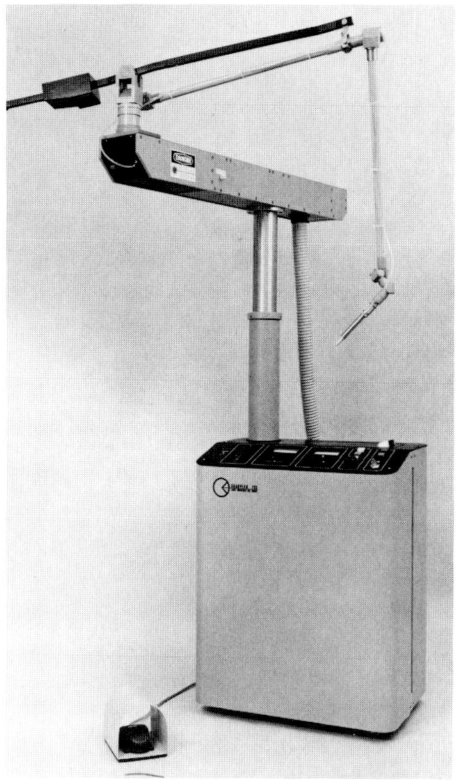

**Fig. 9.2.** Laser with twin-beam aiming system.

The laser head is mounted horizontally on a telescopic column (Fig. 9.2) and houses, besides the $CO_2$ laser, a power detector, an electromechanical beam shutter, and a patented twin-beam HeNe-laser–aiming system. This system is designed to aid the surgeon in aiming the invisible $CO_2$ laser beam both prior to and during its application in free-hand and in microsurgery. The HeNe laser emits a low power (2 mW) visible red beam. The patented optical system splits this red beam and positions the resulting two beams on two sides of the main $CO_2$ laser beam. These beams are directed into a mirrored articulated arm that facilitates maneuverability of the beam in a radius of 2 m around the main cabinet.

This concept is utilized since optical fibers for 10.6-$\mu$m radiation (at the powers required for surgery) are not available.

## Laser Attachments

For free-hand surgery, various penlike focusing handpieces can be attached to the articulated arm. These contain a lens that focuses the $CO_2$ laser beam and refracts the HeNe laser beams to intersect at the precise focus of the $CO_2$ laser beam. The surgeon thus has a three-dimensional, continuously visible indication of the incision point. Standard focal lengths are 50 mm and 125 mm, with focal beam spot diameters of 0.1 mm and 0.23 mm, respectively. The focusing handpiece is also fitted

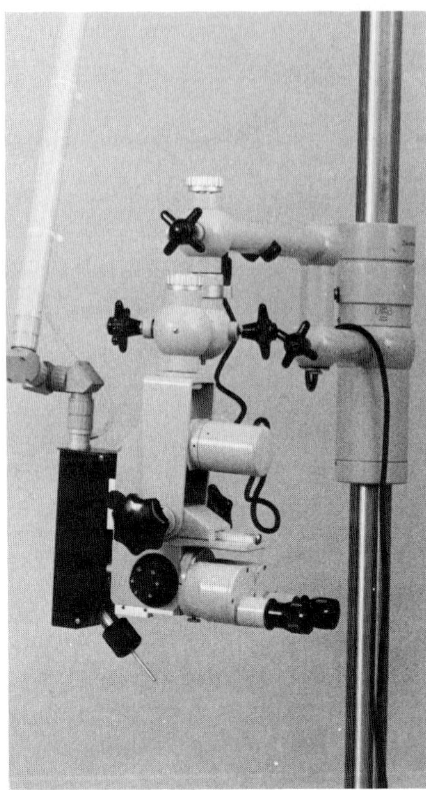

**Fig. 9.3.** Micromanipulator for aiming laser beam onto microscope to aid surgeon in maneuvering beam.

with a mechanical operating guide which can be removed for noncontact surgery. Upon actuation of the main beam, dry nitrogen gas is passed through the handpiece to the incision area to retard oxidation and blow away fumes. It also serves to cool the lens.

For microsurgery, two different Microslad microscope attachments have been developed which can be simply installed on standard operating microscopes requiring no modification of the microscope. These attachments are designed to reflect both the $CO_2$ laser beam and the aiming beam onto the microscope field of view and to facilitate maneuver of the beam by the surgeon. In one version, this is accomplished through a patented mechanical micromanipulator with 7× angle magnification (Fig. 9.3). In another version, electrically activated gimbals with mirror are used. The beam in this version is controlled by a "joy stick" placed on a remote control console. Both Microslad units are equipped with quick-change lenses (for 200-mm and 400-mm microscope objective lenses) and two-stage defocusing capability. Focal spot diameters of $CO_2$ laser beam are 0.45 mm and 0.8 mm, respectively.

Additional attachments to the Sharplan system have been designed as custom items for specialized research programs. These include a laser cystoscope fitted with a Hopkins telescope and a ventilation bronchoscope.

### Simplicity of Design

The Sharplan system is designed for simple operation and control by the nontechnical surgeon. It is ready for use within 20 s of initial switch-on. Once the appropriate power is set and monitored, the surgeon must choose the mode of operation, either continuous or pulsed.

In the continuous mode, laser radiation is emitted for as long as the foot switch is pressed. In the pulse mode, each foot switch depression emits a preset "dosage" of radiation at pulse lengths of 10 ms to 0.5 s.

Medical laser systems must comply with BRH regulation (21 CFR 1040.10). The Sharplan incorporates all the required safety devices and, in addition, has a panel to indicate malfunction, which even reminds the surgeon to open the gas cylinder.

## THE CARBON DIOXIDE LASER IN PRACTICE

The Sharplan $CO_2$ surgical laser is now in routine use in more than 30 countries throughout the world, in every field of surgery without exception. We ourselves have performed over 600 surgical procedures of various kinds and believe that certain definite statements can now be made as to the application of this modality in clinical surgery and its advantages over others.

### Anticipated Significant Blood Loss

The risk of severe blood loss exists in practically every surgical specialty, but is particularly well demonstrated in orthopedic and plastic surgery in which the excisions are mostly large. Mastectomies, mammaplasties, lipectomies, and other procedures of a similar nature have been performed by us and by others with the laser. In addition, orthopedic procedures, such as spine fusions and hip replacements, have been performed in many centers with gratifying results.

It is worth mentioning that not only is the saving of blood impressive in these cases, but the fact that the use of a tourniquet can be avoided reduces postoperative morbidity.

### Surgery Performed in Highly Vascular Areas of the Body

Perhaps the best examples of this are partial hepatectomies and partial nephrectomies, the performance of which have been reported by such surgeons as Christensen (1976), Glantz (1976), and others. In our unit, tongue surgery and surgery of the scalp have been performed routinely by means of the $CO_2$ laser with impressive results (Ben-Bassat et al., 1978).

**Extirpation of Highly Vascular Tumors.** Cavernous hemangioma, Kaposi sarcoma, and hemangiosarcoma have been extirpated by us and others on many occasions. Heppner and Ascher have reported impressive results in dealing with meningiomas, and the advantage of the $CO_2$ laser in conservative myomectomies has been well established by Toaff (1978), Thoms (personal communication), and others.

**Surgery Performed on Patients with Bleeding Tendencies.** Perhaps one of the most dramatic applications of the $CO_2$ laser lies in surgery performed in hemophiliac and thrombocytopenic patients. Farin et al. have reported major orthopedic procedures performed on patients suffering from hemophilia, in whom not only the reduction of blood loss and the postoperative morbidity has been noted, but the striking reduction in expenditure involved in the preparation of antihemophilia factors has been stressed (Kaplan, 1976). Our own experience in this connection in association with such institutions as the Wadley Institute in Dallas, Texas, as well as that of others, has confirmed these findings not only with regard to hemophilia and thrombocytopenia, but also in patients who have been treated with heparin and coumarin.

## Surgery for Malignant Disease

It is universally accepted by surgeons that the surgery of cancer should be performed with minimal opening of blood vessels and lymphatics and minimal manipulation of tissue, together with maximal visualization. The $CO_2$ laser seals the blood vessels and lymphatics during surgery, while at the same time permitting the performance of an almost nontouch extirpation. Moreover, the hemostatic effect enables the surgeon to distinguish accurately between pathologic and normal tissue. Hence the laser's application in cancer surgery is obvious. Those of us who have this modality at our disposal are using it routinely for the excision of accessible malignant disease, in spite of the fact that clinical follow-up is still too short to be able to reach definite conclusions regarding its applicability. Considerable experimental evidence exists, however, to indicate that the hypotheses upon which the laser's introduction in cancer surgery is based is well-founded [Frishman et al. (1974); Peled et al. (1976); Oesterhuis et al. (1976)].

Aronoff, Friedman, Glantz, and many others (Kaplan, 1976, 1978) have reported on their work in dealing with the surgical removal of cancer of various kinds and in various anatomic sites using the $CO_2$ laser. We have performed well over 100 wide excisions of malignant melanomas, with primary skin grafting, and have had no reason to regret having introduced this modality as a routine in our department.

## Operations Performed through Highly Infected Tissue

Excisions of burns, synergistic gangrene, and decubitus ulcers are examples par excellence of the application of the $CO_2$ laser in this connection. Work in this field has been well documented by Fidler et al. (1975), Glantz, Jackson, and others, whereas our experience confirms the advantage reported by them. Gratifying results are also reported by Merashovsky of the Albert Einstein Hospital in São Paulo, Brazil, in the treatment of osteomyelitis (Kaplan 1976, 1978).

## Operations Performed on Organs Requiring Simultaneous Monitoring

The laser is especially useful in surgery for patients for whom monitoring is necessary. This has been well demonstrated by the work of Dittrich in Germany and of Heppner and Ascher, of the Neurosurgery Clinic in Gratz, Austria. The fact that the heart and the brain can be monitored during laser surgery without interfering with the monitor has shown to be of great advantage. In our hospital, the laser is used instead of electric cautery in surgery performed on patients with pacemakers.

## Cavitational Surgery

The use of the $CO_2$ laser together with microscopic attachments and its advantages over other modalities is well established as a result of the pioneering work in this field performed by Strong et al. (1973), Verschueren and Oldhoff (1975), and others.

In our hospital, surgery of the uterine cervix has been performed with gratifying results with the $CO_2$ laser combined with a colposcope (Kaplan et al., 1973). Moreover, rectal surgery has also been shown to be practical. Urologic surgery employing a cystoscope is, as yet, in the experimental stage, but there is every reason to believe that its clinical application will be established in the near future. Microneurosurgery is being conducted with enthusiasm by Heppner and Ascher, and there is no doubt that this technique will be universally accepted in the near future (Kaplan, 1978).

## Specific Tissues Best Incised by Means of the $CO_2$ Laser

Examples par excellence of this application are incisions performed through the sclera and spinal meninges. In the former, the laser prevents increase in intraocular pressure and hemorrhage into the vitreous; in the latter, manipulation of the spinal cord with resultant damage to the nerve roots is avoided. When one considers that extirpative surgery performed with the $CO_2$ laser on a clinical basis was commenced only 7 years ago (Kaplan and Ger, 1973), one cannot help feeling that its application in surgery will become more and more universal as more surgeons introduce this modality into their armamentarium.

The ability to transmit the beam through a fine tube opens possibilities in such fields as stereotactic surgery, whereas its application in specific clinical conditions such as Osler's disease, onychogryposis (Ben-Bassat et al., 1978), and superficial telangiectasia (Kaplan and Peled, 1975) has already been demonstrated, and as time passes, more and more applications will surely be demonstrated.

## SUMMARY

The Sharplan systems are complete $CO_2$ surgical laser systems incorporating the following features:

1. An efficient powerful single-mode ($TEM_{00}$) $CO_2$ laser
2. A compact self-contained power supply with a highly human engineered control console for both ease of operation and safety
3. A balanced, highly maneuverable articulated arm to facilitate free-hand surgery
4. Mechanical and electromechanical micromanipulators attached to standard operating microscopes for precise microsurgery
5. Remote control console
6. Patented twin-beam aiming system indicating precise focus of the invisible $CO_2$ laser beam, in both free-hand and microsurgery
7. Built-in power meter to facilitate application of preset laser "dosages" on tissue
8. Malfunction indicator console
9. Full adherence to BRH standard for the safe use of laser instruments

The Sharplan system, conceived by the joint efforts of Prof. I. Kaplan of Beilinson Hospital and Engineer U. Sharon, has benefited both in its initial design (1972) and in its continuing development from what we believe is an excellent example of mutual productive fertilization between the technical and medical professions.

## REFERENCES

Aronoff BL (1976) In: Kaplan (ed) Laser Surgery. Academic Press, Jerusalem.
Ben-Bassat M, Kaplan I, Levy R (1978) Treatment of hereditary haemorrhagic telangiectasia of the nasal mucosa with carbon dioxide laser. Br J Plast Surg 31:157–158.
Ben-Bassat M, Kaplan I, Shindel Y, Edlan A (1978) The $CO_2$ laser in surgery of the tongue. Br J Plast Surg 31:155–156.
Christensen I (1976) In: Kaplan (ed) Laser Surgery. Academic Press, Jerusalem.
Dittrich H (1976) Personal communication.
Farin I (1976) In: Kaplan (ed) Laser Surgery. Academic Press, Jerusalem.
Fidler JP, Law E, MacMillan BG, Fox SH, Rockwell RJ Jr (1975) Comparison of carbon dioxide excision of burns with other thermal knives. In: Proceedings of the 1st International Symposium on Laser Surgery, Israel, 5–6 Nov., 1975, pp. 90–94.
Friedman E (1976) In: Kaplan (ed) Laser Surgery. Academic Press, Jerusalem.
Frishman A, Gassner S, Kaplan I, Ger R (1974) Excision of subcutaneous fibrosarcoma in mice. Isr J Med Sci 10:6.
Glantz G (1976) In: Kaplan (ed) Laser Surgery. Academic Press, Jerusalem.
Heppner F, Ascher P (1977) Personal communication.
Jackson H (1976) Personal communication.

Kaplan I (ed) (1976) Laser Surgery. Academic Press, Jerusalem.
Kaplan I (1978) Laser Surgery II. Academic Press, Jerusalem.
Kaplan I, Ger R (1973) The carbon dioxide laser in clinical surgery. Isr J Med Sci 9:79–83.
Kaplan I, Sharon U (1976) Current laser surgery. Ann NY Acad Sci 267:247–253.
Kaplan I, Peled I (1975) The carbon dioxide treatment of superficial telangiectases. Br J Plast Surg 18:214.
Kaplan I, Goldman J, Ger R (1973) The treatment of erosions of the uterine cervix by means of the $CO_2$ laser. Obstet Gynecol 41:795–796.
Merashovsky I (1978) Personal communication.
Oesterhuis JW, Eibergen R, Verschueren RCJ, Oldhoff J (1976) The continuous wave $CO_2$ laser compared with conventional methods in experimental tumor surgery. Ned Tijdschr Geneeskd 120:45.
Peled I, Shohat B, Gassner S, Kaplan I (1976) Excision of epithelial tumors: $CO_2$ laser versus conventional methods. Cancer Letters 2:41–46.
Strong MS, Jako J, Polyani T, Wallace RA (1973) Laser surgery in the aerodigestive tract. Am J Surg 126:529–533.
Thoms G (1976) Personal communication.
Toaff A (1978) In: Kaplan (ed) Laser Surgery II. Academic Press, Jerusalem.
Verschueren RCJ, Oldhoff J (1975) The carbon dioxide laser: A new surgical tool. Arch Chir Neerl 25:197–205.

# 10

# Laser Surgery in Gynecology

*Helmut F. Schellhas*

## INSTRUMENTATION

The availability of one carbon dioxide laser surgical system, in which the beam can be applied both through the operating microscope (colposcope) for microsurgery and through the articulated handpiece of a so-called laser scalpel for tissue resection or tumor vaporization in major surgical procedures, is very desirable. Most gynecologists manage clinically intraepithelial mucosal lesions of the female genital tract that are of microscopic dimensions, as well as large benign and, to some extent also, malignant tumors. In gynecology departments of universities and large medical centers, subspecialized experts in colposcopy, gynecologic oncology, tubal reconstructive surgery, and conventional gynecologic surgery all may want to apply the laser beam in their sophisticated fields. The option to convert expediently the modus of operation of a surgical carbon dioxide laser from microsurgical application through an operating microscope to a hand-held thermal scalpel, therefore, should be available for all surgical laser models. Some microsurgical carbon dioxide systems, unfortunately, are designed for colposcopy only. In some of these, a short mounting stand prohibits intraabdominal applicability, as for instance in microsurgery on the fallopian tube. In medical centers, surgical lasers should be shared by several departments for cost-efficiency and cross-use if one laser should be out of service.

The Sharplan laser, which utilizes the laser tube to bridge the distance between the console and the operating table, is excellent for major surgery (Fig 10.1). Although the articulated arm is somewhat unyielding, it is adequate to reach into the pelvic and abdominal cavities. The handpiece allows all manipulations we desire to carry out in major laser surgery. A persisting problem is the occasional bumping of the articulated arm against the surgical lights, which could damage

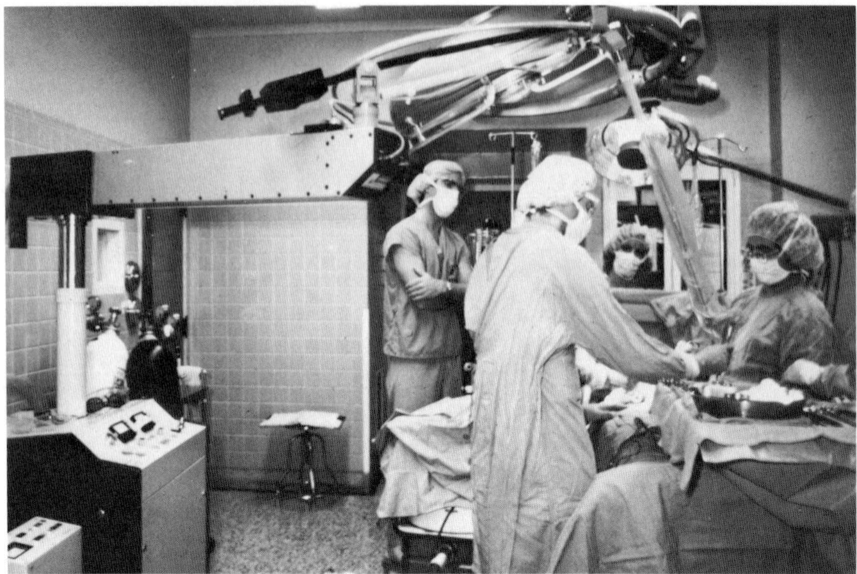

**Fig. 10.1.** The Sharplan laser, which utilizes the laser tube to bridge the distance between console and operating table, is excellent for major abdominal surgery.

the fine mirror system and disalign the laser beam. The surgical team must guard the sensitive laser arm. A pliable fiber-optic cable would be more ideal if it could be made workable for the $CO_2$ laser beam.

# TUMOR-VOLUME REDUCTION THROUGH TISSUE VAPORIZATION

## Tumors of Microscopic Dimensions

Lesions of microscopic dimensions in the female genital tract are detected by cytologic screening and confirmed by tissue biopsy. In many instances, they can be accurately delineated through an operating microscope (colposcope) by a trained physician. The possibility of destroying a neoplastic epithelial lesion by tissue vaporization under direct microscopic vision with a $CO_2$ laser beam has many clinical advantages. Most frequently, intraepithelial neoplastic disease is found in the cervix uteri. Although cervical lesions can be adequately dealt with by means of other thermal surgical procedures, the $CO_2$ laser has been found very advantageous in the control of localized and diffuse vaginal intraepithelial neoplastic lesions. A power output of 10–15 W was sufficient for our work using the 400 $CO_2$ surgical laser of the Coherent Medical Division with a 2-mm-diameter focused beam. Colposcopy has so far been the main field of laser application in gynecology. It is discussed in detail by Dr. Masterson in Chapter 11.

## Radiation-resistant Malignant Tumors and Large Benign Tumors

The greatest advantage of the carbon dioxide laser in gynecologic oncology is the possibility of reducing the volume of unresectable solitary malignant lesions or preferably to remove the tumors entirely. With the Sharplan laser we have vaporized tumors attached to the bony pelvis and in the groin (Fig. 10.2) (Schellhas, 1978). These lesions had already received radiation therapy or were radiation-resistant. The power density provided by the Sharplan 791 He laser was adequate, but the required lasing time was very long. High-power-output $CO_2$ lasers providing 100 or 200 W are probably more efficient for large-volume tumors or subclinical tumors extending over large surfaces.

## Combined Cryogenic and Laser Surgery

Hemorrhage has been a prohibiting problem in the application of the $CO_2$ laser for volume reduction of squamous carcinomas of the cervix metastatic to the vagina and urinary bladder. The tumors had formed large vesicovaginal fistulas through which the patients had hemorrhaged. In January 1978, we employed for the first time a combination of cryosurgery and laser surgery for the control of bleeding (Schellhas, 1979). The tissue to be lased was first frozen with a cryosurg-

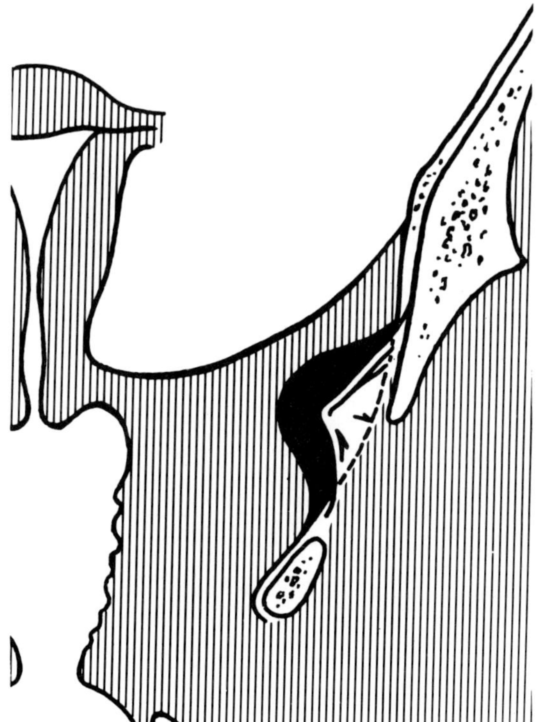

**Fig. 10.2.** Isolated recurrent tumor *(dark field)* developed on the posterior ischial spine following previous surgery and radiation therapy. Laser vaporization is at present the best surgical means to remove tumor tissue attached to bones. (Schellhas HF, Laser surgery in gynecology. Surg Clin North Am 58:151–166, 1978.)

ical unit; $CO_2$ was used as a cryogen in the first patient and liquid nitrogen in subsequent patients. The freezing provides stasis of the microvessels and also freezes frank blood. Vaporization of the frozen tissue was then achieved without undue blood loss.

Carbon dioxide as the refrigerant, applied through a cryoprobe, is able to produce a −25°C isotherm to a depth of 2–3 mm. Liquid nitrogen with a boiling temperature of −195.6°C is a better refrigerant than carbon dioxide gas, which produces a cold of −79°C. It is, however storable for only a short time, whereas $CO_2$ is a storable cryogen. Liquid nitrogen can freeze a large tumor surface faster and deeper as an open spray than through a cryoprobe (Zacarian, 1977). A cryoprobe is more precise in small lesions.

The ischemic frozen tissue absorbs the focused laser beam to a depth of approximately 0.2 mm, in which zone the tissue is then boiled to 100°C and vaporized. Continuous application of the laser beam to greater depth naturally opens functioning blood vessels, with resulting diffuse oozing of blood. The $CO_2$ laser beam is absorbed by blood before its impact can affect microvascular coagulation and is inefficient for further tumor vaporization. Repeat freezing of blood and underlying tumor makes the tissue attainable again for laser application. Continuous alternat-

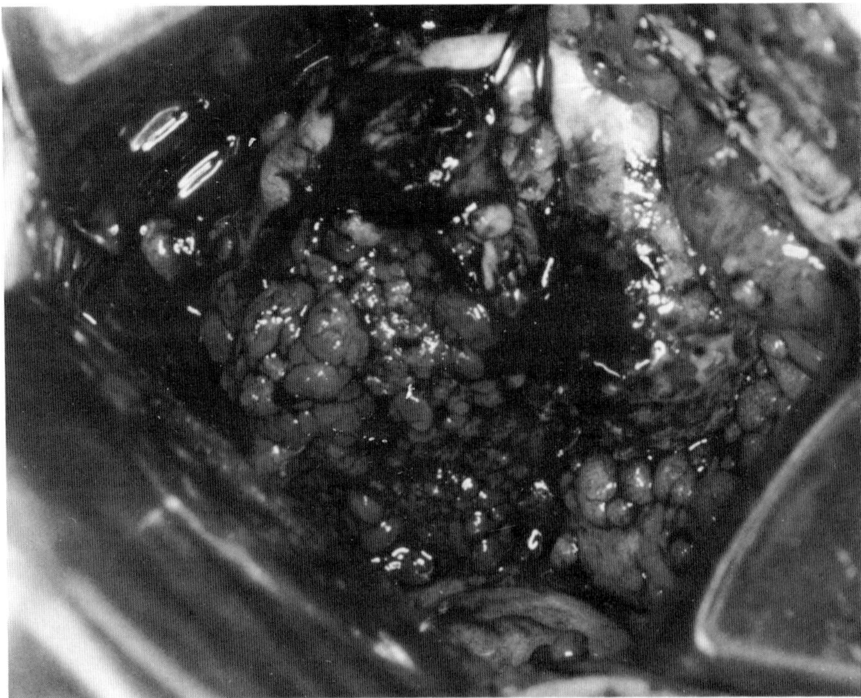

**Fig. 10.3.** Many unresectable malignancies have a widespread diffuse pattern involving serosal surfaces. A laser beam emitting a wavelength specifically absorbed by tumor cells could be used for their selective destruction.

ing administration of both opposite thermal principles eventually can result in the bloodless destruction of vascular tumor tissue. Most solitary tumors can be resected with the $CO_2$ laser alone, with little blood loss. For uncontrollable bleeding, however, it is advantageous to have a cryosurgical unit available. The destruction of vascular tumors should be planned with a freezing-lasing cycle.

### Selective Tumor Destruction

For abdominal cancer surgery, it is desirable to have a $CO_2$ laser available as a standby. In occasional patients, isolated tumors can be vaporized that otherwise are not resectable. The chance for a cure is better with a small tumor volume. Most unresectable malignancies, however, have a widespread diffuse pattern involving the surfaces of bowel, bladder, liver, and peritoneum (Fig. 10.3). To vaporize each small tumor nodule with the $CO_2$ laser is, in most instances, an impossible task.

A laser beam emitting a wavelength specifically absorbed by tumor cells and leading to their selective destruction is needed. A special staining method for the tumor tissue could be used: for instance, brush application of eosin which absorbs selectively the blue-green beam of the argon laser. Another example might be to fluorochrome the nucleic acids of malignant cells with acridine orange, which then transforms ultraviolet light into visible light so that the tumor nodules appear crimson-red (Sani et al., 1964). The different absorption or fluorescence spectra for the nucleic acids of proliferating malignant cells and differentiated benign cells should be exploited. Hematoporphorphyrin derivatives (HPD) are also used for laser-induced fluorescence for diagnosis and therapy. Systemic immune fluorescence methods might be more ideal.

## ABLATIVE SURGERY WITH THE CARBON DIOXIDE LASER SCALPEL

Incisional carbon dioxide laser surgery can be performed with the focused continuous wave $CO_2$ laser beam delivered through the multiarticulated arm of the surgical laser. The penetration depth is determined by the power density of the beam and the time of application. Our incisional technique employs an average of 25 W and a beam spot size of 1 mm, but the power density of the beam can be regulated according to the surgeon's needs.

An incision is made by continuous irradiation with rapid sweeping movements. The $CO_2$ laser beam is fully absorbed in the first millimeters of tissue, and therefore, repeat focused vaporization along the incisional line is necessary. The base of the incision develops a superficially charred layer (carbon deposit) that subsequently stops the laser beam. Further lasing would thermally damage the underlying tissue without the desired vaporization effect. For that reason, immediate debridement by a quick wipe with a moist sponge is done, and this is followed by another wipe with a dry sponge; otherwise, the moisture will partially absorb the laser beam. Prior to laser application, the surgeon should check, on a tongue blade or similar device, the center of the focal point of the laser beam relative to the handpiece of the hand-held laser. The speed of the incision determines the depth of the thermal damage in adjacent tissues and must therefore be optimal (Verschueren, 1979).

The operative field must be dry, as blood and moisture will absorb the laser beam. Small vessels up to 0.5 mm are usually controlled when the blood flow has been compressed. Small bleeders can often be stopped by coagulation with the unfocused laser beam. Most bleeding vessels should, however, be conventionally clamped with a hemostat and ligated. Some laser surgeons direct the unfocused laser beam to the tissue next to the tip of the clamp for hemostasis, but in our experience, this procedure is most ineffective. Coagulation of tissue by heating the tip of the clamp with an unfocused beam is a questionable technique. The beam

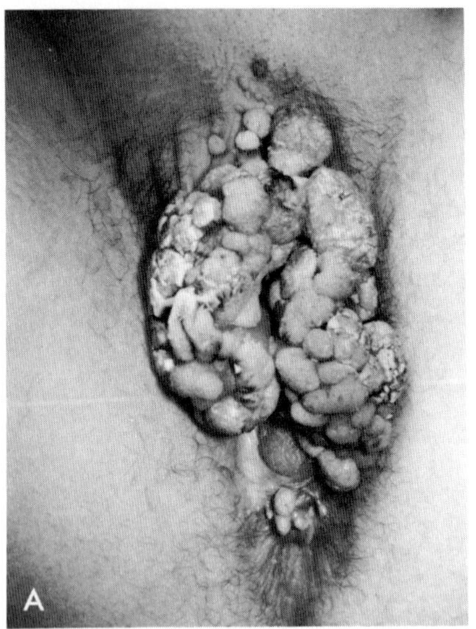


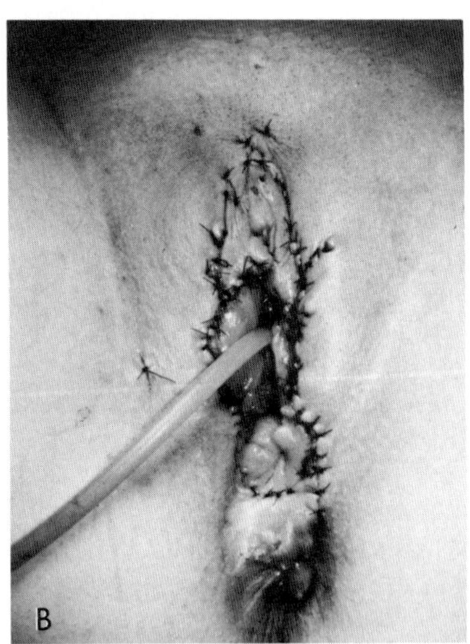


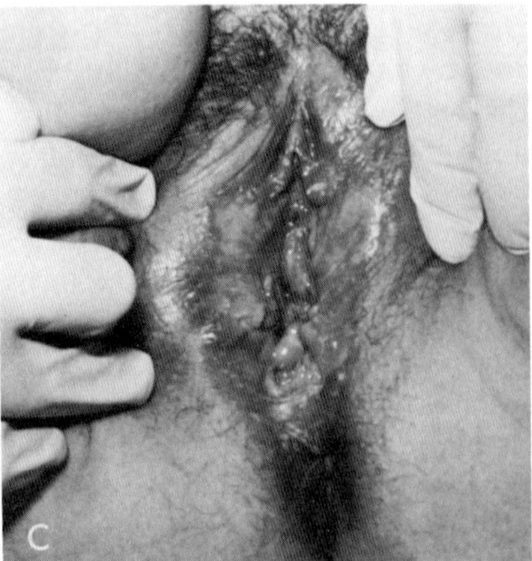


**Fig. 10.4.** Giant condyloma acuminatum in pregnancy. **A.** Before $CO_2$ laser scalpel excision. **B.** After laser scalpel excision. **C.** Appearance of vulva 6 weeks after operation. (Schellhas et al., Resecting vulvar lesions with the $CO_2$ laser. Contemp Obstet Gynecol 6:35–39, 1975.)

will reflect from the surface of the metal and the instrument itself may be damaged. The tissue should be in good tension. The margins of the surgical fields should be shielded with moist gauze. The fumes produced during surgery are removed by a vacuum pump.

Clinically, we have resected giant condyloma acuminata of the vulva in pregnant and nonpregnant patients with minimal blood loss, excellent healing, and no recurrence in a follow-up period of several years (Fig. 10.4) (Schellhas et al., 1976; see also Chapter 11). We have occasionally resected invasive carcinomas of the vulva by performing radical vulvectomy or wide local excision for special medical indications. The $CO_2$ laser may find a permanent place in vulvar surgery for malignancy if the impression that lymphatics are being sealed by the laser beam is experimentally and clinically confirmed. A power output of 25 W is sufficient for tissue dissection, but a higher power output might be advantageous.

## MICROSURGICAL TISSUE DISSECTION AND WELDING

The most challenging microsurgical procedures in gynecology are presently performed in the reconstruction of the fallopian tubes for restoration of fertility. Specially talented and trained gynecologic surgeons developed fine precision instruments which are tediously manipulated under visual control through an operating microscope (Phillips, 1977). For hemostasis, electric current is partially employed.

For tissue dissection as well as for hemostasis, a $CO_2$ laser beam directed through the optical system could be more efficient in the reduction of instrumentation and operating time. A small diameter of the focal point of the laser beam would be most feasible for this type of microsurgery. The heat conduction induced by the focused laser beam creates tissue damage in the incisional margins, which causes edema and impaired healing. A small diameter of the focused laser beam not only can improve the delicate microsurgical dissection but probably also decreases the extent of tissue injury in the hands of a skilled laser surgeon. Among the presently marketed various $CO_2$ lasers, the advertised smallest focal points range between 2 mm and 0.1 mm.

In most interesting animal experiments, Klink et al. (1978) have developed a special $CO_2$ laser technique. For end-to-end anastomosis, the tubal parts were precisely approximated and the serosa and subserosa were coagulated. Sutures were not used for the anastomosis, obviating foreign-body reaction and saving considerable operating time. In these animal experiments, reanastomosis of the tubes was found to be optimal with a power density of 64 $W/cm^2$. The coagulation necrosis of the serosa and subserosa provided sufficient stability for good healing of the muscularis and mucosa. The investigators achieved an uncomplicated pregnancy rate of 79% in the group of animals so treated. Klink et al. (1979) reported the successful application of this technique in humans. Sutures for anastomosis were applied at 6 and 12 o'clock.

## SUMMARY

Carbon dioxide laser surgical techniques will find increasing application in gynecology. The principal uses are in the vaporization of microscopic and also voluminous tumors, in microsurgical tissue dissection and probably welding, in the resection of vascular tissue, and possibly in some radical tumor resections. Fine focal laser beam points and a high-power output are desirable. Versatility and adaptability of the laser instruments for various surgical tasks are important. The combined application of tissue freezing and lasing is of help in the controlled vaporization of vascular tumors. Selective destruction of diffuse malignant tissue implants by special tumor-staining methods and selective laser-beam absorption is a future goal.

## REFERENCES

Klink F, Grosspietzsch R, Klitzing Von L, et al. (1978) Animal in vivo studies and in vitro experiments with human tubes for end-to-end anastomatic operation by a $CO_2$ laser technique. Fertil Steril 30:100–102.

Klink F, Grosspietzsch R, Klitzing Von L, et al. (1979) Erste Erfahrungen zum Einsatz eines $CO_2$ Lasers bei der Gynäkologischen Mikrochirurgie. Laser 1979, International Congress, Munich.

Phillips JM (1977) Microsurgery in Gynecology. American Association of Gynecologic Laparoscopists Publication.

Sani G, Citti U, Quinto P (1964) Fluorescence Microscopy in Cyto-diagnosis of Cancer. Charles C Thomas, Springfield, Illinois.

Schellhas HF (2978) Laser surgery in gynecology. Surg Clin North Am 58:151–166.

Schellhas HF (1979) Cryogens and carbon dioxide laser in cyclic combination for volume reduction in vascular tumors. In: Kaplan I (ed) Laser Surgery III, vol I. Academic Press: Jerusalem.

Schellhas HF, Fidler JP, Rockwell RJ (1976) The carbon dioxide laser scalpel in the management of vulvar lesions. In: Kaplan I (ed) Laser Surgery. Academic Press, Jerusalem, pp. 133–135.

Verschueren RC (1979) International Medical Laser Symposium. Detroit, Michigan.

Zacarian SA (1977) Cryosurgical Advances in Dermatology and Tumors of the Head and Neck. Charles C Thomas, Springfield, Illinois.

# 11

# Techniques of Laser Colposcopic Surgery

*Byron J. Masterson*

Although the laser principle was proposed in 1958 by Schawlow and Townes, the carbon dioxide laser was not developed until approximately 8 years later. Jako (1972) coupled the $CO_2$ laser with the microscope, taking advantage of the properties of the laser that make it clinically attractive. The ability to project the beam into a cavity was foremost in this application. The development of the micromanipulator made precise beam guidance and controlled depth of destruction available in a clinically useful fashion. Subsequent simultaneous projection of a helium-neon (HeNe) laser directly on the tissues to be treated made the $CO_2$ laser beam more easily identifiable prior to treating the tissues. Kaplan et al. (1973) first used the laser in gynecologic surgery in 1973. Bellina (1977), Carter et al. (1978), Schellhas (1978), and Stafl et al. (1977) all presented papers on the subject. The early clinical experiments have given way to clinical experience, and the use of the laser is now well established in gynecology.

## CLINICAL EXPERIENCE

A $CO_2$ laser was obtained for use on the Gynecologic Oncology Service at the University of Kansas in 1975. The period from 1975 to 1980 has seen a restriction of its application to a more specific group of lesions and a continuing refinement of technique and application. Early application of the $CO_2$ laser to nonspecific vulvitis, recurrent herpes, nonsymptomatic and histologically benign adenosis, and chronic cystic cervicitis and the $CO_2$ laser's use for biopsies have been abandoned.

# EQUIPMENT

## Carbon Dioxide Laser

A carbon dioxide laser beam of approximately 25 W in power with a spot size less than 1 mm will provide a power density of 4000 W/cm$^2$ (Sharplan Technical Manual). Such calculations are not precise, as most operators move the laser over tissues in a continuous fashion. The rapid destruction of tissues with the laser, however, requires a power density of this level or greater. The quality of the beam provided by each laser unit commercially available, as well as its beam mode, should be reviewed prior to use by the operator. The clinical prerequisites of treatment described herewith presume a quality laser beam.

## Colposcope

The use of the projected laser beam directed by a micromanipulator via the colposcope presumes an experienced colposcopist. *Few situations could be better designed to produce clinical disaster than an unskilled colposcopist occasionally treating ill-diagnosed conditions with a laser.* The proper use of the laser directed through the colposcope for treatment requires one both skilled in colposcopy and trained in the clinical use of the laser. In our current investigational scheme for the patient with an abnormal cytologic smear (Fig. 11.1), one never treats a patient with the laser in gynecology without a tissue diagnosis. An adequate volume of material to maintain clinical skills in these areas is an additional requirement. In laser surgery, as in so many other clinical situations, practice perfects.

## Ancillary Equipment

Colposcopic materials, including swabs, endocervical specula, cytologic sampling materials, vaginal specula of various sizes, biopsy jars, sharp biopsy forceps (Tischler), endocervical curets and skin hooks, disposable vulvar biopsy kits (Baker), and suction endometrial biopsy kits (Masterson), are needed. Solutions of aqueous povidone-iodine (Betadine), 3% acetic acid, Lugol's solution, tissue fixative, and toluidine blue stain should be available in the examining room. An effective smoke evacuator employing either wall suction or a separate unit is needed as well.

# SAFETY PRECAUTIONS

Chapter 3 should be reviewed by all those considering use of the laser in gynecologic surgery. Eyeglasses should be provided for all personnel, to absorb any reflected beam. Shiny instruments ought to be avoided, although a skilled operator will rarely misdirect the beam. Only aqueous solutions are to be used; any flammable substances might be ignited by the laser. Paper drapes or other materials that might ignite must be avoided. The most common accident in clinical use is a brief firing of the laser by accident. Stepping on the firing pedal during the placement of the speculum or attempts to improve exposure of some difficult vaginal

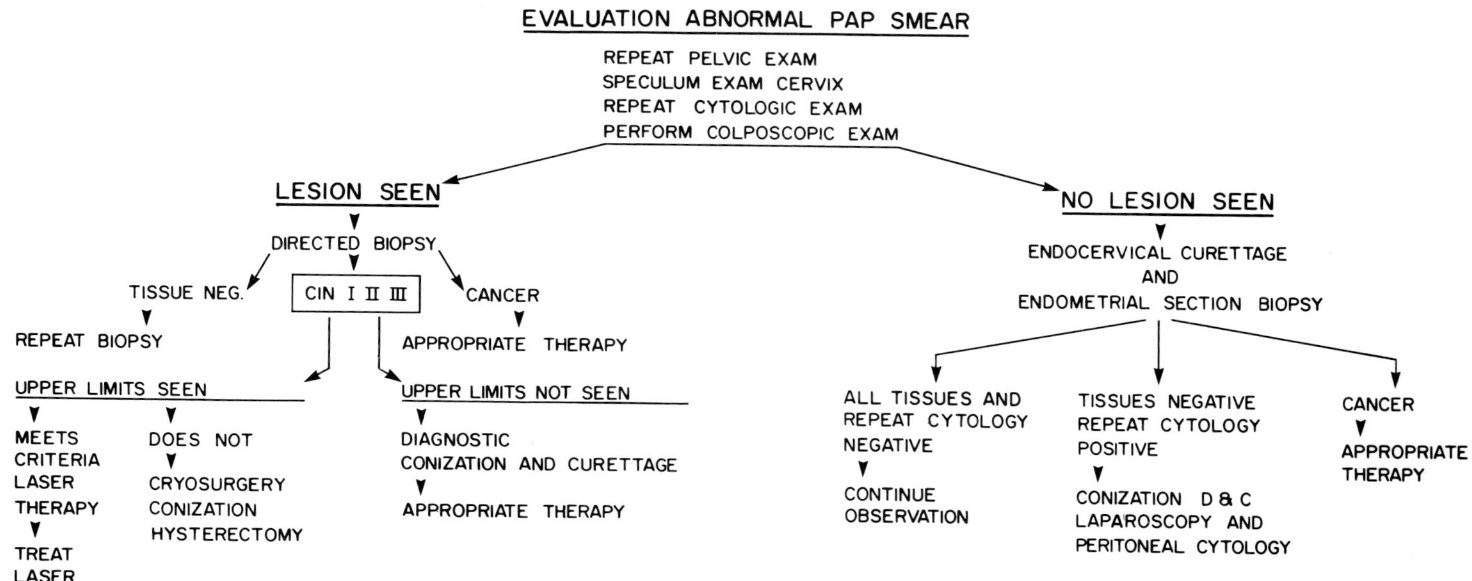


**Fig. 11.1.** Schema for evaluation and management of abnormal cervical cytology. Competent interpretation of cytologic, histologic, and colposcopic findings is an absolute requirement to avoid errors in clinical management. The laser is incorporated as indicated.

recess are the occurrences most commonly associated with such misfires. As the hand of the operator is the area most frequently hit and this is not at the focal point of the beam, little damage is done except to the operator's ego.

Safety manuals provided with the laser equipment should be carefully studied by the operator. Compliance with all safety requirements is essential. The time interval allowing all capacitors to discharge in the unit should be fully observed. It should be self-evident that one does not inspect the interior of a laser while it is connected to its electrical current, nor does one operate ungrounded electrical equipment.

## PERSONNEL

The most significant single factor in the efficient operation of any gynecologic laser clinic is the nurse in charge. Responsibility for laser maintenance and safety, colposcopes, and biopsy equipment, as well as for adequate provisioning of supplies and other materials, must be specifically delegated. Provision and handling of photographic film, videotape, television equipment, cameras, and correlation of cytologic and biopsy materials and reports, as well as record retrieval, must be coordinated to facilitate smooth operation of the laser unit.

Detailed pretreatment discussions with the patient, informational videotapes, explanation of informed-consent forms, and a sympathetic manner greatly improve patient acceptance of any new modality like the laser. The phoning of any biopsy reports to the patient, of course, is helpful as well.

## SPECIFIC TREATMENT PROGRAMS

### Cervical Intraepithelial Neoplasia

The most common use for the $CO_2$ laser in gynecology is the treatment of cervical intraepithelial neoplasia. In the candidate for laser therapy, the lesion should be seen in its entirety with the colposcope, be of known histologic type, and occur in a patient who is likely to be reliable in attendance for follow-up examination. Lesions extending into the endocervical canal should be excluded from laser therapy and treated by other appropriate means. Patients with possible microinvasion or with invasive cancer are likewise not candidates for laser therapy.

Original treatment programs begun in 1975 specified treatment of the lesion alone to a depth of tissue weeping, approximately 1–2 mm. Later protocols were expanded to include the entire transitional zone at the initial treatment. Figure 11.2 illustrates the difference in the two protocols. Some studies of recurrence rates correlated with the depth of excision demonstrated that 5 mm of tissue should be excised (Masterson et al., 1980). This depth of excision will include almost all of the cervical glands that might contain downgrowth of epithelium and extensions of cervical intraepithelial neoplasia. Current techniques include the excision of the entire transitional zone to a depth of 5–7 mm. Our own material has been reviewed by Dr. K. M. Hassanein, Professor and Chairman of Biometry, University

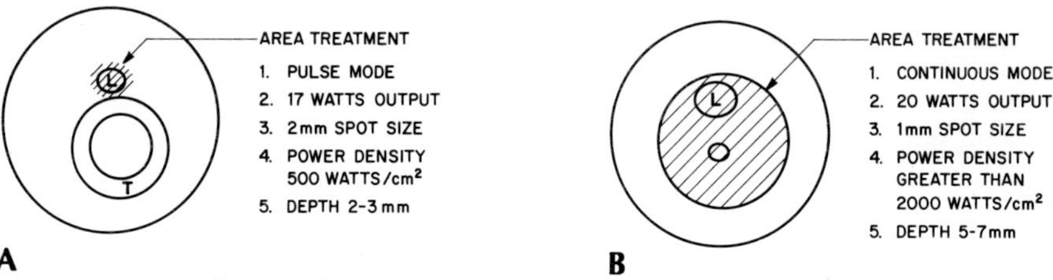


**Fig. 11.2.** Original **(A)** and current **(B)** treatment programs for cervical intraepithelial neoplasia at the University of Kansas Medical Center.

of Kansas. Thus far, chi-square analysis has not shown a difference in recurrence rates. However, until firm data are available, the reader is advised to use the deeper and more extensive treatment plan.

**Technique of Treatment.** The patient is placed in the lithotomy position after a thorough pretreatment explanation and the signing of informed-consent forms for laser therapy. The speculum is placed and the cervix visualized. 3% Acetic acid is sprayed into the cervix, and the surface is carefully restudied. Previous colposcopic examination records and biopsy reports are reviewed. Criteria for acceptability for laser treatment are again established. Any pretreatment photographs are taken at this time.

The laser is set to produce 25 W of power on continuous mode where the spot size is 0.8 mm. This spot size will produce a power density of greater than 4000 $W/cm^2$ (Sharplan Technical Manual, 1979) and will promote rapid destruction of cervical tissue. The smoke evacuator is started after all safety measures have been reviewed and completed. The laser guide light is directed onto the cervix, and an initial burst of laser energy is released. Once the accuracy of the aiming lights is again reaffirmed, laser surgery may begin. If all systems are working acceptably and safety measures are completed, the operator outlines the lesion to be excised. A 2-mm margin of normal-appearing epithelium between the lesion and the outlining laser beam should be included. In a stepwise fashion, the beam is moved from right to left. All the tissues included in the transitional zone are then excised to a depth of 5–7 mm. Continuous evacuation of smoke must accompany this procedure. The patient is reassured during the procedure, and inquiries are made as to her comfort.

The operator measures the depth of the excision with a small segment of plastic millimeter rule held in an intrauterine dressing forceps. Any ridges or incomplete areas of excision are removed, and the area is inspected again for complete excision. Any carbonized areas that obscure this examination should be removed, and a detailed examination is made as to the completeness of tissue destruction.

**Follow-up and Results.** The patient will have noted little pain during the procedure, and effective smoke removal will minimize odor and aid patient acceptance. Povidone-iodine (Betadine) vaginal gel is prescribed, and the patient is advised to avoid intercourse for at least 3 weeks. The use of condoms in the ensuing

3 weeks is also advised. Bleeding after laser surgery is rare, and the profuse watery discharge seen in cryosurgery does not occur.

Masterson and Calkins (in press) noted that results of cytologic studies in 90% of patients indicated a return to normal with laser management of cervical intraepithelial neoplasia and in no patient in their series of 230 did the lesion progress to invasive cancer.

## Condyloma

Increasing numbers of patients with condyloma acuminata are being seen throughout the United States (Powell, 1978). This increase has been observed in intraurethral, vaginal, cervical, vulvar, and anal condyloma. Goldman and Rockwell (1971) reported the use of the laser in skin lesions, and McBurney (1978) and Powell (1978) have reported clinical observations in the efficiency of the laser in condyloma acuminata.

**Diagnosis.** In the past, clinical observation alone was sufficient to establish a diagnosis of condyloma acuminata. The warty appearance of these lesions is certainly characteristic and well known to the experienced observer.

A cause for concern is the increasing number of patients in the age group at which condyloma usually occurs who have Bowen's disease clinically appearing as condyloma (Lupulescu et al., 1977). Pincus et al. (1977) described the histologic findings in five such cases.

Buschke-Lowenstein condyloma may be clinically confusing in the early stages of its development. Its progressive nature and local invasion make the early diagnosis of this difficult lesion clinically important. Wide local excision is vital in the management of this lesion, and the role of the laser in such cases is currently limited. Remember Buschke-Lowenstein in the patient whose symptoms resemble those of a routine case of condyloma acuminata but who fails to respond to usual treatment methods. Goltz's syndrome, with vulvar and perianal angiofibroma, may clinically appear as condyloma as well. Therefore, the selection of two of the more active-looking condylomas for biopsy is advisable. Such lesions have no nerve supply and can be excised without the discomfort of local infiltration in most instances. The patient should return after histologic diagnosis becomes available. A vaginal smear should also be obtained prior to treatment, as many patients have associated cervical intraepithelial neoplasia as well. When cytologic examination is confused by the exfoliation of cells from condyloma, careful colposcopic examination of the cervix will usually distinguish the source of such cells.

The laser is most effective in the management of small, multiple lesions occurring in the vagina, cervix, and vulva. When the laser is chosen to manage lesions in the anal canal, the operator must always be cognizant of the explosive properties of methane gas. The author is personally aware of two explosions with the use of cautery. In such circumstances, the laser is also capable of igniting methane gas.

**Technique of Treatment.** The areas to be treated are cleansed with aqueous povidone-iodine (Betadine) solution after the patient has been placed in the lithotomy position. The base of the vulvar lesions and those in the lower one-half of the vagina are infiltrated with a 1% solution of lidocaine. Observing through the colposcope at low magnification, the operator directs the laser toward the upper lesions. With a 15–20 W setting, continuous mode, and all safety measures accomplished, destruction of the condyloma is carried out in a clockwise fashion from below upward. The patient may attempt to observe what is being done, and by simply raising her head in some instances, she could cause the laser beam to strike her eyes directly. She must have safety glasses and be warned not to look downward at the procedure as it is being performed. The laser beam is always directed in a downward fashion when the upper vulva is undergoing treatment to minimize the chance of such an occurrence. Removal of the condyloma with the laser continues until the skin appears normal. Rarely will a patient have any significant bleeding. Any carbonized material is removed to make certain that the base of the condyloma has been carefully treated. Calkins and Masterson (in press) have noted an 81% success rate with one treatment program as described here.

Other methods of management should be used in concert with the laser to produce the most effective treatment programs. 5-Fluorouracil is useful for intraurethral lesions, and trichloroacetic acid may be used locally as well. In contrast to podophyllin, trichloroacetic acid produces no abnormalities on absorption. Podophyllin, though widely used clinically, does produce significant distortions of histologic appearance, reducing the value of biopsy considerably for 4–6 weeks. Absorption of this product from the vagina in large amounts produces neurologic lesions in the patient and significant defects in any developing fetus (Moher and Maurer, 1979).

Vaccines are useful in chronic, recurring condyloma. Such vaccines are usually manufactured locally in the hospital treating the patient and have been reported as effective by Albin and Curtis (1974) and by Abcarian et al. (1976). Our experience has shown them to be beneficial in recurring cases. Patients who have significant immunosuppression are probably best not treated with immunologic therapy until further clinical data are available.

### Herpes Simplex

The difficult problem of herpes simplex and its distressing symptoms, in which the lesions are multiple and in the area of the urethra, remains a clinical dilemma. The lesions may be easily removed with the $CO_2$ laser. However, such management does little to stop the proliferation of the virus in the perineural sheath and the recurrence of lesions at a time when some other inciting event occurs (Kibrick, 1980). I do not recommend the use of the $CO_2$ laser in the treatment of herpetic lesions of the vulva. Other local measures are as effective and much less expensive.

## SUMMARY

The use of the $CO_2$ laser directed through the colposcope is a significant contribution to clinical medicine. It is now the method of choice in the management of cervical intraepithelial neoplasia, intraepithelial neoplasia recurring in the vaginal cuff after surgery, and the intraepithelial neoplasia that extends out into the vagina. It is clinically effective in the management of condyloma acuminata, and these lesions will be commonly treated with the laser in the future.

The requirements for the safe use of the laser in gynecology are as follows:

Operator
1. Is a skilled colposcopist
2. Is knowledgeable in neoplastic disease
3. Has reviewed all cytologic and biopsy data.
4. Knows precise extent and histologic type disease present
5. Is familiar with equipment being used
6. Observes all laser safety precautions

Patient
1. Is well informed about laser
2. Is well informed about other options for treatment
3. Has signed informed consent
4. Is available for follow-up examination

Lesion
1. Is noninvasive
2. Is entirely visible
3. Has been thoroughly studied and sampled
4. Is appropriate for laser therapy

Laser equipment
1. Is appropriate for task to be performed
2. Has been properly maintained and is in good working order
3. Incorporates proper safety features

The widespread use of the laser in gynecology awaits a cheaper, structurally smaller unit, which will greatly increase acceptance of this method of treatment. New lasers with characteristics different from those of $CO_2$ will be adapted into clinical gynecologic surgery as they become available.

## REFERENCES

Abcarian H, Smith D, Sharon N (1976) The immunotherapy of anal condylomata acuminata. Dis Colol Rectum 19:237–244.

Albin RJ, Curtis WW (1974) Immunotherapeutic treatment of condylomata acuminata. Gynecol Oncol 2:446–450.

Bellina JH (1977) In: Win RM (ed) Carbon dioxide laser in gynecology. Obstet Gynecol Ann 390–391.

Calkins J, Masterson BJ (submitted for publication) Management of condyloma acuminata with the carbon dioxide laser.

Carter R, Krantz KE, Hara GS, Lin F, Masterson BJ, Smith S (1978) Treatment of cervical intraepithelial neoplasia with the carbon dioxide laser beam. Am J Obstet Gynecol 131:831–836.

Goldman L, Rockwell RJ Jr (1971) Lasers in Medicine. Gordon and Breach Science Publishers, New York.

Jako GL (1972) Laser surgery of the vocal cords. Laryngoscope 82:2204–2216.

Kaplan I, Goldman J, Ger R (1973) The treatment of erosion of the uterine cervix by use of the $CO_2$ laser. Am J Obstet Gynecol 41:795–796.

Kibrick S (1980) Herpes simplex infection at term: What to do with mother, newborn, and nursery personnel. JAMA 243:157–160.

Lupulescu A, Mehregan AH, Rahbari H, Pincus H, Birmingham DJ (1977) Venereal warts vs. Bowens disease. A histologic and ultrasfructure of five cases. JAMA 237:2520–2522.

Masterson BJ, Calkins J (submitted for publication) Management of cervical intraepithelial neoplasia with the carbon dioxide laser: A five year experience.

Masterson, BJ, Jordan JA, Bellina JH (1980) The laser in gynecology. ACOG Update 5 (No. 10), May.

McBurney EI (1978) Carbon dioxide laser treatment of dermatologic lesions. South Med J 71:795–797.

Moher LM, Maurer SA (1979) Podophyllin toxicity: Case report and literature review. J Fam Pract 9:237–240.

Pincus H, Lupulescu A, Mehregan AH, Rahbari H (1977) Venereal disease vs. Bowens disease. JAMA 238:2496.

Powell CL, Jr (1978) Condyloma acuminatum: Recent advances in development, carcinogenesis, and treatment. Clin Obstet Gynecol 21:1061–1079.

Schawlow AL, Townes CH (1958) Infrared and optical masers. Physical Rev 112:1940–1949.

Schellhas HF (1978) Laser surgery in gynecology. Surg Clin North Am 58:151–166.

Sharplan Technical Manual (1979) Laser Industries Ltd., Tel Aviv, Israel.

Stafl A, Wilkinson EJ, Mattingly RJ (1977) Laser treatment of cervical and vaginal neoplasia. Am J Obstet Gynecol 128:128–136.

# 12

# Laser Eye Instrumentation: Diagnostic and Surgical

*Maurice B. Landers, III*
*Myron L. Wolbarsht*

The uses of lasers in ophthalmology may be considered under the headings Diagnosis, Therapy, and Research. There is enough overlap among the classifications, however, that research can be discussed with the other two. In both diagnosis and research, the spatial and temporal coherence properties of the laser are often of value. In therapy it is not yet evident that these special properties are necessary.

The eye is a highly specialized part of the body and, as such, is subject to many types of pathology that in other organs of the body would be minor. Because of the close interaction of ocular parts, however, such disorders lead to major disturbances of function. When the eye is considered as an optical instrument (Fig. 12.1), the cornea is the major refracting element, whereas the lens (named for its resemblance in shape to a lentil bean rather than for its supposed function as an optical element) has only one-third or less of the total refracting power. Possibly the most delicate structures in the eye are the retina and the blood vessels near its inner surface. The retina functions both as a light detector and as part of the brain in performing the initial stages of information analysis on the neuronal signals from the photoreceptors.

## DIAGNOSIS

In diagnosis the most usual functional test is the measurement of visual acuity with a letter chart or some similar target. This method tests not only the possibility that the optical elements properly focus the image on the retina, but also the ability of the photoreceptors in the retina to detect the image focused on the retina and of the later neural elements to analyze this information in proper sequence. However, because an eyechart type of visual acuity test can indicate only an overall degra-

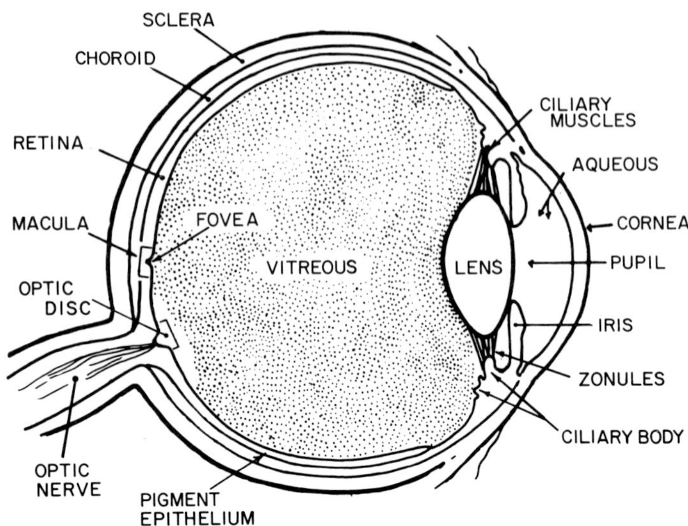


**Fig. 12.1.** Cross section of human eye. The cornea-air interface is the main refractive element; the lens index of refraction is not much higher than that of the fluid surrounding it. The fovea is on the optical axis of the cornea and lens for best image formation. Change of focus for near objects is accomplished by relaxation of tension of the zonules on the lens, which allows the anterior lens surface (next to the pupil) to have a smaller radius of curvature. A frequent cause of ocular complaints is loss of clarity by the lens, which progresses to translucence (cataract) or even opacity. The vitreous is a jellylike material; the aqueous is waterlike. The retina is a transparent tissue lining the inner surface of the eyeball. For sources of oxygen supply to the retina, see Figure 12.5.

dation of function, several supplementary tests are necessary before the part of the system responsible for any improper function can be located and the proper therapy chosen to rectify the problem. In contrast, the use of a laser in an initial screening test can indicate whether it is the optical system or the neural system that is at fault.

## Laser Refraction of the Eye

The speckle pattern of the laser (Fig. 12.2) has been suggested as a way of analyzing the eye's optical system almost independently of the resolving function of the retina (Sinclair, 1965; Knoll, 1966; Ingelstam and Ragnarsson, 1972). In essence, the interference pattern formed by laser light reflected from some nonspeckled surface is projected onto the retina. If the reflecting surface and the retina are confocal with each other, slight relative movements between the reflecting and diffusing surfaces of the eye will not cause the image on the retina to move. However, a difference in the focus will produce movement of the retinal image. The direction of this movement tells whether the retinal plane is in front of the focal plane or behind it in a way similar to that of out-of-focus movements used in retinoscopy. From an optical standpoint, at least, this technique might almost be considered a form of self-retinoscopy. This method is applicable to mass screening techniques, as large numbers of people could be tested with the same projection of a laser image. It is also possible to construct an automatic refractometer that registers the reflection from the retina while the focal length is changed in order to arrive at the null point for the movement of the retinal image. The speckle pattern test ensures that the eye is properly refracted and that an image will be in focus on the retina insofar as the optical system can accomplish it. An examination of the optical pathway for irregularities of refraction or unusual scattering properties will, of course, supplement the speckle test to ensure the optimal optical performance of the eye.

The laser speckle pattern has also been used to measure the range of focus of the eye (Hennessy and Liebowitz, 1972), or the changes in the lens with accommodation (Ukrai and Ohzu, 1976). The most difficult part of this test is the measurement of the amount of astigmatism and especially its diurnal variation. The speckle test has been adapted to measure this variation (Ohzu, 1976; Ronchi et al., 1978), but the procedure is useful for research purposes only at the present time. In the future, diagnostic tests based on the same principle will certainly be devised. For example, small changes in lens elasticity that might predate the initial development of visible cataracts would cause a subtle change in astigmatism with

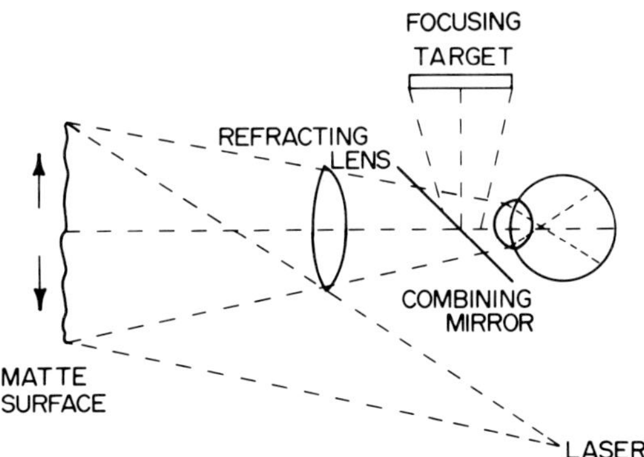


**Fig. 12.2.** Experimental arrangement for measurement of refraction (or accommodation) using the laser speckle pattern (adapted from Ohzu, 1976). The matte surface *(at left)* moves slowly in the direction indicated by the arrows. The focusing target overlays the speckle pattern by means of the combining mirror. The power of the focusing lens is changed by the subject until the speckle lateral motion is stopped. This indicates that the matte surface is in focus, and at that time, the speckle pattern may move randomly; a residual oblique motion is indicative of ocular astigmatism. For more precise refraction, a cylindrical lens can be added to neutralize the speckle oblique motion (Ronchi et al., 1978). In another adaptation of this method, the chromatic aberration of the eye may also be studied by means of lasers of different wavelengths. With this technique Ohzu (1976) showed that the chromatic aberration of the eye from 477 to 633 nm differs by approximately 1 diopter; furthermore this 1-diopter difference remains constant over approximately 4 diopters of accommodation.

accommodation. Thus, a clinical test of this type might reveal an early, and possibly reversible, stage in cataractogenesis.

## Laser Analysis of the Neural Components in Vision

After the eye has been properly refracted, the resolving power of the neural portions of the visual system must be determined. Properly, this must be done without regard to the refractive apparatus or the optical parts. In other words, the purpose of the second part of the laser test protocol is to find out how well the retina can analyze the image that is placed upon it by the cornea and lens. As mentioned earlier, defects in the cornea or lens are difficult to measure by conventional visual acuity tests, as these tests do not specify in which part of the eye the difficulty lies or even whether several parts may each contribute to the overall degradation of the resolution of the visual system.

The use of bandlike interference patterns (most easily generated by a laser) allows a direct test of the resolving power of the retina (LeGrand, 1935; Campbell and Green, 1965). The interference patterns of various spatial frequencies are projected onto the retina, more or less independent of the dioptics of the eye, to provide a companion test to the use of speckle patterns to evaluate the optics alone. An interferometer (Jamin type) in which the path length of one beam is changed by a wedge is shown in Fig. 12.3. This projects a sinusoidally modulated band interference pattern into the eye. The spacing of the bands depends upon the amount of wedge. By determining the minimum resolvable spacing, an estimate can be made of the resolving power of the retina. The refraction of the eye is not important; a deformed or roughened corneal surface, or a deranged or cataractous

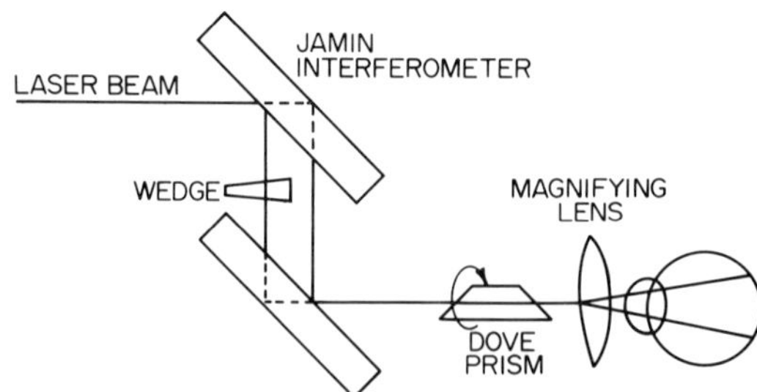


**Fig. 12.3.** Bar pattern generation in the retina by interferometry. The laser beam is separated into two paths by the front and rear reflections from a thick second-surface mirror and recombined by a similar mirror. A length difference between the pathways was introduced by a wedge placed in one beam. A dove prism rotates the orientation of the interference bands and can produce either a slowly rotating pattern or discrete and separate positions. A magnifying lens of variable focal length can change the spacing of the band to indicate the best pathway of the eye. The pattern produced by this type of interferometer is a grating whose contrast between dark and light is lessened by the amount of light scattering in the optical pathway. Variations on this basic schema can produce other patterns besides bars. Also, it is possible to produce, by moiré fringes, a similar but higher contrast pattern in black and white (Lotmar, 1979).

lens can still transmit sufficient light to form a sharply defined pattern on the retina, although the contrast is lowered by any light scattering.

There are other ways of by-passing the optics to project an image on the retina: moiré patterns, x-ray fluorescence, and transillumination, to name a few. In all, the principle is much the same, in that the optics of the eye are nullified to give an independent test of retinal (and particularly macular) function. None of these have been useful clinically, because they lack either the desired degree of resolution or are too difficult to administer. Lotmar's attempts (1980a) to use moiré fringes have been the closest to clinical success in this group. Even the interference pattern method has its difficulties, in that the fringes are not always recognized by the patient (Green and Cohen, 1971). Attempts to enhance recognition and give a sharper endpoint by moving or rotating the pattern, in which the patient indicates the direction of rotation or orientation of the bands, have achieved some success (Ohzu, 1976).

It has been the clinical experience of ophthalmologists testing the many variations of the interference fringe method that if the cataract or visual disturbance is in only one eye while the other eye has good visual capability, the measurements are very successful (Goldmann and Lotmar, 1969). However, if the patient is not able to compare a pattern that is clearly seen with one eye with the somewhat degraded pattern in the defective eye, the results are not so good. That is, the test is less predictive of the possible function of the retina after the optical system is restored by some operation, such as cataract removal, corneal transplant, vitrectomy, etc. In the future it might be possible to use more sophisticated forms of this test with more clinical success. For example, some nonuniform type of path length change could produce fringes shaped to be easily appreciated by the patient. Possibly the use of microscopic letters on a bleached photographic film, in which the thickness of the film is proportional to the density of the original silver image, might create fringe shapes to suggest familiar letters or patterns to the patient.

## Holographic Techniques

**Glaucoma Diagnosis.** Another use of the laser in diagnosis is in relation to glaucoma. The enormous amount of detail that can be recorded in a hologram has a great fascination for those who wish to document the changes in the eye (Van Ligten et al., 1966), especially changes indicative of glaucoma, such as increased cup/disk ratio (Vaughn et al., 1973; Calkins, 1976). As a hologram of the retina can give a three-dimensional view, successive holograms at different time intervals would document the changes in the cup depth very precisely.

Other methods may be superior to holograms for this purpose, i.e., the stereochronographs or chronostereoscopy of Lotmar (1980b). Nevertheless, many attempts have been made to produce holograms clinically usable for glaucoma diagnosis (see Ohzu, 1976, for review). Holography has many possible merits, but to date, its disadvantages have prevented widespread clinical acceptance. The low quality of the image due to the speckle pattern is only one factor; safety considerations based on the high-power levels of the lasers used and the requirements for mechanical stability are as important.

**Other Applications of Holography.** In addition to the applications of holography in glaucoma research, there are many other applications for it in research on the eye, such as documentation of the shape, size, and location of suspected tumors or foreign bodies. Holographic interferometry can demonstrate changes in the position of the vitreous body or the retina. Holographic techniques should also be useful in determining the changes in the curvature of the cornea as a function of intraocular pressure (Ohzu, 1976). For example, holographic interferometry of the cornea should furnish a way of documenting the intraocular pressure, especially if used in conjunction with the air puff tonometer which produces a depression of the cornea by a known force. To some extent, the elasticity of the sclera around the nerve head has been studied in this manner in an enucleated eye (Matsumato et al., 1978). However, the technique in the living eye would be difficult, and there is a question of whether the additional information that it gives is sufficient to render it useful as a clinical tool. The laboratory value certainly could be great, as the differential deformation of the cornea with external force can be studied. This would fully document any changes in corneal elasticity attendant upon the development of increased intraocular pressure. The changes in the lens surface with accommodation could also be examined by the same technique. Because of the greater chance to optimize the optical conditions in research, it is in that field that high-acuity holograms of the eye may soon be available, but there will certainly be a long delay before the same quality is also produced clinically.

Holography is a photographic process, and it is appropriate to mention here other possible photographic uses of lasers. For example, multiwavelength lasers could produce colored holograms. In another approach, the use of a laser to project a bright, easily recognized spot on the retina for reference purposes in focusing techniques has also been suggested (Wolbarsht et al., 1978).

### Light Scattering

The picosecond range pulses available from mode-locked lasers and the development of sophisticated electronics allow a novel use of the laser in analyzing the light-scattering properties of the eye. For example, the development of cataracts can be followed by putting ultrashort laser pulses into the eye and then, with high resolution, measuring the time required for the reflected and scattered light to return (Bruckner, 1977). This lidar (optical radar) method allows a calculation of the location of the scattering centers (or layers) within the lens and their relative magnitude. The use of tunable lasers can give the wavelength dependence function of the scattering, and from this an estimate of the size of the scattering particles can be made.

## THERAPY AND SAFETY

Therapy and safety are inexorably linked, since the therapeutic uses of the laser depend principally on its ability to cause damage. The physical and biologic effects of laser pulses are many. At lower energy and power levels, thermal effects predominate; but at high peak powers, other so-called nonlinear interactions are found, such as two photon, Brillouin scattering, frequency doubling, etc. The site of the interaction is often enlarged by physical amplification (steam generation, shock-wave disruption). Further amplification, of a biologic nature, usually follows after a latent period—often as long as a day. This type of amplification often is a result of cell death with release of histamine-like agents (Hayes and Wolbarsht, 1968).

Superficially at least, safety research coincides with the main therapeutic application of lasers in ophthalmology, which is to create a thermal lesion on the retina to control various types of retinal dysfunction.

## Glaucoma

For glaucoma, a laser is often used to induce a thermal lesion in and around the trabecular meshwork to open a pathway into Schlemm's canal (Krasnov, 1973; Wickham et al., 1977; van der Zypen et al., 1979), or, alternatively, to shrink the trabecular meshwork and thus assist Schlemm's canal in remaining patent. Attempts have also been made to use the nonthermal effects of laser pulses to overcome the low absorption of this tissue. The rapid rise times and high electromagnetic fields of ultrashort laser pulses can generate phonons or initiate electron avalanche with plasma formation. These can all act to create a shock wave sufficient to disrupt a very localized area of the trabecular meshwork and thus open additional outflow to Schlemm's canal (van der Zypen et al., 1979). As yet, with either of these methods, no long-term follow-ups are available of patients treated although some successful cases are several years old. However, at present, it seems that these procedures are helpful.

## Safety

The safety aspects of laser usage are highly important in ophthalmology because the eye is the most vulnerable target organ (Chapter 3). The attempts to work out the mechanisms of injury so that proper extrapolations can be made to cover new laser types also aid in the understanding of the proper therapeutic use.

## Patterned Photocoagulation

An unusual approach to the problem of performing controlled pattern photocoagulation for safety research (and also for therapy) has been advanced by Madeiros et al. (1979). They propose to use the Fourier transform properties of the delivery optical system to introduce several discrete and precisely located retinal exposures simultaneously with a known ratio between the power levels. This scheme requires that a diffraction screen be placed between the laser source and the eye (Fig. 12.4). The appropriate diffracting screen is made by holographic techniques, and the process is a relatively simple one. The laser exposure gives an intensity distribution at the retina that is essentially the Fourier transform of the intensity distribution

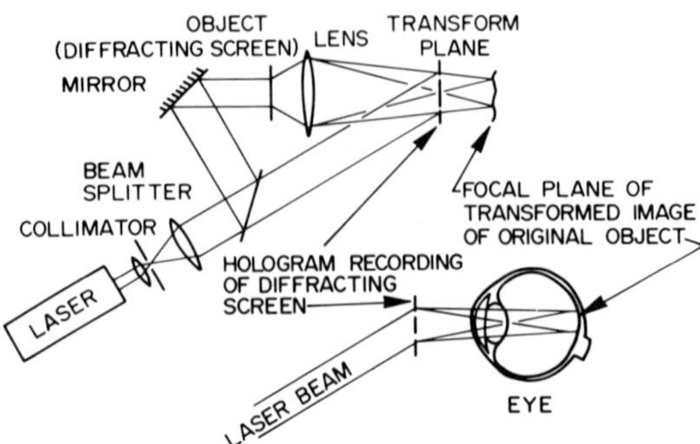


**Fig. 12.4.** Optical diffraction geometry. The intensity distribution in the focal plane at the retina, formed by the cornea, lens, and pupil, is essentially the Fourier transform of the intensity distribution in the diffracting screen. This type of image has been used to form a series of retinal exposures with a known energy relation to each other. This situation allows a quick and easy assessment of the threshold energy level for retinal damage by a given laser. Its therapeutic usefulness may also be similar in that a central lesion can be placed with satellites of known energy relation around it. A series of diffracting screens could be used for different modes of treatment. To date, only Ronchi gratings have been used to form the diffracting screen, but more complex functions will probably be tested in the future (based on Madeiros et al., 1979).

of the diffraction screen formed by the limiting aperture. This screen can be produced by holographic techniques to give any arbitrary function.

## Photocoagulation Therapy for Proliferative Diabetic Retinopathy

A good example of the use of lasers in therapeutic ophthalmology is the treatment of proliferative diabetic retinopathy by photocoagulation. Photocoagulation is the only widely accepted use of lasers in medical therapy and, as such, it deserves extensive discussion.

The major problem in diabetic retinopathy is a proliferation of retinal vessels along the surface of the retina and into the vitreous cavity. These new vessels, because of their fragility, give rise to hemorrhages. Also, occasionally, retraction of the vitreous around the new blood vessels pulls the retina away from the pigmented epithelium.

Several large-scale clinical trials have demonstrated the value of pan-retinal photocoagulation in controlling retinal-vessel proliferation. Often 2000 or more laser lesions are placed in the peripheral retina. However, the lesions are not necessarily directly on the unwanted blood vessels, and the rationale behind the therapeutic use of laser photocoagulation for proliferative diabetic retinopathy has been questioned [see Wolbarsht and Landers (1979) for review]. Originally, the argon laser was selected by L'Esperance (1968) because its wavelength was well matched to the absorption of hemoglobin. He intended that the laser photocoagulation would be used to occlude single vessels by heating the blood within them. Although this focal vessel coagulation was not very effective therapeutically, the coherent radiation argon laser photocoagulator developed at Stanford Research Institute still had wide acceptance clinically. This instrument seemed effective for scatter or panretinal lesion formation; it was also an easily managed, well-engineered instrument.

The initial cause of the growth of new retinal vessels in diabetics is not known for certain, although the first clinical sign is blockage of part of the vascular bed. It has been suggested that these vessels grow in response to a tissue factor X (Wise, 1956), or tumor angiogenesis factor (Patz et al., 1978) secreted by the diabetic ("sick") retina. It has also been suggested that destruction by photocoagulation of a sufficient amount of the diabetic retina is followed by a replacement with scar tissue that does not secrete the tissue factor X. This decreased secretion of factor X allows new vessel growth to cease (Patz et al., 1978).

Other workers have suggested that replacing the retina with scar tissue lowers the metabolic requirements of the retina for oxygen (Blach and Hamilton, 1978). In this case the lower oxygen tension from the loss of vessels in the diabetic retina is thought of as the stimulus to growth. Neither of these models is exactly consistent with the details of laser photocoagulation, and an alternative model has been proposed that takes into account the site of the lesion and the physiology of the microcirculation (Wolbarsht and Landers, 1979).

The new model does not assume that there is a tissue factor X; rather it assumes that mechanical factors control growth, thus chronic dilatation of blood vessels is followed by growth, whereas constricted or even the normal-sized vessels are inhibited from growing. For this model, the efficacy of photocoagulation depends upon the dual blood supply of the retina. The retinal vessels supply oxygen to the inner half, and the choroidal vessels to the outer half (Fig. 12.5). The retinal vessels change their size and flow rate to keep a constant level of tissue oxygen availability. On the other hand, the choroidal vessels have a very high rate of flow which saturates the surrounding tissue with oxygen at all times. Moreover, they do not regulate their flow regardless of changes in the surrounding tissue oxygen demand.

As mentioned earlier in this review, in diabetic retinopathy, many of the smaller retinal blood vessels become inoperative. It may be that the remaining retinal vessels dilate in an effort to supply oxygen to the now hypoxic portions of the inner retina. The photocoagulation lesion is in the pigment epithelium and the photoreceptor layer, which forms the outer retina. This is the portion of the retina that gets its oxygen from the choroidal circulation. Thus, destruction of the photoreceptors, the rods and cones, would have no effect on the oxygen demand of the inner retina, nor should this destruction change the output of tissue factor X since the inner retina would not be affected at all by the laser lesion. However, the rods and the cones have the majority of the mitochondria in the retina. This indicates they also have the highest metabolic rate, and indeed the outer retina does utilize the majority (perhaps as much as 80%) of the retinal oxygen (Bill, 1975). When large portions of the outer retina are replaced with scar tissue following photocoagulation, the oxygen normally used in the outer retina now diffuses into the inner retina (Fig. 12.6). As a result of this additional oxygen, all dilated (and growing) vessels are constricted and are no longer stimulated to grow. In deriving this conclusion, it is assumed that it is the dilatation of the vessel itself (rather than the low tissue oxygen) that is the key factor in causing vessels to grow, i.e., chronic dilatation stimulates vessel growth, whereas normal or constricted vessels do not grow. Even further, a constricted new vessel may be resorbed.

Thus, the action of photocoagulation is indirect: It destroys the part of the retina that depends upon the choroidal circulation, the oxygen balance within the retina is changed, and the retinal vessels no longer attempt to supply oxygen to parts of the retina in which the vessels disappeared as a result of the diabetic disease process. On the basis of this model, it would seem that the wavelength of the laser photocoagulation should be selected to match the absorption of the pigment granules while any action on the fragile retinal vessels is avoided. Possibly a yellow or red CW laser might be the answer.

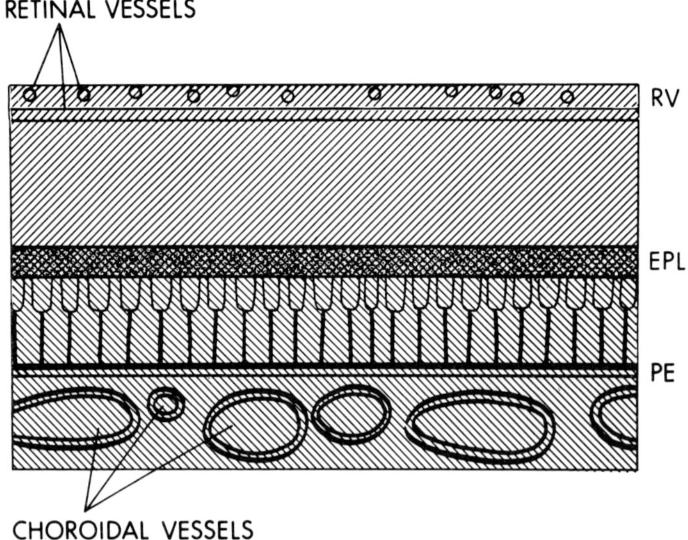


**Fig. 12.5.** Schematic cross section of the retina showing the sources of oxygen consumed by the various layers under normal conditions. Retinal vessels supply the inner part of the retina. One retinal vessel runs longitudinally in the plane of illustration. The outer half of the retina (*(lower part of figure)* is supplied from choroidal vessels. The oxygen supply from the two sources overlaps in the outer plexiform layer. Choroidal and retinal circulations react differently to changes in oxygen requirements of tissues or to changes in oxygenation in blood. Retinal vessels constrict and change their flow pattern to maintain a constant tissue-oxygen availability. Choroidal vessels do not change significantly with oxygen demands of tissue or oxygen content of blood. Blood flow through the choroid is very large; under normal conditions only 4% of oxygen carried by hemoglobin is removed. Thus, venous oxygen concentration is almost as high as arterial. The majority of oxygen in the retina is consumed by the rods and cones, as over 90% of mitochondria are located in this region between the pigment epithelium (*PE*) and the external plexiform layer (*EPL*).

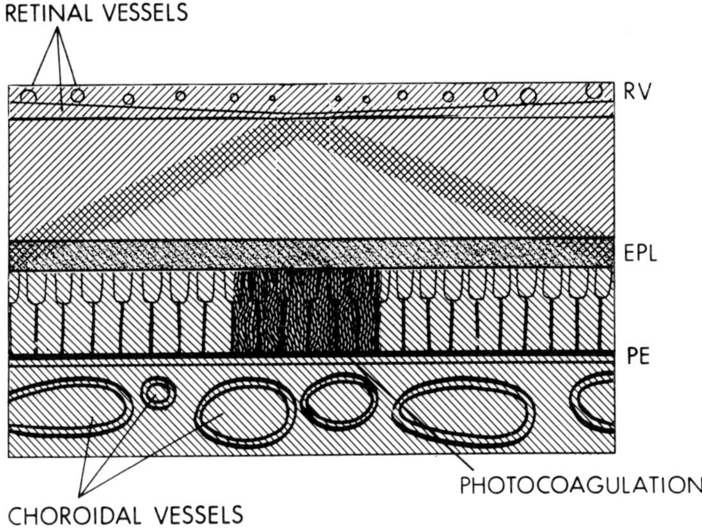


**Fig. 12.6.** Schematic cross section of the retina showing the source of oxygen consumed by the various retinal layers around a moderate photocoagulation lesion. The blood has the same oxygen tension as shown in Figure 12.5. Destruction of the rods and cones (which consume the majority of oxygen supplied by the choroid) allows more oxygen to reach the inner layers of the retina. Retinal vessels constrict to maintain oxygen availability around them at the normal level. In diabetic retina, vessels are dilated to supply additional oxygen to hypoxic areas where vessel dropout has removed circulation. A longitudinal vessel is shown constricting when it comes into the zone of high oxygen availability. Thus, increased oxygen supply around the lesion in a localized portion of the retina affects higher choroidal blood oxygenation in the retina. When laser lesions are extensive, as in panretinal photocoagulation, all retinal vessels will be normal size or constricted to give more or less normal flow pattern as result of generalized increase in oxygen availability from choroidal circulation to the inner layers of the retina. This inhibition of dilatation of retinal vessels will also inhibit neovascularization or new vessel growth in the diabetic retina (see text).

## Surgery with a Carbon Dioxide Laser

There is a possibility that a $CO_2$ laser can be developed for both external and internal surgery on the eye, in addition to the argon, Nd, and ruby lasers that are currently in use. The $CO_2$ laser vaporizes tissue, particularly the water in tissue. Thus, attempts to remove the lens or the vitreous or to cut a circle upon the cornea for corneal grafts have all been under investigation, but none as yet have reached the clinical stage.

Carbon dioxide laser surgery on the external eye is probably no different from that in other parts of the body except for the miniature size of the eye and the importance of function, such as movement of the lids and, to a lesser degree, the globe. However, the use of the $CO_2$ laser for surgery inside the eye is a more difficult matter. The $CO_2$ laser acts by vaporizing water and its associated tissue elements. The large expansion that takes place with steam formation might be explosive in nature within an enclosed space such as the eye. Indeed, the use of any laser inside the eye for ablative surgery is quite difficult. A $CO_2$ laser with an optical-fiber delivery system has the further difficulty that its action may take place directly at the exit port. This would probably ruin the exit port. However, it has been suggested that a variation of the standard pars plana vitrectomy operation might solve both problems (Landers, unpublished report). The eye would be filled with air (or nitrogen), and optical-fiber probes would be inserted through the pars plana to allow the $CO_2$ laser radiation to vaporize the vitreous or lens. Extra hollow probes would be used for exhaust, while still arranged to keep the eye completely pressurized when the laser is not operating. The air-filled eye presents some optical problems. However, these are not insurmountable, and it would seem that in the not-too-distant future there will be $CO_2$ surgery inside the eye. This, of course, might offer many technical advantages over other types of intraocular surgery, especially with regard to the vitreous.

## Diagnosis of a Melanoma: A Proposal to Localize Photoacoustical Spectroscopy

One of the most difficult conditions to diagnose in ophthalmology is an intraocular malignant melanoma. The difficulty is differentiating the malignant melanoma from a nevus (pigmented mole). Although such a mass can be seen and although it may cause loss of function, it may still be a benign mass—a nevus. The signs that are usually examined are growth rate and metabolism. Both are higher in the melanoma as compared to the nevus. The rate of growth can only be determined with accurate records. Unfortunately, none of the accepted tests for metabolic rate—such as radioactive phosphorus ($^{32}P$) uptake—can be used optimally on an intraocular mass. A biopsy would be very helpful, but the fear of spreading the melanoma eliminates that possibility. Inside the eye, the melanoma is within the eye's analog of the blood-brain barrier. Every care is taken to avoid breaching this natural containment of the cancer because it is commonly thought that any breaks in this barrier will allow metastases. Thus, there is no easy way to ascertain the identification of a reasonably large pigmented mass, especially without a previous history.

However, there is an approach, in theory at least (Wolbarsht, 1979), to differentiate between these two masses, even though the pigmentation and external appearance are very much the same. The rate of metabolism, the relative oxygenation, or perhaps even the amount of mitochondria may be grounds for differentiating the melanoma from the nevus. In theory, these factors can be differentiated by laser-induced photoacoustical spectroscopic imaging (LIPASI).

**Photoacoustical Spectroscopy.** Photoacoustical spectroscopy is one of the newest techniques used to investigate nearly transparent objects with low absorption. The technique depends upon the absorption of light somewhere in an object, the degradation of light into heat that spreads through the object, and the translation of this heat into bulk expansion of the material followed by a sound wave generated at the surface. First described by A. G. Bell and S. Tainter in 1880, it was largely ignored until its revival in recent years. Largely based on Rosencwaig's theoretical analysis (1975), the technique has been highly refined. The sensitivity of the technique is increased by chopping the light beam so that only signals in phase with the light beam need be amplified and integrated. Averaging techniques and higher chopping rates increase the signal-to-noise ratio by a tremendous amount. As the wavelength of light is changed, a plot of the differential absorption is obtained, proportional to the height of the photoacoustical signal. In many situations the specimen is not homogeneous, and it is desirable to know the differential absorption of different absorbing parts. This cannot be accomplished easily by conventional photoacoustical spectroscopy, as both a scanning beam and a low chopping rate are needed (Wang et al., 1979), but in principle at least, a combination of photoacoustical spectroscopy and ultrasonic methods will give this localization.

Ultrasonic localizations (ultrasonograms) consist of the input of a test ultrasonic pulse, as in sonar, which is then reflected (or echoed) differentially from each change in the sonic index of refraction in the specimen. The source of the echo is localized by computer processing of the signals from an array of detectors and is displayed by giving the distance away from the detectors in the radar B- and C-scan modes [see Havlice and Taenzer (1979) for review]. The usual photoacoustical signal is not suitable for this type of processing. It is not localized and, as it results from bulk heating and cooling of the material, has only low-frequency components—less than 10 kHz. Moreover, it is air-coupled to the receiver, further minimizing any possibility of ultrasonic components. However, there is another approach to photoacoustical spectroscopy: A short laser pulse can generate an ultrasonic pulse directly from the absorbing site (Cleary, 1977; Felix, 1974).

**Laser-induced Photoacoustical Spectroscopic Imaging.** The laser-induced photoultrasonic signal can be detected and displayed as an ultrasonogram. If various laser wavelengths are used for stimulation, we have a new technique: laser-induced photoacoustical spectroscopic imaging (LIPASI). If a laser pulse is used for excitation, the recording situation differs from an ordinary ultrasonogram in that all absorbing sites are excited at essentially the same time, for the speed of light is so much greater than the speed of sound. The recording conditions are presented in Figure 12.7. The display of this photoacoustical ultrasonogram could be interlaced with a conventional ultrasonogram, which would give more familiar landmarks to allow location of the photoacoustical absorbing sites. The height of the laser-induced photoacoustical pulse would be attenuated by the law of inverse squares so this must be taken into account when relative absorption is figured as a function of density. There will also be attenuation by the various reflecting surfaces, which can be corrected for a comparison with a conventional ultrasonogram. Each type of display would then assist in the interpretation of the other.

The technique of LIPASI is best suited to characterizing absorbing sites in a transparent medium. The human body is not transparent, yet it is not too far away from this in the infrared, at least. Few organic compounds absorb strongly in the near infrared, and the main optical activity of biologic tissues is scattering. How-

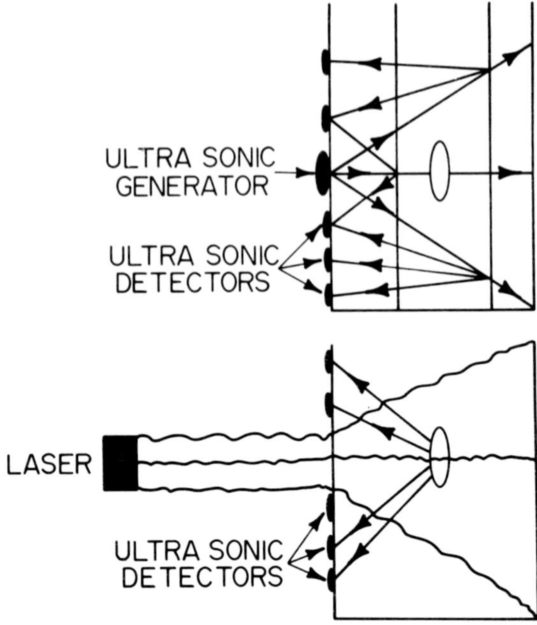


**Fig. 12.7.** Ultrasonic imaging and laser-induced photoacoustical spectroscopic imaging (LIPASI). *At top*, in normal ultrasonic imaging, the sound pulse from the ultrasonic generator is reflected from boundaries of the various layers within the tissue. Echoes are detected by an array that was the phasing, to give relative distances from reflecting sites. This allows analysis and three-dimensional imaging of reflecting surfaces. *At bottom*, in LIPASI, laser pulses absorbed by particular portions of the tissue emit ultrasonic pulses detected by an array, as in usual ultrasonic imaging at top. However, in LIPASI, the image will be interlaced with the three-dimensional picture from conventional ultrasonic imaging. Multiple reflections from the various interfaces in both diagrams, however (not shown), will certainly pose a problem for rejection, but careful timing can probably assist in proper selection of data for display.

ever, two metabolic systems of great biologic importance show differential absorption in the near-infrared region, as a function of their oxidative states, hemoglobin and cytochrome c oxidase (cytochrome a, $a_3$) (Jöbsis, 1977, 1979). From this difference, tissues could be characterized by their oxidation state. In the eye, for example, a melanoma might have a more active tissue metabolism, with relative hypoxia during its growth phase as compared with a nevus.

Even if LIPASI does not work in the eye, it may be possible to apply it to other parts of the body. The heart would also be a good target. The laser pulse could be timed to occur at certain phases of the cardiac cycle, thus maintaining a relatively constant distance from the absorbing site to the detectors. The localization of infarcts would be possible. Also, over a period of time, any revascularization of the infarct site could be observed and the prognosis modified accordingly.

The theory is sound. However, effectuating this technique has many pitfalls.

Indeed, whether it is even possible in the laboratory, much less in the clinic, still remains to be demonstrated.

## AIDS TO THE BLIND

It may be that when no further ophthalmic therapy is available, the laser cane may furnish the "terminal" eye care. The laser cane, in its commercial version (Typhlocane, Bionic Instruments, Bala Cynwd, Pennsylvania), is a device to aid mobility in the blind. It has three gallium-arsenide infrared-emitting laser diodes whose beams scan the environment as the cane is rotated toward obstructions, ground-level dips, and/or changing obstacles. Tone pitches and finger vibrations are generated to indicate which type of hazard is encountered.

## SUMMARY

The possible applications of lasers in opthalmology are many; the present clinical applications are few. Even the research projects have barely begun to take advantage of the very real renaissance in optics started by lasers. It is not the lasers themselves. It is, rather, a new attitude and the new family of technologies fostered by them that furnish the means for a revolution. Nevertheless, ophthalmology is on the verge of a great change, and the laser will play a key part in it.

## REFERENCES


Bill A (1975) Ocular circulation. In: Moses RA (ed) Adler's Physiology of the Eye, 6th ed. C.V. Mosby, St. Louis, pp. 210–229.

Blach R, Hamilton AM (1978) The techniques and indications for photocoagulation in diabetic retinopathy. I. Principles of photocoagulation. Int Opthalmol 1:19–29.

Bruckner AP (1977) Picosecond light scattering measurements in the cataractous lens. In: Proceedings of the Technical Program in Electro-Optics/Laser 77 Conference and Exposition, Anaheim, California, pp. 473–479.

Calkins J (1976) Fundus camera holography. In: Greguss P (ed) Holography in Medicine. IPC Science and Technology Press, Ltd. Surrey, England, p. 85.

Campbell F, Green D (1965) Optical and retinal factors affecting visual resolution. J Physiol (London) 176:576–593.

Cleary SF (1977) Laser pulses and the generation of acoustic transients in biological material. In: Wolbarsht ML (ed) Laser Applications in Medicine and Biology, vol. 3. Plenum Press, New York, pp. 175–219.

Felix MP (1974) Laser-generated ultrasonic beams. Rev Sci Inst 49:1106–1108.

Goldmann H, Lotmar W (1969) Beitrag zun Problem der Bestimmung der "retinalen Sehschärfe" bei Katarakt. Klin Monatsbl f Augenheil 154:324–329.

Green DG, Cohen MM (1971) Laser interferometry in the evaluation of potential macular function in the presence of opacities in the ocular media. Trans Amer Acad Opthalmol and Otolar 75:629–637.

Havlice JF, Taenzer JC (1979) Medical ultrasonic imaging: An overview of principles and instrumentation. Proceedings of Institute of Electron and Electrical Engineers 67:620–641.

Hayes JR, Wolbarsht ML (1968) Thermal model for retinal damage induced by pulsed lasers. Aerospace Medicine 39:474–480.

Hennessy RT, Leibowitz H (1972) Laser optometer incorporating the Badal principle. Behav Res Meth Instrum 4:237–239.

Hochheimer BF (1974) Lasers in opthalmology. In: Wolbarsht ML (ed) Laser Applications in Medicine and Biology, vol. 2. Plenum Press, New York, pp. 41–75.

Ingelstam E, Ragnarsson SI (1972) Eye refraction examined by the aid of speckle pattern produced by coherent light. Vis Res 12:411–420.

Jöbsis F (1977) Noninvasive, infrared monitoring of cerebral and myocardial oxygen sufficiency and circulatory parameters. Science 198:1264–1267.

Jöbsis F (1979) Oxidative metabolic effects of cerebral hypoxia, In: Fahn S et al. (eds) Advances in Neurology, vol. 26. Raven Press, New York, pp. 299–318.

Kak AC (1979) Computerized tonography with x-ray, emission and ultrasound sources. Proceedings of Institute of Electron and Electrical Engineers. 67:1245–1272.

Knoll H (1966) Measuring ametropria with a gas laser. A preliminary report. Amer J Optom and Arch Amer Acad Optom 43:415–418.

Krasnov MM (1973) Laseropuncture of anterior chamber angle in glaucoma. Amer J Ophthalmol 75:674–678.

LeGrand Y (1935) Sur la mesure de l'acuité visuelle au moyen de franges d'interférence. C R Acad Sci (Paris) 200:490.

L'Esperance FA Jr (1968) An ophthalmic argon laser photocoagulation system: Design, construction, and laboratory investigations. Trans Amer Ophthalmol Soc 66:827–994.

Lotmar W (1980a) Apparatus for the measurement of retinal visual acuity by Moiré fringes. Invest Ophthalmol Vis Sci 19:393–400.

Lotmar W (1980b) Rapid detection of changes in the optic disc. Stereochronoscopy. Int Ophthalmol 2:169–174.

Madeiros JA, Borwein B, McGowan JW (1979) Application of optical transform techniques to laser irradiation of the eye. Invest Ophthalmol Vis Sci 18:602–613.

Matsumato T, Nagata R, Salshin M, Matsuda T, Nakao S (1978) Measurements by holographic interferometry of the deformation of the eye accompanying changes in intraocular pressure. Appl Opt 17:3538–3539.

Ohzu H (1976) Application of laser in ophthalmology and vision research. Mem Waseda Univ Sch Sci Eng 40:1–28.

Patz A, Bram S, Finkelstein D, Chen E, Lutty G, Bennett A, Coughlin W, Bardner J (1978) A new approach to the problem of retinal neovascularization. Trans Amer Acad Ophthalmol Otolaryngol 85:626–637.

Ronchi L, Serra A, Meucci C (1978) Intraradian changes in accommodative astigmatism recorded by a modified version of Badal's optometer. Proc Int Symp Ophthalmol Opt (Tokyo) 15–18.

Rosencwaig A (1975) Photoacoustic spectroscopy of solids. Physics Today 22–30.

Sinclair DC (1965) Demonstration of chromatic aberration in the eye using coherent light. J Opt Soc Amer 55:575.

Ukrai K, Ohzu H (1976) Measurement of accommodation by observing speckles. Optica Act 1:66.

Van der Zypen E, Bebie H, Fankhauser F (1979) Morphological studies about the efficiency of laser beams upon the structures of the angle of the anterior chamber: Facts and concepts related to the treatment of the chronic simple glaucoma. Int Ophthalmol 1:109–122.

Van Ligten RF, Lawton K, Grolman B (1966) The hologram and its ophthalmic potential. Amer J Opt 43:351.

Vaughn K, Laing R, Wiggins R (1974) Holography of the eye: A critical review. In: Wolbarsht ML (ed) Laser Applications in Medicine and Biology, vol. 2. Plenum Press, New York, pp. 77–132.

Wang TT, McDavid JM, Lee SS (1979) Photoacoustic detection of localized absorption regions. Appl Opt 18:2354–2355.

Wickham MG, Worthem DM, Binder P (1977) Physiological effects of laser trabeculotomy in rhesus monkey eyes. Invest Ophthal 16:624–628.

Wise GN (1956) Retinal neovascularization. Trans Amer Ophthalmol Soc 54:729–826.

Wolbarsht ML (1980) Ophthalmic uses of lasers. In: Hillenkamp F, Sacchi C, and Pretesi R (eds) Lasers in Medicine and Biology, A NATO Advanced Study Institute. Plenum Press, New York, pp. 401–420.

Wolbarsht ML, Landers MB III (1979) Lasers in opthalmology: The path from theory to application. Appl Opt 18:1518–1526.

Wolbarsht ML, Bessler M, Hickingbotham D (1978) A manual or automatic method for focusing a fundus camera independent of image quality. Proc Int Symp Ophthalmol Opt (Tokyo) 111–113.

# 13

# Laser Doppler Velocimetry in the Measurement of Retinal Blood Flow

*Charles E. Riva*
*Gilbert T. Feke*

Alterations of blood flow in the retinal vascular system, whether associated with specific ocular diseases such as retinal-vessel occlusion, or whether resulting from systemic diseases such as diabetes or systemic hypertension, may lead to serious impairment of visual function and, often, to blindness. To increase the chances for successful treatment, it is important that such alterations in blood flow be detected as early as possible in the course of a disease.

Laser Doppler velocimetry (LDV) is the only known noninvasive technique that can provide quantitative measurements of retinal blood flow. In its current stage of development, the technique can be used to obtain absolute and continuous measurements of the maximum speed of red blood cells (RBCs) in individual retinal vessels of human subjects with clear ocular media and adequate target fixation. The technique thus stands at the threshold of clinical applicability where no other means exists for routine measurement of retinal blood flow.

A generalized block diagram of a retinal laser Doppler velocimeter (RLDV) is shown in Figure 13.1. An observer directs the attenuated beam from a helium-neon (HeNe) laser onto a chosen measurement site along a retinal vessel by means of input optics. The beam divergence at the cornea is adjusted to illuminate the entire cross section of the vessel. The major retinal vessels typically range from 80 to 200 $\mu$m in diameter. A portion of the Doppler-shifted scattered light that emerges from the eye is directed onto the cathode of a photomultiplier tube (PMT) by means of collecting optics. The resulting photocurrent, which contains the

This work was performed at the Eye Research Institute of Retina Foundation, Boston, Massachusetts, and was supported by PHS Grant 2 RO1 EYO-1303 from the National Eye Institute Research Career Development Award EY-00120 (C. E. Riva), by Research to Prevent Blindness, Inc., and by the Adler Foundation, Inc. The authors thank D. G. Goger who provided technical assistance during the experiments and in the preparation of the figures.

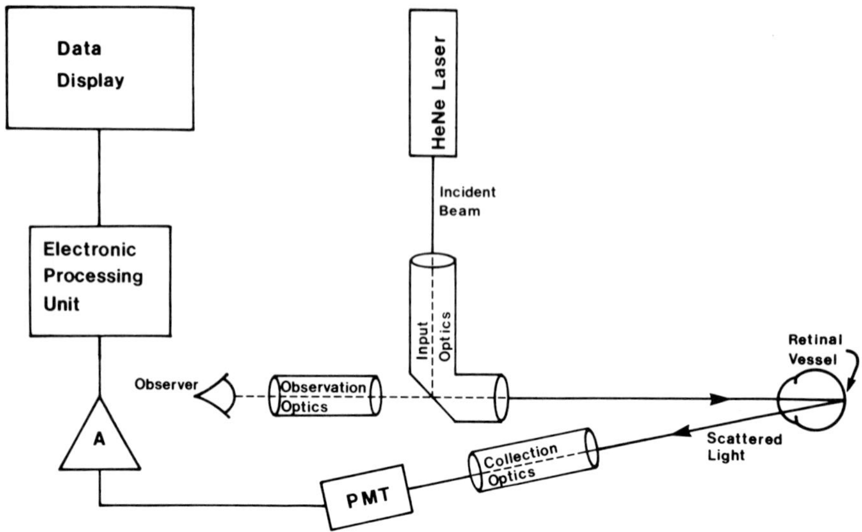


**Fig. 13.1.** Generalized block diagram of retinal laser Doppler velocimeter.

desired information on RBC speed, is processed by means of a spectrum analyzer, an autocorrelator, or a frequency-to-voltage converter. The output of the processing unit is displayed in a form adequate for determining the RBC speed.

In the ensuing sections of this chapter, we examine in detail the principle of operation of an RLDV. The limitations and constraints inherent to the technique as well as the limitations arising from this particular application of the LDV technique will emerge from our presentation. We then discuss some of our experimental methods which point the way to clinical applicability.

## PRINCIPLES OF RETINAL LASER DOPPLER VELOCIMETRY

### The Characteristics of the Scattered Electric Field Incident to the Photodetector Surface

We begin our discussion with an examination of the illuminated volume from which the scattered light is collected. In a simple model (Fig. 13.2), the incident laser light, $\vec{E}_o \cos \omega_o t$, illuminates the entire cross section of a retinal vessel. The scattered light, $\vec{E}_s(\vec{r},t)$, at a distance $(\vec{r})$ from the illuminated scattering volume, consists of light scattered by the flowing RBCs as well as light scattered by the vessel wall. In general, the light scattered at a particular angle by a collection of RBCs all flowing with a velocity $\vec{V}_n$ is Doppler-shifted in frequency by an amount:

$$\Delta f_n = \frac{1}{2\pi} (\vec{K}_n - \vec{K}_o) \cdot \vec{V}_n \tag{1}$$

where $\vec{K}_o$ and $\vec{K}_n$ are, respectively, the wave vectors of the incident light and of the light scattered by the RBCs flowing with velocity $\vec{v}_n$.

$$|\vec{K}_n| \approx |\vec{K}_o| = \frac{2\pi n}{\lambda}$$

where n is the refractive index of the medium and λ is the wavelength *in vacuo* of the incident laser light. λ = 632.8 nm for the HeNe laser.

A range of RBC velocities is present in a retinal vessel, however, so that the scattered light contains a corresponding range of Doppler-shifted frequencies. Since RBCs at typical blood concentrations are known to exhibit Poiseuille flow in glass tubes with diameters larger than 100 μm (Goldsmith, 1968), it is reasonable to assume that Poiseuille flow also exists in the large retinal vessels. In this case, the range of RBC velocities is described by a parabolic profile as a function of the radial distance, R, from the axis of the vessel of radius $R_o$:

$$V(R) = V_{max}\left[1 - \left(\frac{R}{R_o}\right)^2\right] \tag{2}$$

As indicated in Figure 13.2B, the RBCs giving rise to a particular Doppler shift, $\Delta f_n$, are all located in a cylindrical shell characterized by a particular velocity $\vec{V}_n$. If we divide the range of velocities into $n_{max}$ equal increments, ΔV, then RBCs with

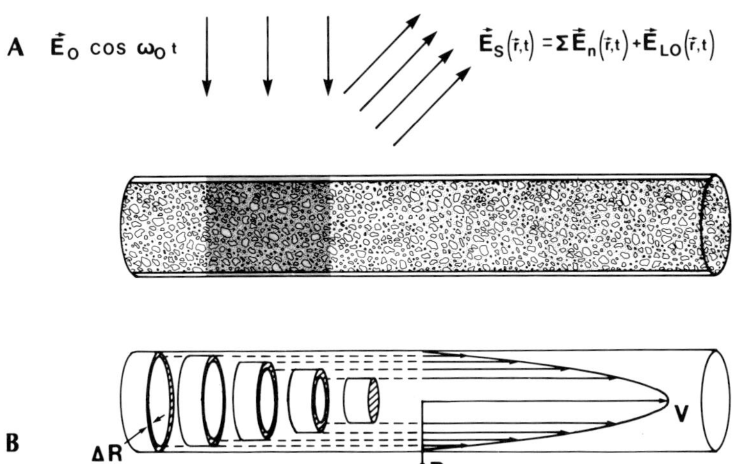


**Fig. 13.2. A.** Schematic representation of illuminated volume of retinal vessel from which scattered light is collected. $E_o$ → cos $\omega_o t$, incident laser light; $E_s$ →(↔), light scattered by flowing red cells and by vessel wall. *Shading* indicates light. **B.** Indication of parabolic velocity profile V(R), and corresponding division of illuminated volume into concentric cylindrical shells, each containing equal numbers of RBCs flowing at each velocity increment.

speeds between V and V + $\Delta V$ are located in a shell of radial thickness $\Delta R$, where from Eq. (2), $\Delta R = R_o^2 \Delta V/2RV_{max}$. As has been shown by Riva et al. (1972), this implies that there are equal numbers of RBCs flowing at each velocity increment.

The scattered light may thus be written as

$$\vec{E}_s(\vec{r},t) = \sum_{n=0}^{max} \vec{E}_n(\vec{r},t) + \vec{E}_{LO}(\vec{r},t) \tag{3}$$

where each $\vec{E}_n$ oscillates at a frequency $2\pi(f_o + \Delta f_n)$. $\vec{E}_{LO}$ is the light scattered from the vessel wall, the outermost cylindrical shell. This unshifted light oscillates at the incident laser frequency $2\pi f_o$, and thus acts as a local oscillator.

If each cylindrical shell were uniformly illuminated, and if only singly scattered light emerged from the illuminated volume, then each $\vec{E}_n(\vec{r},t)$ would possess the same amplitude. This would be the case for a dilute suspension of non-light-absorbing particles. This is not the case, however, for blood in which multiple scattering has a pronounced effect on the characteristics of the scattered light. These phenomena will be discussed later in this chapter. For the moment, we will return to our model and assume that each $\vec{E}_n(\vec{r},t)$ does have the same amplitude:

$$\vec{E}_n(\vec{r},t) = \vec{A}(\vec{r}) \cos 2\pi(f_o + \Delta f_n)t \tag{4}$$

For $\vec{E}_{LO}(\vec{r},t)$, we write accordingly

$$\vec{E}_{LO}(\vec{r},t) = \vec{A}_{LO}(\vec{r}) \cos 2\pi f_o t \tag{5}$$

Therefore the optical field scattered at a particular angle from the illuminated volume is

$$\vec{E}_s(\vec{r},t) = \vec{A}_{LO}(\vec{r}) \cos 2\pi f_o t + \vec{A}(\vec{r}) \sum_{n=0}^{max} \cos 2\pi(f_o + \Delta f_n)t \tag{6}$$

The spectral density of the scattered light, $S_E(f)$, obtained by applying Fourier analysis is:

$$S_E(f) = \frac{A_{LO}^2}{2} \delta(f - f_o) + \frac{A_{LO}A}{2} \tag{7}$$
$$\text{for } f_o \leq f \leq f_o + \Delta f_{max}$$

where $\delta(f - f_o)$ is the delta function at the incident laser frequency. Thus, for our model, the optical spectral density function consists of a delta function at $f_o$, followed by a flat portion of magnitude $A_{LO}$ $A/2$ from $f_o$ to $f_o + \Delta f_{max}$. It is zero beyond $f_o + \Delta f_{max}$; $\Delta f_{max}$ is the frequency shift corresponding to the maximum RBC velocity, $V_{max}$. A measurement of the optical spectral density would thus be sufficient for determining the RBC speed. However, since $f_o$ is approximately 5

$\times 10^{14}$ Hz, and a typical $\Delta f_n$ is of the order of several kilohertz, the required resolution, ($\Delta f / f_o \approx 10^{-11}$), if far beyond the capability of conventional spectroscopic techniques. However, by detecting the scattered field with a PMT, the information contained in the optical spectral density function can be translated down to sufficiently low frequencies, where adequate resolution can be obtained. The technique by which such a translation is achieved is known as optical mixing spectroscopy.

## The Characteristics of the Heterodyne-detected Resultant Photocurrent

**The Stochastic Nature of the Photocurrent.** The scattered field $\vec{E}_s(\vec{r},t)$ given by Eq. (6) is directed onto the photocathode of a detector. The current density $j(\vec{r},t)$ produced by the electric field acting at a point $\vec{r}$ on the photocathode is proportional to the instantaneous intensity evaluated at $(\vec{r},t)$. The proportionality constant includes a quantum efficiency that is the ratio of the number of emitted photoelectrons to the number of incident photons. In general, one may write:

$$j(\vec{r},t) = \beta |\vec{E}_s(\vec{r},t)|^2 \tag{8}$$

Although Eq. (8) predicts a well-defined continuous current density, in reality the PMT current consists of pulses corresponding to the emission of single photoelectrons from the photocathode. Since the emission process is random, $j(\vec{r},t)$ is a fluctuating quantity whose appropriate description is a statistical one.

In the application of the general formalism of Lastovka (1967) to our model, calculation of $j(\vec{r},t)$ requires specification of the probability that $j(\vec{r},t)$ has a given value when the photocathode is illuminated by the field $\vec{E}_s(\vec{r},t)$. Designating this probability as $P[j(\vec{r},t)]$, one can define an ensemble average[1] of $j(\vec{r},t)$:

$$< j\,(\vec{r},t) > = \int j(\vec{r},t) P[j(\vec{r},t)] d[j(\vec{r},\, t)] \tag{9}$$

It can be shown that

$$< j(\vec{r},t)> = \beta |\vec{E}_s(\vec{r},t)|^2 \tag{10}$$

so that the information on RBC speeds, contained in the frequency content of $\vec{E}_s(\vec{r},t)$, is also present in $< j\,(\vec{r},t) >$. The photocurrent measured, however, is the total current $< i(t) >$, and is given by the integral of the current density over the illuminated photocathode area, S:

$$< i(t) > = \int_S < j(\vec{r},t) > dS = \beta \int_S |\vec{E}_s(\vec{r},t)|^2 dS \tag{11}$$

[1]Since the statistical processes we are dealing with here are stationary random processes in the wide sense, the ensemble averages are equal to the time averages.

**The Power-Spectral Density of the Photocurrent.** The most convenient way to determine the frequency content of $< i(t) >$ is first to compute its autocorrelation function $R_i(\tau)$:

$$R_i(\tau) = \ll i(t + \tau)i(t) \gg \tag{12}$$

The power-spectral density of the photocurrent is then determined by evaluating the Fourier cosine transform of $R_i(\tau)$ (Reif, 1965):

$$S_i(\omega) = \frac{1}{2\pi} \int_{-\infty}^{\infty} R_i(\tau) \cos \omega\tau d\tau \tag{13}$$

From Eqs. (11) and (12),

$$R_i(\tau) = \int_S \int_{S'} \ll j(\vec{r}_2,t_2)j(\vec{r}_1,t_1) \gg dS_1dS_2 \tag{14}$$

To evaluate $R_i(\tau)$, it is necessary to consider the joint probability distribution which specifies the probability that *n* photoelectrons are emitted at time $t_2$ in the time interval $\Delta t_2$ per unit area at $\vec{r}_2$ and that *m* photoelectrons are emitted at time $t_1$ in the interval $\Delta t_1$ per unit area at $r_1$.

It can be shown that

$$< j(\vec{r}_2,t_2)j(\vec{r}_1,t_1) > = \begin{cases} \beta^2|\vec{E}_s(\vec{r}_2,t_2)|^2|\vec{E}_s(\vec{r}_1,t_1)|^2; & t_2 \neq t_1 \text{ or } \vec{r}_2 \neq \vec{r}_1 \\ \beta e|\vec{E}_s(\vec{r}_1,t_1)|^2; & t_2 = t_1,\ \vec{r}_2 = \vec{r}_1 \end{cases} \tag{15}$$

where e is the charge of an electron.

Letting $t_1 = t$, $t_2 = t + \tau$, $\vec{r}_1 = \vec{r}$ and $\vec{r}_2 = \vec{r} + \vec{\rho}$; and using Eq. (11) for $< i(t) >$ gives

$$R_i(\tau) = \beta^2 \int_S \int_{S'} < |\vec{E}_s(\vec{r} + \vec{\rho}, t + \tau)|^2|\vec{E}_s(\vec{r},t)|^2 > d^2\vec{r}d^2\vec{\rho} + e \ll i(t) \gg \delta(\tau) \tag{16}$$

The last term is the so-called shot-noise term and arises from the discrete nature of the emission process. In this expression, $\ll i(t) \gg$ is the total dc photocurrent which is produced by $\vec{E}_s(\vec{r},t)$. From Eq. (6):

$$\ll i(t) \gg = \beta S\,[\tfrac{1}{2}|\vec{A}_{LO}(\vec{r})|^2 + \tfrac{1}{2}|\vec{A}(\vec{r})|^2] \tag{17}$$

Again, using Eq. (6):

$$|\vec{E}_s(\vec{r},t)|^2 = |\vec{A}_{LO}(\vec{r})|^2 \cos^2 \omega_o t + 2\,[\vec{A}_{LO}(\vec{r}) \cdot \vec{A}(\vec{r})] \cos \omega_o t \sum_{n=0}^{max} \cos (\omega_o + \Delta\omega_n)t + |\vec{A}(\vec{r})|^2 \sum_{n=0}^{max} \sum_{j=0}^{max} \cos^2 (\omega_o + \Delta\omega_{nj})t \qquad (18)$$

A similar expression is obtained for $|\vec{E}_s(\vec{r} + \vec{\rho}, t + \tau|^2$.

Let us assume now that $\vec{A}_{LO}(\vec{r}) \gg \vec{A}(\vec{r})$; i.e., the amplitude of the light scattered by the vessel wall, $\vec{E}_{LO}(\vec{r},t)$, is much larger than any of the amplitudes of the waves of $\vec{E}_n(\vec{r},t)$. Such a condition defines the so-called heterodyne mixing process. With this assumption, it follows from Eqs. (16)–(18) that

$$R_i(\tau) = \frac{\beta^2 S^2}{4}[|\vec{A}_{LO}(\vec{r})|^2 + |\vec{A}(\vec{r})|^2]^2 + \frac{e\beta S}{2}[|\vec{A}_{LO}(\vec{r})|^2 + |\vec{A}(\vec{r})|^2]\delta(\tau) + 4\beta^2 \int_S \int_{S'} \langle[\vec{A}_{LO}(\vec{r} + \vec{\rho}) \cdot \vec{A}(\vec{r} + \vec{\rho})]\,[\vec{A}_{LO}(\vec{r}) \cdot \vec{A}(\vec{r})]\rangle d^2\vec{r}\, d^2\vec{\rho} \times \cos \omega_o\tau \sum_{n=0}^{max} \cos (\omega_o + \Delta\omega_n)\tau \qquad (19)$$

We can rewrite our expression for $R_i(\tau)$ by defining a spatial correlation function for the local oscillator portion of the scattered light as

$$T_{LO}(\vec{r},\vec{\rho}) = \frac{1}{|\vec{A}_{LO}(\vec{r})|^2} \vec{A}_{LO}(\vec{r} + \vec{\rho}) \cdot \vec{A}_{LO}(\vec{r}) \qquad (20)$$

and a spatial correlation function for the Doppler-shifted portion of the scattered light as

$$T(\vec{r},\vec{\rho}) = \frac{1}{|\vec{A}(\vec{r})|^2} \vec{A}(\vec{r} + \vec{\rho}) \cdot \vec{A}(\vec{r}) \qquad (21)$$

These functions describe the amplitude and phase behavior of the local oscillator and Doppler-shifted scattered fields as a function of position $\vec{\rho}$ on the detector relative to a fixed reference point $\vec{r}$. Eq. (19) thus becomes:

$$R_i(\tau) = \frac{\beta^2 S^2}{4}[|\vec{A}_{LO}(\vec{r})|^2 + |\vec{A}(\vec{r})|^2]^2 + \frac{e\beta S}{2}[|\vec{A}_{LO}(\vec{r})|^2 + |\vec{A}(\vec{r})|^2]\delta(\tau) + 4\beta^2 |\vec{A}_{LO}(\vec{r})|^2 |\vec{A}(\vec{r})|^2 \cos \omega_o\tau \sum_{n=0}^{max} \cos (\omega_o + \Delta\omega_n)\tau \cdot \int_S \int_{S'} T_{LO}(\vec{r},\vec{\rho}) T(\vec{r},\vec{\rho})\, d^2\vec{r}\, d^2\vec{\rho} \qquad (22)$$

Eq. (22) illustrates clearly that the optical heterodyne mixing process involves both the *spectral* and *spatial* characteristics of the local oscillator and the Doppler-shifted scattered light.

The expression can be further simplified if we note that the double surface integral in Eq. (22) has a maximum value of $S^2$. We can then define a dimensionless spatial factor [B] as

$$[B] = \frac{1}{S^2} \int_S \int_{S'} T_{LO}(\vec{r},\vec{\rho}) T(\vec{r},\vec{\rho}) d^2\vec{r} d^2\vec{\rho} \tag{23}$$

If we assume that the intensities of both the local oscillator scattered light and the Doppler-shifted scattered light are uniform over the illuminated photocathode area S, then $T_{LO}(\vec{r},\vec{\rho})$ and $T(\vec{r},\vec{\rho})$ are both independent of $\vec{r}$, so that

$$[B] = \frac{1}{S} \int_S T_{LO}(\vec{r}_o,\vec{\rho}) T(\vec{r}_o,\vec{\rho}) d^2\vec{\rho} \tag{24}$$

where $\vec{r}_o$ is a fixed reference point on S.

To evaluate the integral in Eq. (24), we must return to our model illustrated in Figure 13.2B. The electric field, $\vec{E}_n(\vec{r},t)$, scattered from each of the cylindrical shells, is spatially coherent on only a portion of S. We may refer to this area as $S_{COH_n}$. In general, the size of a coherence area on the detector surface is inversely proportional to the spatial extent of the source, so that the largest $S_{COH_n}$ is associated with the cylinder containing the RBCs moving at $V_{max}$ at the center of the retinal vessel. The smallest $S_{COH_n}$ is associated with the cylindrical shell containing the slowest moving RBCs at the periphery of the vessel. The coherence area associated with the local oscillator field, $S_{COH_{LO}}$, is even smaller since it arises from the vessel wall. As a result, $T_{LO}(\vec{r}_o,\vec{\rho})$ decreases toward zero faster than $T(\vec{r}_o,\vec{\rho})$. In first approximation, $T(\vec{r}_o,\vec{\rho})$ equals unity in the region where $T_{LO}(\vec{r}_o,\vec{\rho})$ is different from zero. If S is larger than $S_{COH_{LO}}$, then

$$[B] = \frac{1}{S} \int_S T_{LO}(\vec{r}_o,\vec{\rho}) d^2\vec{\rho} = \frac{S_{COH_{LO}}}{S} \tag{25}$$

where

$$S_{COH_{LO}} = \int_{\text{all } \rho} T_{LO}(\vec{r}_o,\vec{\rho}) d^2\vec{\rho} \tag{26}$$

We see that when the local oscillator arises from the vessel wall, [B] is independent of $S_{COH_n}$. For a given detector area, it depends only upon the size of the coherence area of the local oscillator.

Having examined the spatial effect of the optical mixing process, we can now rewrite our expression for $R_i(\tau)$ in Eq. (22) as:

$$R_i(\tau) = \frac{\beta^2 S^2}{4}[|\vec{A}_{LO}|^2 + |\vec{A}|^2]^2 + \frac{e\beta S}{2}[|\vec{A}_{LO}|^2 + |\vec{A}|^2]\delta(\tau) + 4\beta^2 S^2 \left[\frac{S_{COH_{LO}}}{S}\right] |\vec{A}_{LO}|^2 |\vec{A}|^2 \cos\omega_o\tau \sum_{n=0}^{max} \cos(\omega_o + \Delta\omega_n)\tau \quad (27)$$

The effect of the optical heterodyning mixing process becomes apparent when expressed as

$$\cos\omega_o\tau\cos(\omega_o + \Delta\omega_n)\tau = \tfrac{1}{2}\cos\Delta\omega_n\tau + \tfrac{1}{2}\cos(2\omega_o + \Delta\omega_n)\tau \quad (28)$$

The second term involves optical frequencies that are beyond the response range of the photodetector, so that our final effective expression for $R_i(\tau)$ is

$$R_i(\tau) = \frac{\beta^2 S^2}{4}[A_{LO}^2 + A^2]^2 + \frac{e\beta S}{2}[A_{LO}^2 + A^2]\delta(\tau) + 2\beta^2 S S_{COH_{LO}} A_{LO}^2 A^2 \sum_{n=0}^{max} \cos\Delta\omega_n\tau \quad (29)$$

The Fourier transform of $R_i(\tau)$ is straightforward and gives, for the power-spectral density of the photocurrent, the following:

$$S_i(\Delta f) = \frac{\beta^2 S^2}{4}[A_{LO}^2 + A^2]^2\delta(\Delta f) + \frac{e\beta S}{2}[A_{LO}^2 + A^2] + \beta^2 S S_{COH_{LO}} A_{LO}^2 A^2 \quad (30)$$

in the range $0 \le \Delta f \le \Delta f_{max}$.

Beyond $\Delta f_{max}$

$$S_i(\Delta f) = \frac{e\beta S}{2}[A_{LO}^2 + A^2] \approx \frac{e\beta S}{2} A_{LO}^2 \quad (31)$$

which is the power-spectral density corresponding to the shot-noise term.

As is illustrated in Figure 13.3, $S_i(\Delta f)$ is an exact replica of $S_E(f)$ as given in Eq. (7), so that the RBC speed may be determined from a measurement of $S_i(\Delta f)$. Since

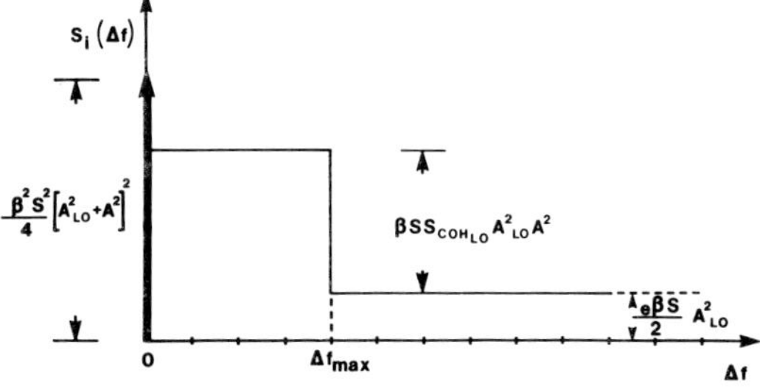


**Fig. 13.3.** Theoretically predicted photocurrent power-spectral density [Eqs. (30) and (31)] explicitly showing dc component at $\Delta f = 0$, signal component extending to $\Delta f_{max}$, and shot-noise component.

the spectrum has been shifted from optical frequencies down to the kilohertz range, the spectral analysis can be done with high resolution.

**The Intrinsic Signal–to–Shot-Noise Ratio.** In practice, the ability to measure $S_i(\Delta f)$ with high resolution requires that the power-spectral density of the signal term be larger than the power-spectral density of the shot-noise term. There is an intrinsic signal–to–shot-noise ratio (SNR), as follows:

$$SNR = \frac{2\beta S S_{COH_{LO}} A_{LO}^2 A^2}{eSA_{LO}^2} \quad (32)$$

The SNR exhibits several interesting features. Since both the signal and shot-noise terms increase linearly with $A_{LO}^2$, the SNR is independent of the intensity of the local oscillator contribution to the scattered light. Similarly, since both the signal and shot-noise terms increase linearly with increased illuminated detector area $S$, SNR remains constant for $S \geq S_{COH_{LO}}$, so that no gain in SNR is obtained by increasing the illuminated area beyond $S_{COH_{LO}}$. Therefore, for a fixed vessel diameter, SNR can be increased only by increasing the intensity of the Doppler-shifted contribution to the scattered light. In practice, this is accomplished by increasing the intensity of the incident light.

## Processing the Photocurrent

The most direct way of obtaining the power-spectral density of the photocurrent is with a spectrum analyzer. This device consists basically of a tuned filter whose center frequency can be continuously shifted. The narrow band filter is followed by a squarer and an integrator so that the output is the time-averaged power associated with the portion of the photocurrent passing through the filter. Recently developed real-time spectrum analyzers and fast Fourier transform (FFT) digital analyzers can simultaneously sample a large number of frequency intervals and provide a complete spectrum in a time approximately equal to the reciprocal of the resolution bandwidth.

The photocurrent can also be processed with a digital autocorrelator which directly computes the function $R_i(\tau)$ (Eq. 29). It was this technique that was first used by Tanaka et al. (1974) to estimate the RBC speed in human retinal vessels.

A third means of processing the photocurrent is by means of an electronic tracking system, which provides a continuous voltage signal that is proportional to the instantaneous maximum RBC speed. This technique is described later in this chapter.

**Illustrative Spectrum from Flowing Spheres.** In a suspension of polystyrene spheres in distilled water flowing through a glass capillary tube of 200-$\mu$m internal diameter, the known maximum speed was 1.44 cm/s. The tube was horizontal, the incident beam was perpendicular to the flow, and the back-scattered light was collected at an angle of 15° with respect to the incident beam. The measurement

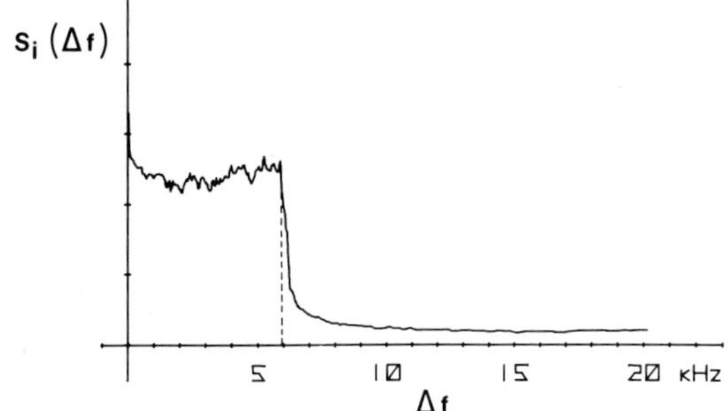


**Fig. 13.4.** Spectrum obtained from 0.1% suspension of 0.312-μm-diameter polystyrene spheres in distilled water flowing through glass capillary tube of 200 μm internal diameter. *Dashed line*, expected $\Delta f_{max}$.

time, using a real-time spectrum analyzer, was 51.2 s. The spectrum (Fig. 13.4) is essentially flat up to about 5.9 kHz and then abruptly falls to the shot-noise level. The expected $\Delta f_{max}$ calculated from Eq. (1) is 5.9 kHz so that the agreement is excellent. Furthermore, the spectrum closely resembles the idealized spectrum of Figure 13.3, a finding that suggests all the assumptions implicit in the derivation of $S_i(\Delta f)$ [Eqs. (30) and (31)] are valid for the case of a dilute suspension of non-light-absorbing particles.

**The Output Signal-to-Noise Ratio.** The experimentally determined $S_i(\Delta f)$ is the time-averaged power associated with the photocurrent. We have seen, however, that the photocurrent is a fluctuating quantity, so there is an uncertainty in the measurement of $S_i(\Delta f)$ when the measurement is performed in a finite time. This phenomenon is illustrated by four spectra obtained using different measurement times from a 0.1% suspension of 1.009-μm-diameter polystyrene spheres flowing at a maximum speed of 3.61 cm/s through a 200-μm-internal-diameter glass capillary tube (Fig. 13.5). As expected, the precision with which $S_i(\Delta f)$ can be determined increases as the measurement time increases. A meaningful index of this precision is the output signal-to-noise ratio (SNR), defined as the ratio of signal power, $I_s$, to the root mean square fluctuation in signal power plus shot-noise power, $I_{sn}$:

$$(SNR)_{out} = \frac{I_s}{\sigma[I_s + I_{sn}]} \tag{33}$$

It can be shown in general (Cummins and Swinney, 1970) that

$$(SNR)_{out} = \frac{I_s}{I_s + I_{sn}} (1 + \Delta\nu T)^{1/2} \tag{34}$$

where $\Delta\nu$ is the resolution bandwidth of the spectrum analyzer and T is the measurement time. Thus, if $\Delta\nu T \gg 1$, $(SNR)_{out}$ is proportional to the square root of the measurement time. The spectra plotted in Figure 13.5 have been normalized so that the mean of $S_i(\Delta f)$ is constant for each spectrum. The measure $\Delta\nu$ = 20 Hz

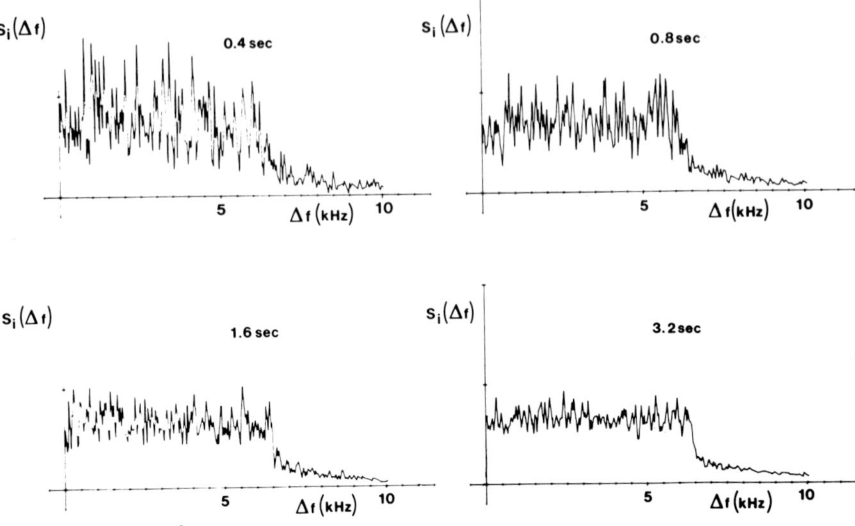


**Fig. 13.5.** Spectra obtained in measurement times of 0.4, 0.8, 1.6, and 3.2 s from 0.1% suspension of polystyrene spheres in distilled water flowing through glass capillary tube. Precision may be observed to increase with increase in measurement time.

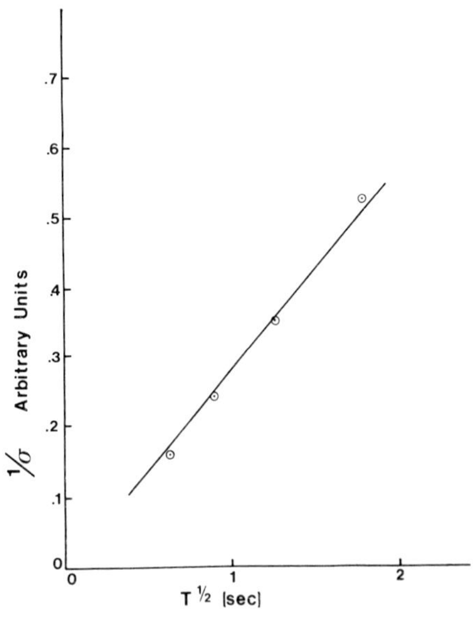


**Fig. 13.6.** Reciprocal of root mean squares of fluctuations in spectra of Figure 13.5, plotted as function of square root of measurement time.

is also constant for each spectrum. In this case, Eqs. (33) and (34) predict that $1/\sigma[S_i(\Delta f)]$ is proportional to $T^{1/2}$. When computed in the range $0 \leq \Delta f \leq \Delta f_{max}$ for each of the spectra shown, $1/\sigma[S_i(\Delta f)]$ was indeed observed to follow a $T^{1/2}$ dependence (Fig. 13.6).

# EXPERIMENTAL METHODS, RESULTS, AND INTERPRETATION

## Spectra Obtained in vitro from Flowing Red Blood Cells

Four spectra were obtained using different measurement times from whole blood (hematocrit, 41%) flowing at a maximum speed of 1.44 cm/s through a glass capillary tube with a 200-$\mu$m internal diameter (Fig. 13.7). The speed and the scattering geometry were the same as those used to obtain the spectrum shown in Figure 13.4, so that the expected $\Delta f_{max}$ is 5.9 kHz. Clearly, the spectrum obtained in 51.2 s does not exhibit the ideal characteristics of a spectrum from a dilute suspension of spheres. There is no discernible cutoff at 5.9 kHz. Also, there is a monotonic decrease in the amplitude, suggesting nonuniform illumination of the various cylindrical shells indicated in the idealized model (Fig. 13.2). The spectral power beyond 5.9 kHz is most likely the result of multiple scattering of the laser light as it penetrates into and exits from the flowing medium (Riva et al., 1972;

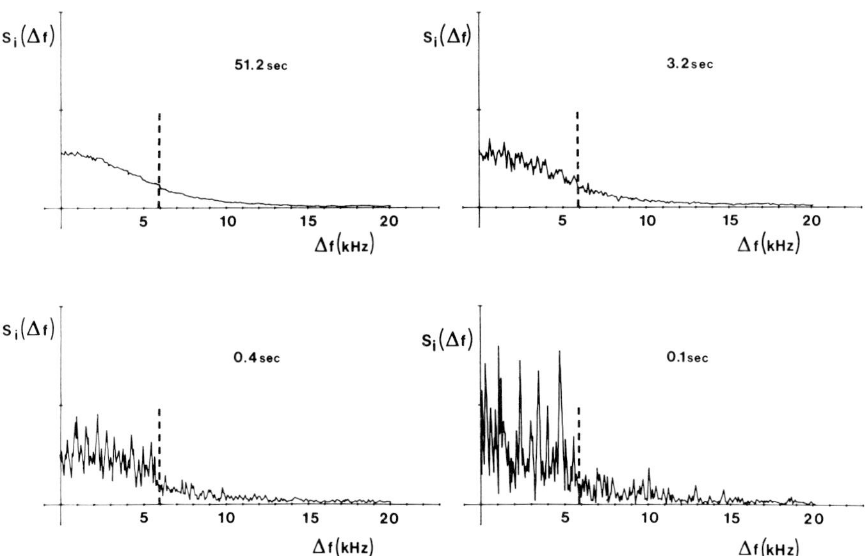


**Fig. 13.7.** Spectra obtained in measurement times of 51.2, 3.2, 0.4, and 0.1 s from whole blood flowing through glass capillary tube. *Dashed lines*, expected $\Delta f_{max}$.

Feke and Riva, 1978). The spectrum obtained in 3.2 s has essentially the same characteristics as the spectrum obtained in 51.2 s (Fig. 13.7). However, since the measurement time is much shorter, the statistical fluctuations in $S_i(\Delta f)$ are increased, as expected. A new characteristic is exhibited in the spectrum obtained in 0.4 s (Fig. 13.7), with a greater increase in the fluctuations in $S_i(\Delta f)$ in the region of the spectrum $\Delta f < \Delta f_{max}$ than in the region $\Delta f > \Delta f_{max}$. The result is that the cutoff at 5.9 kHz begins to become discernible. The spectrum obtained in 0.1 s shows a clear break in the magnitude of the fluctuations around 5.9 kHz (Fig. 13.7).

An explanation for this phenomenon can be hypothesized when one first considers that in the region of the spectrum $\Delta f < \Delta f_{max}$, the spectral power arises primarily from single scattering, whereas in the region $\Delta f > \Delta f_{max}$, the spectral power arises only from multiple scattering. One then assumes that in addition to the usual statistical fluctuations in $S_i(\Delta f)$, there are fluctuations introduced by fluctuations in the number of RBCs giving rise to a particular $\Delta f$. Considerably fewer RBCs are involved in single scattering than in multiple scattering; therefore, the fluctuations in the region $\Delta f < \Delta f_{max}$, which may be termed $\Delta f_s$, are much greater than in the region $\Delta f > \Delta f_{max}$, which we denote $\Delta f_m$. The functional dependence upon measurement time, *T*, of the fluctuations in $S_i(\Delta f)$, $\sigma_N^2[S_i(\Delta f, T)]$, arising from fluctuations in the number, *N*, of RBCs giving rise to a particular frequency shift, $\Delta f$, is considered explicitly in Appendix A. It is shown that the ratio

$$\frac{\sigma_N^2[S_i(\Delta f_s, T)]}{\sigma_N^2[S_i(\Delta f_m, T)]}$$

increases as the measurement time, *T*, decreases, which is the experimentally observed phenomenon. We see, therefore, that even though the spectra from flowing RBCs are not ideal, the cutoff frequency corresponding to the maximum RBC speed may be identified by using optimal measurement times.

## Spectra Obtained in vivo from Human Retinal Vessels

**The Experimental Arrangement.** Spectra have been obtained in vivo from human retinal vessels using the optical and electronic arrangement shown schematically in Figure 13.8. The optical fiber collects the scattered light (Riva and Ben-Sira, 1975). The linearly polarized beam emerging from a Spectra Physics 133 HeNe laser impinges on the subject's eye after being reflected by a small mirror mounted in front of the ophthalmoscopic lens of the camera. The beam is focused onto a retinal vessel. Prior to being aimed into the eye, the intensity of the beam is attenuated with a rotatable polarizer to a level well below the maximum permissible for continuous irradiance of 0.1 $W/cm^2$ (Sliney and Freasier, 1973). Eye movements are minimized by having the subject fixate a target with the eye that is under measurement. The target is the exit aperture (diameter 100 $\mu m$) of a fiber optic which is illuminated by a light source (LS). The retina is illuminated with green light for observation and centering of the incident beam on the vessel.

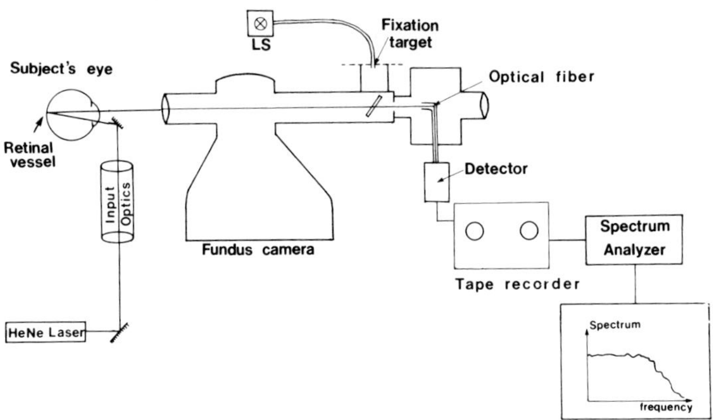


**Fig. 13.8.** Schema of optical and electronic arrangement used to measure spectra from human retinal vessels. Basic optical component is standard fundus camera modified with laser input optics, internal fixation target, and an optical fiber mounted in a scanning ocular.

The portion of the light scattered by the RBCs and accepted by the entrance pupil of the camera is collected by an optical fiber mounted in a scanning ocular. The entrance aperture of this fiber is located in an image plane conjugated to the retina. The collected light is transmitted to an RCA 8645 photomultiplier tube mounted adjacent to the ocular. The output photocurrent is recorded on magnetic tape with a Revox A77 stereo tape recorder. It is subsequently analyzed by means of a Federal Scientific UA 500 real-time spectrum analyzer, which provides the square root of $S_i(\Delta f)$ at its output. The output is squared by an analog module, and the resultant $S_i(\Delta f)$ is plotted on an X-Y recorder.

**Measurements from Retinal Vessels.** In a typical measurement obtained from a human subject (Fig. 13.9), the photocurrent arising from the light scattered from a site along a retinal vein was recorded. Spectra obtained from a portion of the tape, using analysis times of 0.1, 0.2, and 0.8 s, showed the effect of decreasing the measurement time. The fluctuations in $S_i(\Delta f)$ in the range of frequencies up to approximately 6.5 kHz increase dramatically as the analysis time is shortened. The characteristics of these spectra are similar to those of the in-vitro spectra shown in Figure 13.7. Thus there is good experimental evidence that $\Delta f_{max}$ corresponds to the frequency where there is a clear break in the magnitude of the fluctuations in $S_i(\Delta f)$.

Successive measurements were obtained from a retinal vein during an experiment where a subject first stopped breathing at time 0 for approximately 48 s and then resumed breathing (Fig. 13.10). The 0.8-s measurement time for each spectrum was longer than optimal so that the estimate of each $\Delta f_{max}$ involves some errors. Nevertheless, $\Delta f_{max}$ clearly increases after the subject has stopped breathing, an indication of increased RBC speed, and then decreases back to normal after the subject has resumed breathing.

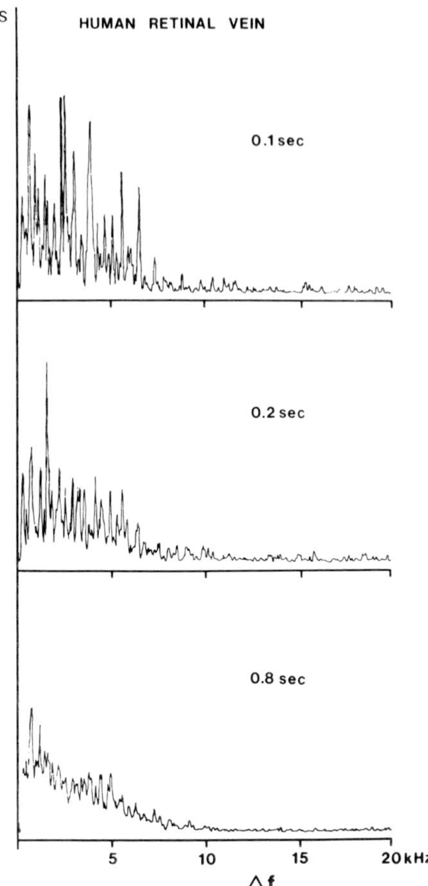


**Fig. 13.9.** Spectra obtained in measurement times of 0.1, 0.2, and 0.8 s from a human retinal vein, demonstrating effect of decreasing measurement time. (Feke GT et al., Blood velocity in human retinal vessels. Electro-Optical Systems Design 10:40–43, 1978.)

Spectra obtained in succession from retinal veins in subjects under normal physiologic conditions exhibit essentially the same cutoff frequency. However, spectra obtained from retinal arteries show that $\Delta f_{max}$, and therefore $V_{max}$, varies synchronously with the cardiac cycle.

## Absolute in-vivo Measurements of the Maximum Red Blood Cell Speed

An absolute measure of the maximum RBC speed could be determined directly from the spectra shown in Figures 13.9 and 13.10 if the intraocular angular orientation of the incident and scattered light beams, with respect to the flow direction in the retinal vessel, were known. This is difficult to achieve with the fundus camera-based optical arrangement illustrated in Figure 13.8. However, a bidirectional measurement technique, which utilizes a standard slitlamp microscope as its basic optical component, has recently been developed (Riva et al., 1979) and solves most of the problems of the intraocular scattering geometry.

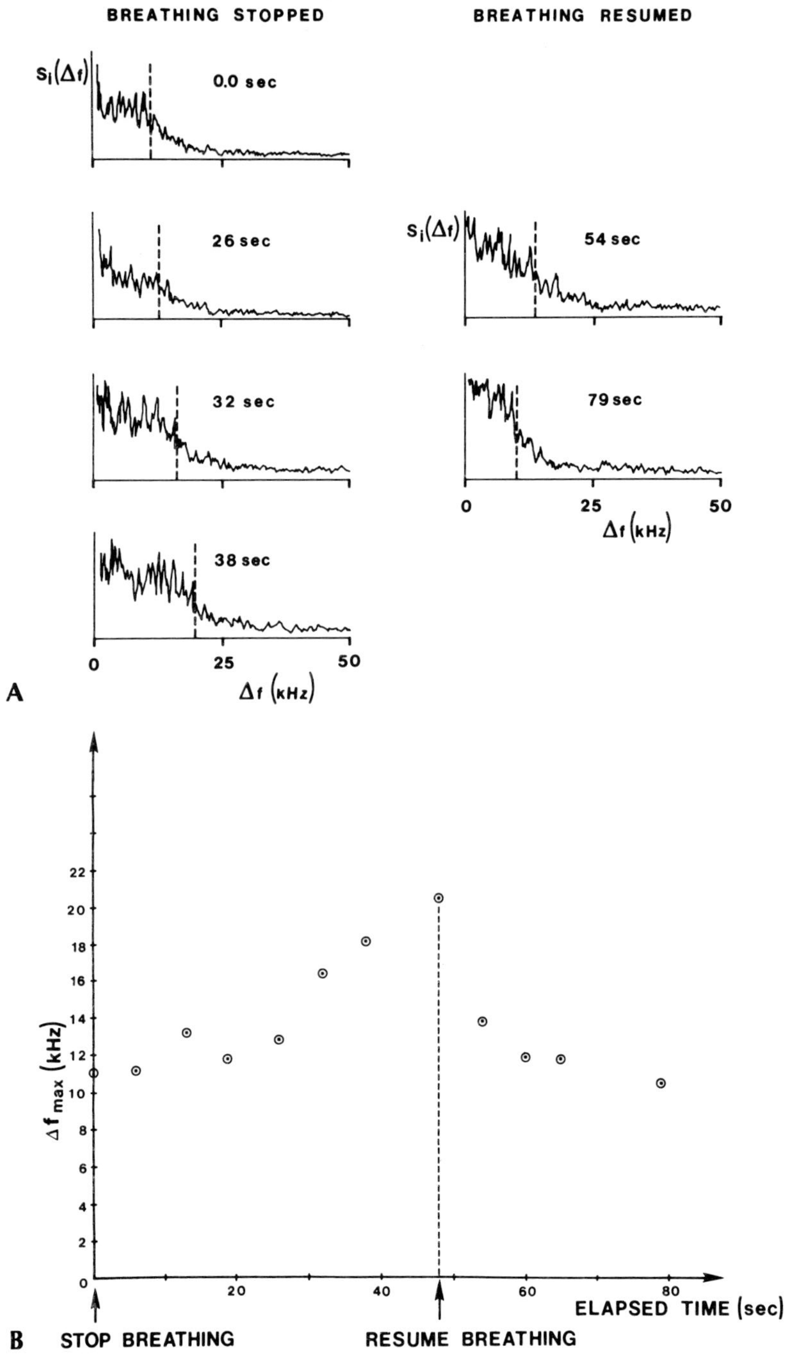

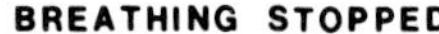


**Fig. 13.10. A.** Representative spectra obtained in measurement time of 0.8 s from human retinal vein in experiment in which subject stopped breathing at time 0.0 s and then resumed breathing 48 s later. Total elapsed times are indicated with each spectrum. *Dashed lines*, estimates of each $\Delta f_{max}$. **B.** Cutoff frequencies, $\Delta f_{max}$, plotted as function of elapsed time.

In this technique, a flat front-surface corneal contact lens, with a refractive index equal to that of the cornea, is used to simplify the scattering geometry. Spectra are obtained for two directions of the scattered light (both in the horizontal plane) while the incident beam direction remains fixed. The maximum RBC speed, $V_{max}$, can then be obtained from the following relation:

$$V_{max} = \frac{\lambda[\Delta f_{max_2} - \Delta f_{max_1}]}{\Delta\alpha' \cos\beta}(1 - Pl) \qquad (35)$$

where $\Delta\alpha'$ is the extraocular angle between the directions of the two scattered beams, $\beta$ is the angle between the direction of the vessel and the horizontal plane, P is the dioptric power of the lens of the eye, and $l$ is the distance in meters between the second principal plane of the lens and the posterior pole of the retina. Data tabulated by Sorsby et al. (1962) may be used to obtain average values of P and $l$ as a function of the ocular refraction of a subject. As shown by Riva et al. (1979), this procedure introduces a statistical uncertainty of only 8% in $V_{max}$.

The bidirectional technique has been applied to measurements of $V_{max}$ in the retinal vessels of an anesthetized owl monkey. A value of $V_{max}$ = 1.8 cm/s was obtained for a 175-$\mu$m-diameter retinal vein. For a 92-$\mu$m-diameter retinal artery, $V_{max}$ ranged from 8.7 cm/s at peak systole to 2.6 cm/s at minimum diastole. These values are in the same range as those measured by Bulpitt et al. (1973), who used a high-speed fluorescein cineangiographic technique.

## Continuous Relative Measurements of the Maximum Red Blood Cell Speed

As has been indicated, measurements from retinal arteries require synchronization with the cardiac cycle. For this, the photocurrent arising from the light scattered from a site along a retinal artery is recorded on one channel of the tape recorder. A pulse coincident with the peak of the pressure wave measured in the subject's finger is simultaneously recorded on the other channel. An electronic gating module is used to activate the spectrum analyzer for a 0.1-s interval following a variable delay with respect to the recorded pulse. Spectra may thus be obtained during consecutive 0.1-s analysis time intervals (Fig. 13.11). The estimated cutoff frequencies, 5.5, 9, 4.5, and 3.5 kHz, indicate that $V_{max}$ varies by about a factor of 3 during the cardiac cycle.

As mentioned earlier, the photocurrent can also be processed by a frequency-to-voltage analog tracking system, as described by Stern et al. (1977). We have used a similar system to obtain a continuous voltage output, $V$, which is proportional to the instantaneous maximum RBC speed. A detailed discussion of this method is presented in Appendix B.

A continuous recording of $V$, obtained from a human retinal artery during several cardiac cycles (Fig. 13.12), confirms the regular systole/diastole variation of $V_{max}$ of the order of a factor of 3 measured by spectral analysis.

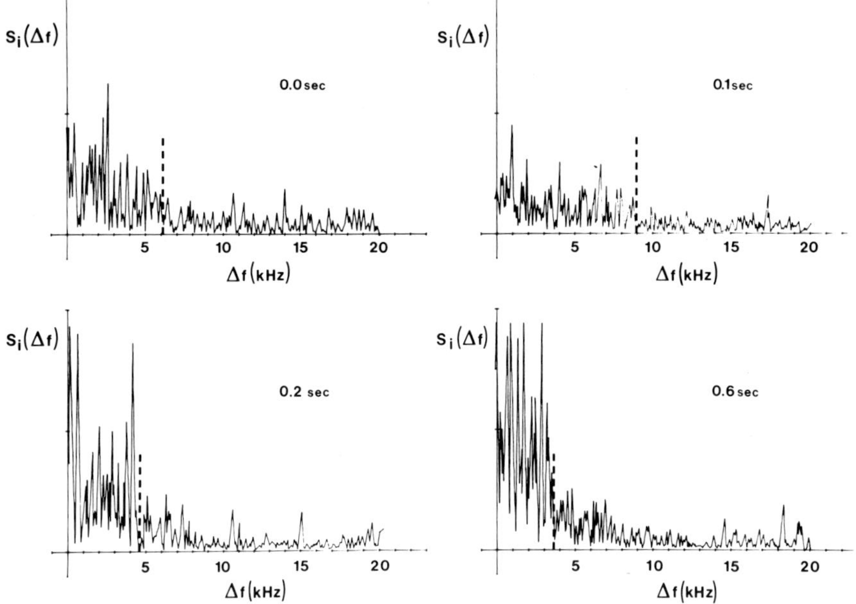


**Fig. 13.11.** Spectra obtained in 0.1–s measurement time intervals from human retinal artery during four portions of one cardiac cycle. Estimated cutoff frequencies are 5.5, 9, 4.5, and 3.5 kHz. Time delay to beginning of each measurement, relative to a trigger pulse synchronized to heart rate is indicated with each spectrum. *Dashed lines*, estimates of each $\Delta f_{max}$.

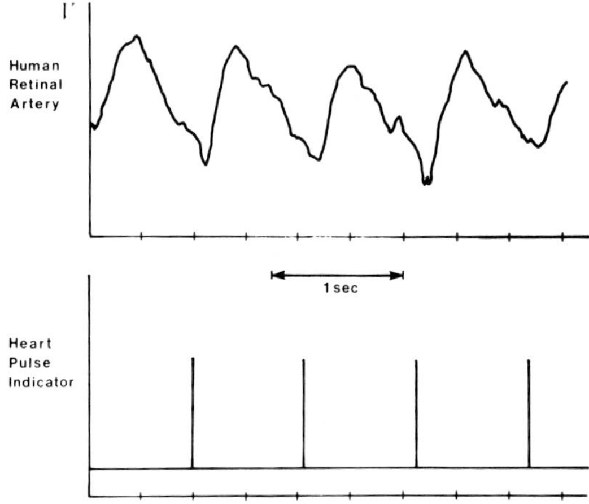


**Fig. 13.12.** Continuous recording, V, of relative systole/diastole variations of $V_{max}$ in human retinal artery during several cardiac cycles. *At bottom*, spikes indicate heart rate and are derived from pressure wave in subject's fingertip.

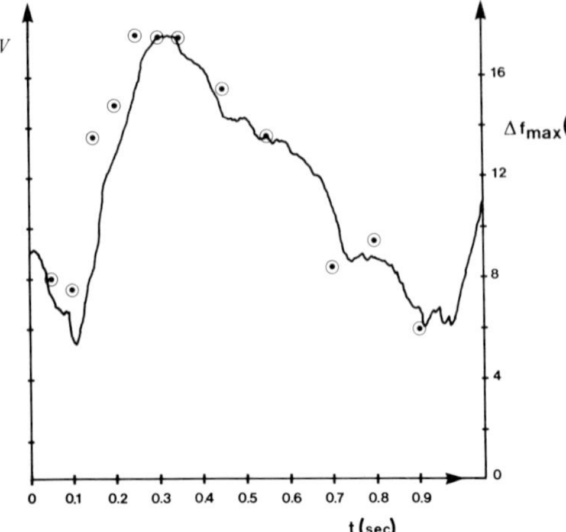


**Fig. 13.13.** Comparison between the continuous recording of V during one cardiac cycle of Figure 13.12 and consecutive cutoff frequencies $\Delta f_{max}$ obtained during the same cardiac cycle in 0.1-s time intervals *(discrete points)*.

In a test of the validity of the technique, the continuous recording of *V* during one of the cardiac cycles of Figure 13.12 was replotted (Fig. 13.13). The cutoff frequencies obtained from spectral analysis of the same photocurrent signal during consecutive 0.1-s time intervals are plotted as points at the appropriate delay times. The excellent agreement suggests that this technique can be used instead of spectrum analysis in processing the photocurrent recorded during experiments involving continuous variations in the RBC speed.

## PRESENT LIMITATIONS OF RETINAL LASER DOPPLER VELOCIMETRY AND THE APPROACH TO CLINICAL APPLICABILITY

Difficulties in obtaining spectra with distinct cutoff frequencies arise when eye movements occur during the measurement, carrying the retinal vessel out of the path of the incident beam. In this case, the light that is collected has been scattered either entirely from the choroid, which underlies the retina, or partially from the retinal vessel and partially from the choroid. The resultant spectra exhibit a rapidly decreasing amplitude, beginning at frequency shifts that are low compared to the expected cutoff frequency.

Although the technique of having the subject fixate a target with the eye under measurement is quite successful in reducing eye movements in trained subjects, an untrained patient population presents more of a problem. A possible automated means of reducing the effects of eye movements involves stabilization of the incident laser beam on the retinal vessel using eye tracking techniques, such as the double Purkinje image eyetracker (Crane and Steele, 1978) or those techniques employing a mirror and contact lens system.

Even under optimal conditions of eye stability, the resolution of the technique depends upon retinal irradiance exposure limits. As discussed earlier in this chapter, in a particular experiment the intrinsic signal-to-noise ratio can be increased only by increasing the intensity of the incident laser light. The measurements on volunteers presented in this chapter were obtained using approximately one-half the maximum permissible level for continuous retinal irradiance [0.1 $W/cm^2$ (Sliney and Freasier, 1973)]. There exists considerable disagreement, however, as to a reasonable limit for continuous illumination. Clearly, more studies are needed on the particular effects of HeNe laser light on the retina.

Finally, routine clinical applicability of retinal laser Doppler velocimetry will occur when an absolute measure of $V_{max}$ may be made with relative ease. Implementation of the bidirectional technique discussed in the section on in-vivo measurement of maximum RBC speed seems, at this writing, to be the best approach.

# Appendix A. The Effects of Fluctuations in the Number of Red Blood Cells Present in the Illuminated Volume

The expression for the power-spectral density of the photocurrent, $S_i(\Delta f)$ Eq. (30), which was derived under the assumptions associated with the model shown in Figure 13.2, is the predicted form of the spectrum for essentially infinite measurement time. As discussed in the section, Principles of Retinal Laser Doppler Velocimetry, because of the stochastic nature of the photocurrent, there are fluctuations in $S_i(\Delta f)$ when the measurement time is finite. The spectra shown in Figure 13.5, obtained from a suspension of 1.009-$\mu$m-diameter spheres, were used to verify the expected relationship Eq. (34) between the fluctuations in $S_i(\Delta f)$ and the measurement time, $T$. Implicit in Eq. (34) is the assumption that fluctuations in the number of scatterers present in the illuminated volume are negligible. Applying this assumption to our model (Fig. 13.2) would require that fluctuations in the number of RBCs present in each cylindrical shell be negligible. In this Appendix, we will assume that the fluctuations in RBC number are not negligible and consider the resultant *additional* effect upon the fluctuations in $S_i(\Delta f)$.

If we consider just the signal component of $S_i(\Delta f)$ (Fig. 13.3), then on the basis of Eq. (30), the measured time-averaged power at a particular Doppler-shifted frequency, $\Delta f_n$, may be written as:

$$S(\omega_n, T) = [\beta^2 S S_{COH_{LO}} A_{LO}^2] \frac{1}{T} \int_0^T A^2(\omega_n, t)dt \tag{A.1}$$

where the quantity in brackets is a constant.

This expression can be simplified if we note from Eq. (11) that $\beta S A^2(\omega_n,t)$ is the photocurrent $i(\omega_n,t)$ originating from the RBCs giving rise to the Doppler-shifted frequency $\Delta f_n$. Therefore, one can write

$$S(\omega_n, T) = K \cdot \frac{1}{T} \int_0^T i(\omega_n, t)dt \tag{A.2}$$

where $K = \beta S_{COH_{LO}} A_{LO}^2$.

We now consider the fluctuations in $S(\omega_n,T)$ due only to the fluctuations in $i(\omega_n,t)$ arising from fluctuations in the number of RBCs producing $i(\omega_n,t)$.

By definition, the variance of the fluctuations in $S(\omega_n,T)$ is

$$\sigma_N^2[S] = < S^2 > - < S >^2, \tag{A.3}$$

where $< >$ represents the ensemble average.

The second term of Eq. (A.3) is

$$< S >^2 = \left[ K \cdot \frac{1}{T} \int_0^T < i(\omega_n,t) > dt \right]^2$$
$$= K^2 < i(\omega_n,t) >^2 \qquad (A.4)$$

since $< i(\omega_n,t) >$ is the time-independent mean value of the photocurrent at $\omega_n$.

The first term of Eq. (A.3) is

$$< S^2 > = K^2 \frac{1}{T^2} \int_0^T dt \int_0^T < i(\omega_n,t) i(\omega_n,u) > du \qquad (A.5)$$

We note that $< i(\omega_n,t)i(\omega_n,u) >$ is the autocorrelation function of the photocurrent at $\omega_n$, which can be written as $R_i(\omega_n,\tau)$, where $\tau = t - u$. We can simplify our analysis by assuming that $R_i(\omega_n,\tau)$, can be written as the sum of a gaussian function and a constant:

$$R_i(\omega_n,\tau) = \sigma^2[i(\omega_n)]e^{-\tau^2/2\epsilon^2} + < i(\omega_n) >^2 \qquad (A.6)$$

where $\epsilon$ represents a characteristic decay time of the autocorrelation function. We see from Eq. (A.3) that $R_i(\omega_n,\tau)$ has its maximum value, $< i^2(\omega_n) >$, at $\tau = 0$ and decays to $< i(\omega_n) >^2$ at large values of $\tau$.

Combining Eqs. (A.3)–(A.6) gives, for the variance of the fluctuations in $S(\omega_n,T)$, the following equation:

$$\sigma_N^2[S(\omega_n,T)] = \frac{K^2\sigma^2[i(\omega_n)]}{T^2} \int_0^T dt \int_0^T \exp\left(-(t-u)^2/2\epsilon^2\right)du \qquad (A.7)$$

If one now substitutes the variables $t' = t/\epsilon$ and $u' = u/\epsilon$, one obtains

$$\sigma_N^2[S(\omega_n,T)] = \frac{K^2\sigma^2[i(\omega_n)]}{(T/\epsilon)^2} \int_0^{T/\epsilon} dt' \int_0^{T/\epsilon} \exp\left(-\tfrac{1}{2}(t'-u')^2\right)du' \qquad (A.8)$$

We now consider $\sigma_N^2[S(\omega_n,T)]$ at two frequencies: $\omega_s$, which is in the region of the spectrum $\Delta f < \Delta f_{max}$ (see Fig. 13.7), the region dominated by single scattering; and $\omega_n$, which is in the region of the spectrum $\Delta f > \Delta f_{max}$, the region of multiple scattering. Since $i(\omega_s)$ is produced only by the RBCs moving in one cylindrical shell, while $i(\omega_m)$ is produced by RBCs moving throughout the total illuminated volume, $\sigma^2[i(\omega_s)]$ is larger than $\sigma^2[i(\omega_m)]$. Also, one can assume that $R_i(\omega_s,\tau)$ will decay more rapidly toward its baseline value than $R_i(\omega_m,\tau)$ as one expects $i(\omega_s)$ to fluctuate more rapidly than $i(\omega_m)$. Accordingly, we denote by $\epsilon_s$ and $\epsilon_m$, with $\epsilon_s < \epsilon_m$, the characteristic decay times of the autocorrelation functions $R_i(\omega_s,\tau)$ and $R_i(\omega_m,\tau)$ respectively.

We will now consider the ratio

$$\frac{\sigma_N^2[S(\omega_s,T)]}{\sigma_N^2[S(\omega_m,T)]}$$

for the two limiting cases: $T/\epsilon \gg 1$, and $T/\epsilon \ll 1$. When $T/\epsilon \gg 1$, the double integral in Eq. (A.8) approaches a constant so that

$$\frac{\sigma_N^2[S(\omega_s,T)]}{\sigma_N^2[S(\omega_m,T)]} = \frac{\sigma^2[i(\omega_s]}{\sigma^2[i(\omega_m)]} \cdot \frac{\epsilon_s^2}{\epsilon_m^2} \qquad \text{(A.9)}$$

When $T/\epsilon \ll 1$, the function $e^{-1/2}\ (t' - u')^2 \approx 1$ within the integration range. Therefore,

$$\frac{\sigma_N^2[S(\omega_s,T)]}{\sigma_N^2[S(\omega_m,T)]} = \frac{\sigma^2[i(\omega_s)]}{\sigma^2[i(\omega_m)]} \qquad \text{(A.10)}$$

We see then that this ratio is larger for very short measurement times than for long measurement times by the factor $\epsilon_m^2/\epsilon_s^2$.

# Appendix B. Continuous Relative Measurements of the Maximum Red Blood Cell Speed

In this Appendix we derive the relation between the continuous voltage output $V$, shown in Figures 13.12 and 13.13, and the corresponding cutoff frequency that appears in the spectrum. We begin by noting that the root-mean-square value of the photocurrent is equal to the square root of the total integrated power in the spectrum of the photocurrent:

$$\mathrm{RMS}(i) = \left[ \int_0^B S_i(\Delta\omega)d\omega \right]^{1/2} \tag{B.1}$$

In this expression the upper limit of integration, $B$, is, in practice, the upper bandwidth limit of a filter at the output of the photodetector. We also note that, in general, the power spectrum of the differentiated photocurrent, $S_i'(\Delta\omega)$, is related to $S_i(\Delta\omega)$ by

$$S_i'(\Delta\omega) = \omega^2 S_i(\Delta\omega) \tag{B.2}$$

Therefore,

$$\mathrm{RMS}(i') = \left[ \int_0^B \omega^2 S_i(\Delta\omega)d\omega \right]^{1/2} \tag{B.3}$$

If one refers to Eq. (30) and to Figure 13.3, the signal component of the spectrum has a constant amplitude, $I_s$, in the range $0 < \Delta\omega \leq \Delta\omega_{max}$; and the shot-noise component of the spectrum has a constant amplitude, $I_{sn}$, throughout the range passed by the filter: $0 < \Delta\omega \leq B$. We assume that the dc component at $\Delta\omega = 0$ is blocked by the filter. If we also assume that the total integrated power in the signal component of the spectrum, $P_s$, remains constant while $\Delta\omega_{max}$ varies in time

$$I_s \int_0^{\Delta\omega_{max}(t)} d\omega = P_s \tag{B.4}$$

we have

$$I_s = \frac{P_s}{\Delta\omega_{max}(t)} \tag{B.5}$$

We note from Eqs. (17) and (31) that $I_{sn}$ is proportional to the mean value of the photocurrent, $\bar{i}$, so that Eq. (B.3) becomes

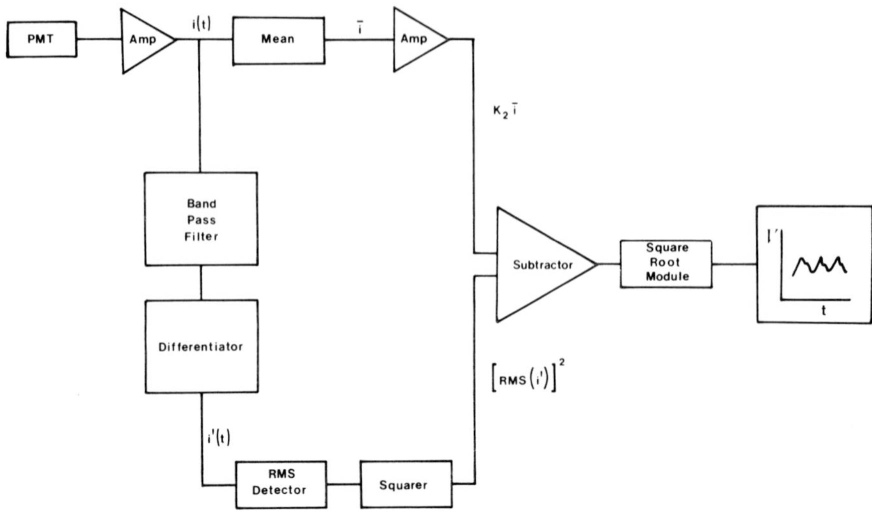


**Fig. 13.14.** Block diagram of analog circuit used to obtain V(t).

$$\text{RMS}(i') = \left[ \frac{P_s}{\Delta\omega_{max}(t)} \int_0^{\Delta\omega_{max}(t)} \omega^2 d\omega + a\bar{i} \int_0^B \omega^2 d\omega \right]^{1/2} \tag{B.6}$$

where $a = \dfrac{e\beta s}{2}$

Performing the integration leads to

$$K_1[\Delta\omega_{max}(t)]^2 = [\text{RMS}\ (i')]^2 - K_2\bar{i} \tag{B.7}$$

where $K_1 = \dfrac{P_s}{3}$ and $K_2 = \dfrac{aB^3}{3}$

Taking the square root gives the following result:

$$K_1^{1/2} \cdot \Delta\omega_{max}(t) = ([\text{RMS}(i')]^2 - K_2\bar{i})^{1/2} \tag{B.8}$$

The righthand side of Eq. (B.8) is the voltage output, *V* (Figs. 13.12 and 13.13). It is proportional to the cutoff frequency, $\Delta\omega_{max}$, which is, in turn, proportional to the maximum RBC velocity, $V_{max}$. A block diagram of the analog circuit used to obtain V(t) (Fig. 13.14). The constant $K_2$ is determined by noting that for a stationary target, $\Delta\omega_{max} = 0$, so that

$$K_2 = \left[ \frac{[\text{RMS}(i')]^2}{\bar{i}} \right]_{\text{stationary}} \tag{B.9}$$

## REFERENCES

Bulpitt CJ, Kohner EM, Dollery CT (1973) Velocity profiles in the retinal microcirculation. Bibl Anat 11:448–452.

Crane HD, Steele CM (1978) Accurate three-dimensional eyetracker. Appl Optics 17:691–705.

Cummins HZ, Swinney HL (1970) In: Wolf E (ed) Progress in Optics, vol. VIII. North Holland Publishing Co., Amsterdam, pp. 133–200.

Feke GT, Riva CE (1978) Laser Doppler measurements of blood velocity in human retinal vessels. J Opt Soc Am 68:526–531.

Feke GT, Riva CE, Eberli B, Benary V (1978) Blood velocity in human retinal vessels. Electro-Optical Systems Design 10:40–43.

Goldsmith HL (1968) The microrheology of red blood cell suspensions. J Gen Physiol 52:5s–28s.

Lastovka JB (1967) PhD thesis, Department of Physics, Massachusetts Institute of Technology (unpublished).

Reif F (1965) Fundamentals of Statistical and Thermal Physics. McGraw-Hill, New York, pp. 585–587.

Riva CE, Ben-Sira I (1975) Two-point fluorophotometer for the human ocular fundus. Appl Optics 14:2691–2693.

Riva CE, Ross B, Benedek GB (1972) Laser Doppler measurements of blood flow in capillary tubes and retinal arteries. Invest Ophthalmol 11:936–944.

Riva CE, Feke GT, Eberli B, Benary V (1979) Bidirectional LDV system for absolute measurement of blood speed in retinal vessels. Appl Optics 18:2301–2306.

Sliney DH, Freasier BC (1973) Evaluation of optical radiation hazards. Appl Optics 12:1–24.

Sorsby A, Leary GA, Richards MJ (1962) Correlation ametropia and component ametropia. Vision Res 2: 309–313.

Stern MD, Lappe DL, Bowen PD, Chimosky JE, Holloway GA Jr, Keiser HR, Bowman RL (1977) Continuous measurement of tissue blood flow by laser-Doppler spectroscopy. Am J Physiol 232:H441–448.

Tanaka T, Riva CE, Ben-Sira I (1974) Blood velocity measurements in human retinal vessels. Science 186:830–831.

# 14

# Technical Problems of Carbon Dioxide Laser Surgery in the Rectum

*Rene C. J. Verschueren*

Malignant tumors of the rectum are an ordeal for the patients. They cause much suffering from bloody diarrhea, secretion of mucus, and anal pain. When the rectal cancer is in the proximity of the anus, an abdominoperineal resection often is required. For very selected cases of rectal cancer, meeting strict criteria, some forms of local therapy offer a good cure rate. Some decades ago, electrofulguration was introduced for the local eradication of these rectal tumors (Klok, 1964; Crile and Turnbull, 1972; Swerdlow and Salvati, 1972). Recently, local endocavitary radiotherapy has been advocated, and very good results were obtained (Sischy et al., 1978).

## LIMITATIONS AND DRAWBACKS OF ELECTROFULGURATION FOR RECTAL TUMORS

The local destruction of sessile polyps and small cancers by means of electrosurgery is based on the thermal effect generated by the electric current while it is passing through the tissues. The procedure is carried out through specially designed rectoscopes by means of spherical electrodes. When the dial of the electrosurgical unit is in the appropriate position, it requires about 5 s of coagulating current before the tissues around the electrode start boiling. The pathologic tissue is vaporized away, step by step. This is a slow process that may take up to an hour for bulky tumors. The electrode is kept at the same spot for a rather long time, and the

Mr. G. T. Prins, chief technician, ENT department (Head Prof. Dr. P. E. Hoeksema) of the University Hospital Groningen, designed and manufactured the rectoscope and the alternate optical system of the micromanipulator.

temperature at the contact surface is kept at about 100°C by the thermostatic effect of boiling water. Therefore, deep penetration of thermal damage as a consequence of heat conduction can be expected. The depth of this thermal damage and the amount of destruction of normal tissue are unpredictable. A first consequence is that the surgeon has to burn deeply in order to be confident about the thoroughness of this procedure. The risk of full-thickness devitalization of the rectal wall requires that this technique be used only in the extraperitoneal part of the rectum, where preoperative or late perforations have no dramatic consequences because that part of the rectum is surrounded by the soft tissues of the pelvis. The anterior part of the rectum in the female is a weak spot since a rectovaginal fistula may develop after full-thickness devitalization of the rectal wall. A very serious drawback of electrofulguration is the amount of necrotic tissue that is left behind. Premature release of this necrotic slough may cause severe postoperative hemorrhage. In the majority of cases this necrotic slough takes weeks to disappear, and healing of the defect is slow. When the patients are seen 6 weeks after electrosurgery, most of them have a slowly healing ulcer. While this so-called secondary healing takes place, an amount of scar tissue is formed. After the defect heals, this scar has the tendency to shrink, thus causing narrowing of the lumen of the rectum. This hazard of rectal stenosis is the reason that electrosurgery is contraindicated when the tumor covers more than one-third of the circumference of the lumen.

The drawbacks of electrosurgery, thus, are as follows: (1) deep penetration of thermal damage, (2) lack of visual control of the extent of the surgery, (3) slow healing, and (4) the hazard of stenosis due to scarring. It is our belief that the $CO_2$ laser, as a substitute for electrosurgery, may not have these drawbacks.

## THE CARBON DIOXIDE LASER IN THE ERADICATION OF RECTAL TUMORS

The $CO_2$ laser emits in the far infrared, and its beam therefore offers the unique advantages for tissue ablation by evaporation. There is strong exponential absorption ($\alpha = 200/\text{cm}$) of this beam in any living tissue, and radiant energy is therefore absorbed at the surface, thus allowing step-by-step tissue evaporation. Thermal damage in the walls of the defect is very limited after laser evaporation and is determined by the exposure time. The thickness of this thermal damage, as investigated by means of enzyme histochemistry, varies between 150 $\mu$m and 800 $\mu$m for exposure times varying between 0.3 and 6 s (Verschueren, 1976). As a consequence of this limited thermal damage, healing is prompt and no late hemorrhages were seen during our preliminary clinical work. The prompt healing after $CO_2$ laser evaporation assures minimal scarring and absence of stenosis.

Rectal surgery with the $CO_2$ laser was started in our institution in 1975. Initially only small polyps were excised or vaporized in situ. Subsequently, as experience and confidence increased, bigger tumors were eradicated. During more recent years, the technique of these procedures has been modified and the instrumentation changed to a certain extent.

## EQUIPMENT REQUIRED FOR CARBON DIOXIDE LASER MICROSURGERY IN THE RECTUM

### The Carbon Dioxide Laser

Any $CO_2$ laser on the market can be used for rectal surgery, whether it is working in the single mode or not. However, the energy output of several available $CO_2$ lasers is rather low for this purpose. The tissue volume to be vaporized in rectal surgery can exceed several cubic centimeters. The average surgical $CO_2$ laser designed for gynecologic or ENT applications has a maximum energy output of about 20 W. These lasers have been designed for the evaporation of small areas of the epithelium of vocal cords or the ablation of the epithelium of the uterine cervix.

The evaporation of larger tissue masses, as in the rectum, may be time-consuming when carried out with $CO_2$ lasers having rather low maximum output. Our initial clinical microsurgery in the rectum was carried out with a Sharplan 791 (Laser Industries, Tel Aviv, Israel) with a maximum output of about 35 W. Subsequently, when an early $CO_2$ laser with a maximum output of 100 W was used, tissue ablation could be achieved in a faster way.

### The Operating Microscope

We have been very pleased with the versatility and reliability of the Zeiss OPMI I operating microscope. The optical system allows the simultaneous use of a motion-picture or television camera and a camera for still photography. The 50-W bulbs give enough light for photographic work. The use of an external xenon light source obviously increases the quality of the visual material.

### The Rectoscope

Tissue that is to be vaporized will be transformed into smoke and vapor. The rectoscopes, therefore, need to have a special suction channel to allow for evacuation of the smoke from the working area. Insufficient evacuation of smoke will obscure vision and render the continuation of the surgery impossible. Several forms of polymethylmetacrylate tubes were tried out in order to find the most appropriate design for a laser rectoscope.

From our preliminary experimental work on dogs, we decided that a laser rectoscope had to meet the following requirements:

1. The internal diameter should be at least 34 mm to allow binocular vision through the operation microscope.
2. The tip should be at a 45° angle with the axis of the rectoscope to make introduction through the anus easier.
3. Removable cold light must be available to provide illumination while the rectoscope is centered around the polyp or tumor.
4. The construction of the rectoscope must allow stable fixation onto the operating table as soon as the instrument is in the appropriate position.

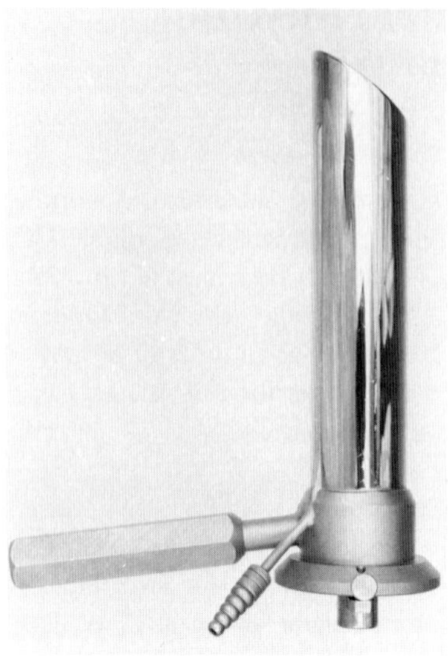

**Fig. 14.1.** Lateral view of the rectoscope.

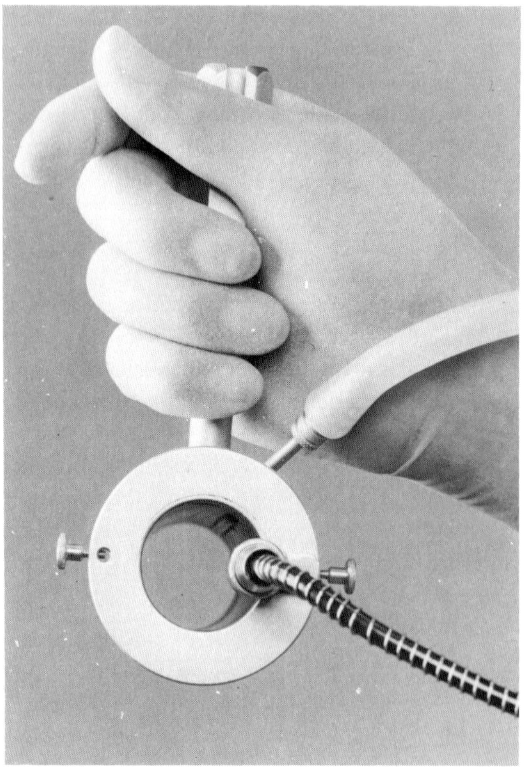

**Fig. 14.2.** Rear aspect of the rectoscope. The suction tube and channel are visible in the right upper quadrant; the removable adaptor for the light fiber is below.

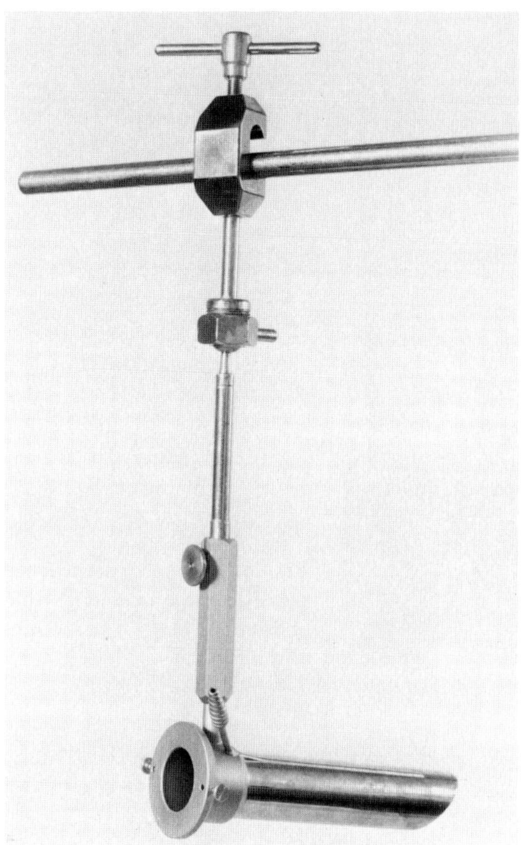

**Fig. 14.3.** The suspension system allowing stable fixation of the rectoscope onto the operating table.

Two rectoscopes meeting these requirements were built for the preliminary clinical work. These long rectoscopes were designed for the removal and evaporation of polyps in the rectum and the rectosigmoid colon, and have been described previously (Verschueren, 1976). Subsequently, when our interest became limited to the lower rectum, a new rectoscope was designed for this purpose (Figs. 14.1 and 14.2). This instrument, manufactured from aluminum, has a length of 20 cm and an external diameter of 38 mm. A suction tube for the evacuation of smoke is built into the inner part of the rectoscope. To avoid closure of this tube by aspirated mucosal tissue, the tube should be shorter than the rectoscope itself. A removable clip allows temporary fixation of a light fiber from an external light source to the rear end of the rectoscope. This is needed to facilitate introduction of the rectoscope through the anus so that the instrument may be positioned around the target tissue. The shaft at the rear end of the rectoscope offers a strong grip for the surgeon during the introduction of the instrument and stable fixation to the operating table as soon as the appropriate position has been obtained. The suspension system on the operating table contains a ball and socket joint, allowing smaller adjustments of the position of the rectoscope (Fig. 14.3).

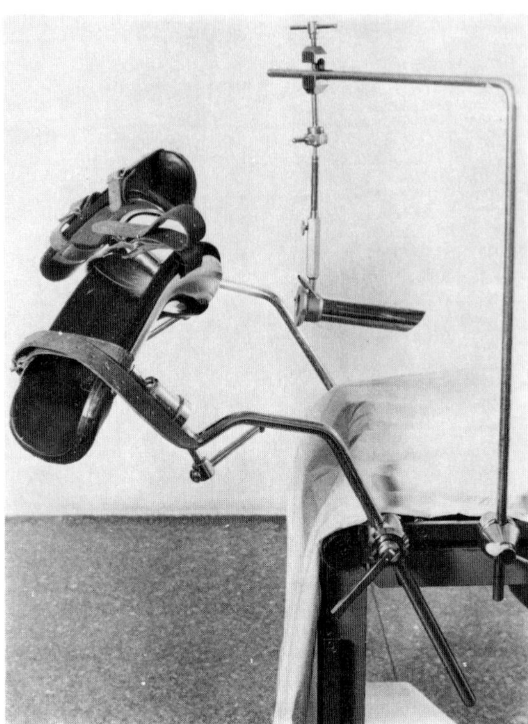

**Fig. 14.4.** The rectoscope is suspended on the operating table, and the leg rests for positioning of the patient.

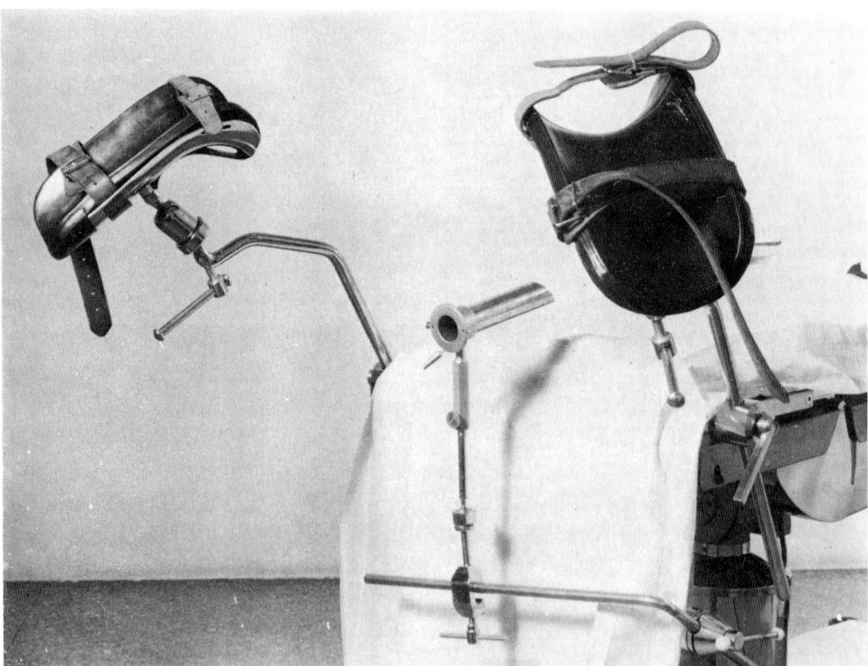

**Fig. 14.5.** The alternate position of the rectoscope, used when dealing with tumors on the anterior aspect of the rectum.

In the majority of cases, the patient is placed in the lithotomy position, and the rectoscope is suspended (Fig. 14.4). The front end of the rectoscope is oblique, and the lumen is open on the side opposite to the handle so that it is easier to turn the rectoscope upside down when treating tumors seated on the anterior aspect of the rectum. In this position the rectoscope is no longer suspended, but stands on the fixation system (Fig. 14.5).

## The Micromanipulator

We have been working with a micromanipulator designed by the American Optical Corporation. The parallel laser beam, after leaving the plasmatube or the manipulator arm, is focused by means of a 400-mm lens. The main part of the micromanipulator is gimbal-mounted mirror positioned at 45° to the incident laser beam and deflecting it along the viewing axis of the microscope. Apertures on both sides of the mirror give room for the visual path of the surgeon's eyes. A fiber-optic system partly catches the illuminating light from the microscope and, via a beam splitter, projects a marker spot in the focal plane of the microscope eyepiece. This beam splitter is situated in the same plane as the laser-beam–reflecting mirror, so that the marker spot can be made to coincide with the impact point of the focused laser beam. The optical system generating this marker spot contains a green lens, a very fortunate choice because the green color makes it easy to identify the target light, even on highly vascular mucosal surfaces or on surfaces partially carbonized during the process of tissue evaporation. Micromanipulators from other companies have a helium-neon (HeNe) laser beam to generate the target light. The red color of this light is hard to identify on highly vascular surfaces. This inspired ENT surgeons I saw working with this system to use a blue lens in front of the microscope, thus making it easier to identify the target light. Unfortunately, the blue lens dimmed the light from the microscope to the extent that the surgeons could work only at low magnification.

In the American Optical micromanipulator, the laser beam reflecting gimbal-mounted mirror can be moved by means of a control stick ("joystick"). Gimbal and control stick are arranged so that (1) the motion of the laser beam and the marker spot are directly proportional and (2) in the sense of the movement of the stick, there is a demagnification of 7:1. The mechanical linkage of the control stick and gimbal makes it possible for the surgeon to move the focal spot with the speed considered appropriate for a particular situation. Micromanipulators with a motor drive are nice pieces of technology but have certain drawbacks. The motion of the control stick is transmitted to small electromotors that turn the mirror in the desired direction at a previously selected speed. I have used a similar device on an asbestos block and felt completely uneasy because of the limited variability of the speed of movement. While I am vaporizing a tumor away, it is my technique to adapt the speed of movement of the focal spot to the effect on the tissue, thus increasing the speed when vaporization penetrates too deeply and slowing down when deep tissue ablation is required. To achieve this, the direct mechanical transmission between control stick and gimbal is a prerequisite.

## PROBLEMS WITH THE SPOT SIZE IN RECTAL SURGERY AND THEIR SOLUTION

In the beam of the single-mode laser, the spatial distribution of the energy is gaussian. This distribution of the energy is the same when the laser beam has been focused. The focal spot of the physicists is, by definition, the circle containing 86% of the radiant energy, and its diameter is determined by the formula

$$d = f\theta$$

where d, diameter of the focal spot in centimeters; f, focal length of the lens in centimeters; $\theta$, divergence of the beam in radians. The surface of the focal spot thus will be

$$\pi\left(\frac{d}{2}\right)^2 \quad \text{or} \quad \frac{\pi f^2\theta^2}{4}$$

The energy density in the focal spot consequently is inversely proportional to the square of the focal length of the lens.

### Focal Spot Effect

The spot size of interest to surgeons depends on the actual effect of the focal spot upon the exposed tissue. When the beam of a particular $CO_2$ laser is focused by means of a particular lens on the surface of a particular tissue for a well-defined exposure time, the diameter of the defect created by laser evaporation will be determined by the output of the laser device. A minimum of energy density ($I_v$) is required for tissue evaporation to take place. At low output of the laser device, this minimal requirement will be met only by the central part of the focal spot (Fig. 14.6). As the energy output increases, the fraction of the gaussian curve containing this threshold energy density becomes larger and the diameter of the resulting tissue defect increases. For the same reason, the diameter of the crater increases with longer exposure times. The consequence is that the "physicist's spot size" of a particular $CO_2$ laser with a particular lens means nothing practical for the surgeon who is interested only in the effect on the tissue—the size of the defect or the width of the incision. Moreover, the resulting effect upon the tissue will also be determined by the water content and the composition of the tissue.

During the first years we used a 400-mm lens on the micromanipulator and a lens with the same focal length on the operation microscope. At the present time, whether we perform buccal or rectal work, we are interested only in vaporizing tissue away. The $CO_2$ laser, therefore, is not used as a "light knife" but as a tissue-vaporizing instrument.

When tumors of polyps that need to be vaporized are only a few millimeters higher than the surrounding normal mucosa, the focused laser beam may be used only at a low energy output to avoid too deep penetration. This tissue is vaporized away by making sweeping movements with the focus of the laser over the tumor.

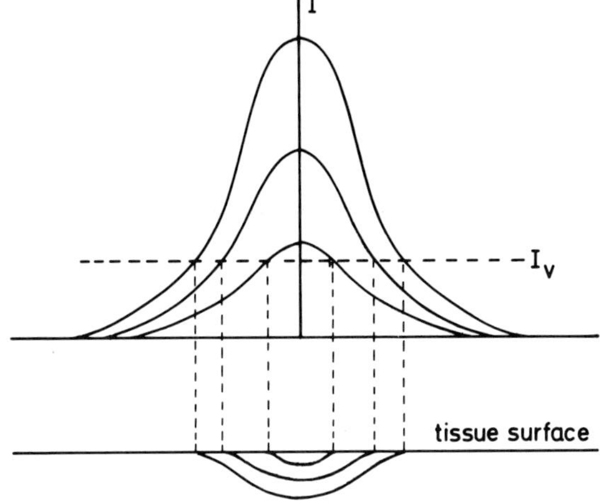


**Fig. 14.6.** Schema depicting the relationship between the focal spot and the crater created in tissues. The vertical axis represents the intensity (I) at the center of the spot. $I_v$ is the threshold energy density required for tissue evaporation to take place.

At high output, the narrow track made by the focused laser beam might reach more deeply than is appropriate, even when the beam is moved very fast. In between the individual narrow tracks, pathologic tissue may be left intact, thus making the procedure less radical. An additional disadvantage of working with the focused beam is that covering an area of several square centimeters at low output proves to be very time-consuming since only a small volume of tissue is vaporized per unit time.

Our problem can be summarized as follows: The active spot of the laser beam should be greater so that tissue may be vaporized away over a broader track at high output of the laser device while too deep vaporization is avoided.

**Solutions to the Focal Spot Problem.** A first solution to this problem was to work with the defocused beam. This could be achieved without effectuating major changes in the optical system of the micromanipulator merely by substituting a 300-mm lens of the microscope for the 400-mm lens. The consequence is that micromanipulator and microscope come 10 cm closer to the patient, and a slightly defocused laser beam is impinging on the tissues (Fig. 14.7). With this plan, microsurgery was carried out and proved to be safe and fast, even with the $CO_2$ laser emitting 100 W. Very shallow step-by-step vaporization could be performed, and deep penetration into underlying tissues was avoided.

## Hemostasis

Hemostasis sometimes was a problem during the performance of $CO_2$ laser microsurgery in the rectum. Until recently, our technique consisted in moving the focused beam over the bleeding vessel with very quick sweeping movements, hoping to dehydrate and shrink the tissues in the vicinity of the bleeding vessel. As a consequence of the small size of the focal spot, hemostasis was sometimes hard to obtain. Even the slightly defocused spot obtained by using the 400-mm lens at a 300-mm distance proved not to be the perfect solution to this problem.

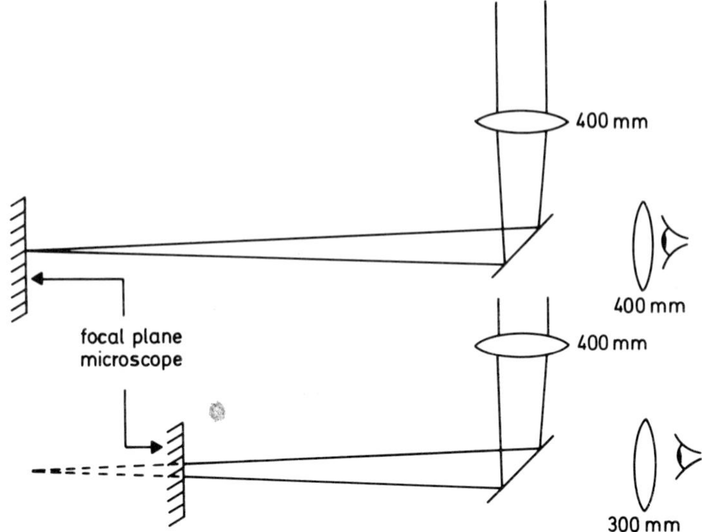


**Fig. 14.7.** Schema of the original optical system of the micromanipulator *(top)* with the system after substitution of the microscope lenses *(bottom)*.

The ideal solution for the hemostasis in $CO_2$ laser microsurgery would be to utilize a spot with a diameter of several millimeters to permit simultaneous exposure of both the bleeding vessel and the surrounding tissues. Consequently, the tissue at the surface will slowly dehydrate and soon even carbonize while the conduction of heat from the surface toward underlying layers will cause shrinking of the tissues and obliteration of the vessel.

To achieve this end, the laser-beam–focusing system of the American Optical micromanipulator was removed, and a tube containing a 500-mm germanium lens (Fig. 14.8) was substituted. The purpose of this lens with a long focus was to attain a large focal spot. The tube was manufactured from aluminum and subsequently anodized. A longitudinal slot in the tube made it possible to move the germanium lens from the focused position in the upper part to an out-of-focus position. With this progressive and stepless defocusing, the diameter of the focal spot could be varied from 1 mm when in focus to 3 mm when the lens was 20 cm out of focus. The diagram in Figure 14.9 depicts how this variation in spot size can be obtained by moving the germanium lens downward in the tube. This new device was only recently introduced in our clinical work, and the first results were very gratifying.

## CONCLUSION

The ideas presented in this article are born of experience with the $CO_2$ laser in one particular area, and there still is a long road to the ideal laser instrumentation for this particular application. The solutions presented here are far from ideal, but minimal technical skill is required to work with this instrumentation.

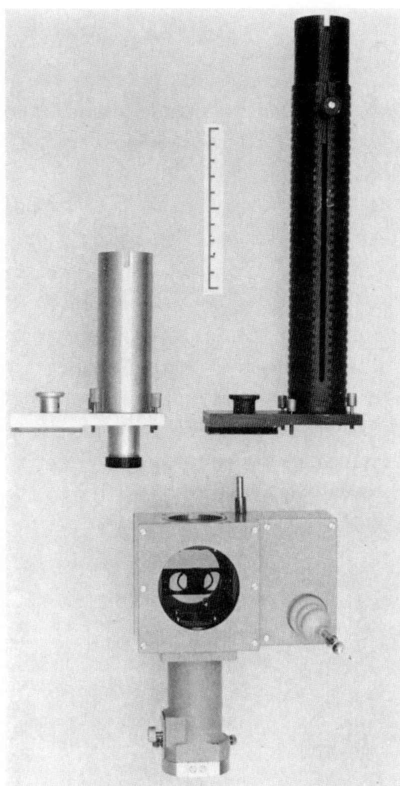

**Fig. 14.8.** The micromanipulator *(bottom)* and interchangeable laser-focusing systems. The original part *(top left)* contains a 400-mm lens. The newly designed system with the movable germanium lens is *at right*.

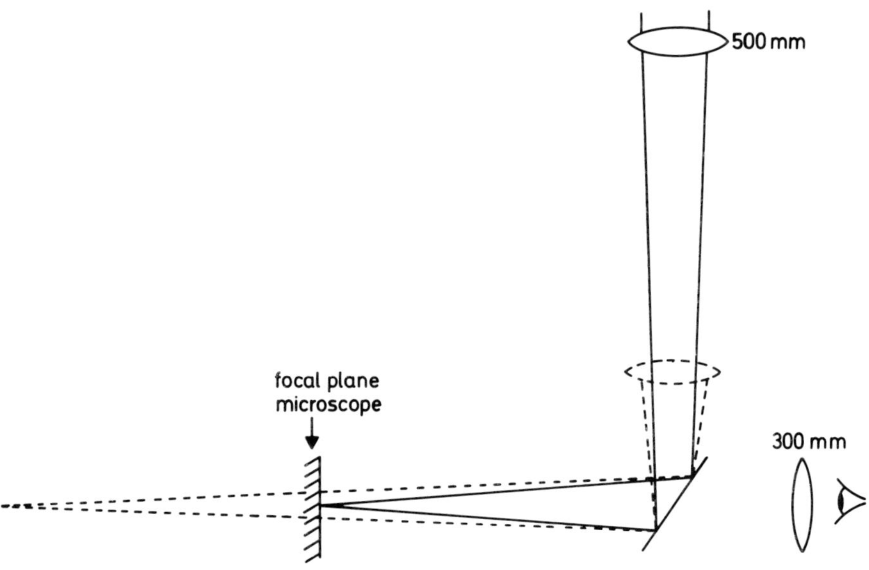


**Fig. 14.9.** Schema of the situation created by combination of a 500-mm germanium lens with a 300-mm lens in the microscope. *Dotted lines*, consequence of bringing laser-focusing lens down.

We hope that other surgeons will be inspired to use the $CO_2$ laser for rectal surgery and that, as a consequence, implement manufacturers become interested to the extent that further improvements and adaptations are developed in $CO_2$ lasers to meet the requirements of this special kind of surgery.

## SUMMARY

The beam of the $CO_2$ laser can be used in conjunction with an operating microscope for precise tissue ablation in cavities. The author used this technique for the vaporization of polyps and tumors of the rectum and rectosigmoid colon. It has clear advantages over electrofulguration. Technical requirements for instrumentation for rectal surgery differ from those required by other surgical specialties. Modifications in the optic system of standard lasers can increase the yield and the reliability of this particular technique.

## REFERENCES

Crile G Jr, Turnbull RB (1972) The role of electrocoagulation in the treatment of carcinoma of the rectum. Surg Gynecol Obstet 135:391–396.

Klok AA (1964) The treatment of some forms of rectal cancer by electrocoagulation. Arch Chir Neerl 16:173–183.

Sischy B, Remington JH, Sobel SH (1978) Treatment of rectal carcinomas by means of endocavity irradiation. Cancer 42:1073–1076.

Swerdlow DB, Salvati EP (1972) Electrocoagulation of colon of the rectum. Dis Col Rectum 15:228–232.

Verschueren R (1976) The $CO_2$ Laser in Tumor Surgery. Van Gorcum, Assen, The Netherlands.

# 15

# Laser Biomedical Engineering: Clinical Applications in Otolaryngology

*Geza J. Jako*

## LASER BIOMEDICAL ENGINEERING IN OTOLARYNGOLOGY

The first lasers, ruby, neodymium-in-glass and argon, were tried experimentally in various areas of biological and medical research. In the field of otolaryngology, Stahle and Hoegberg (1965) used pulsed lasers for inner-ear irradiation, Conti and Bergomi (1966) for irradiation of the posterior labyrinth, and Sataloff (1967) for experimental irradiation of otosclerotic stapes. Kelemen et al. performed studies on the effects of massive irradiation in the ears of mice using pulsed ruby and neodymium lasers. In 1965, with Dr. M. Polanyi at the American Optical Company, I studied the possibility of cutting into the vocal cords with the laser. Human cadaver specimens were used for the initial study, with a high-output pulsed neodymium-in-glass laser operating at 1.06 $\mu$m (Fig. 15.1). The limited tissue absorption of the wavelength of this laser was increased by painting the specimen with a 5% copper sulfate solution. With rather high energy levels, only small lesions could be affected in the vocal cords. Histologic studies demonstrated tissue destruction. Experiments with these high-output short-pulsed lasers were performed by various researchers in the mid-1960s. They soon realized that these lasers created explosive effects in tissue. After irradiation of experimental tumors, scattered cells and tissue fragments could be found in the operative area. Naturally, this ruled out the use of lasers, especially in tumor surgery.

In 1965, K. M. Patel built the first carbon dioxide laser which worked in the continuous-wave mode. Polanyi realized the possibility of using this infrared laser, with the output at 10.6 $\mu$m, for surgical applications. In 1966, he and his team developed the first $CO_2$ surgical laser system. In 1967, at Polanyi's laboratory, I started applying the $CO_2$ laser to human tissue, first evaporating tissue from the

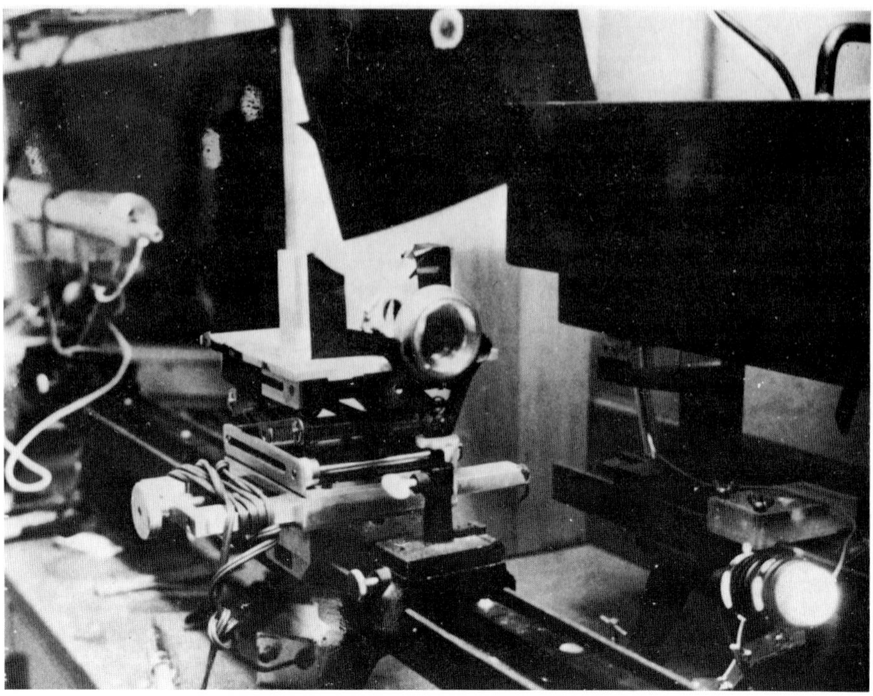

**Fig. 15.1.** Neodymium-in-glass laser with human laryngeal specimen, 1965.

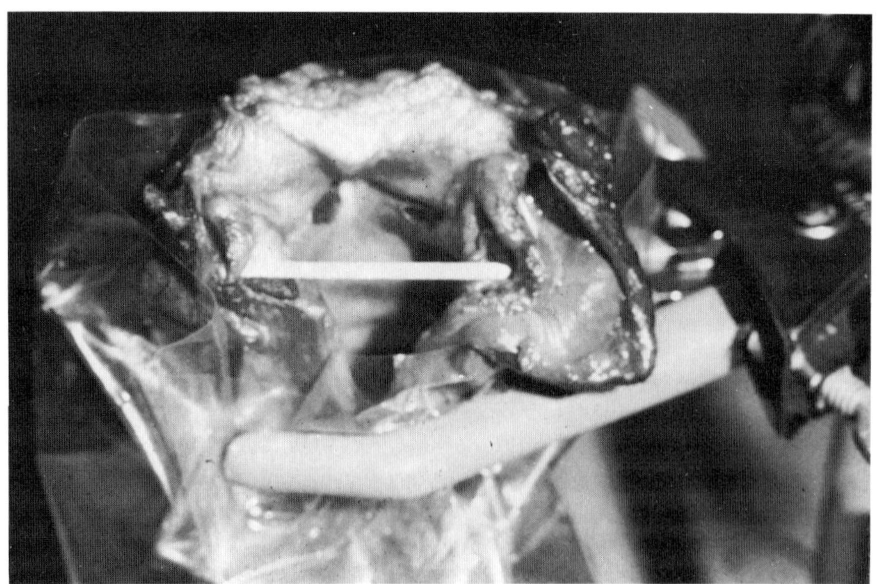

**Fig. 15.2.** Experimental excision of human vocal-cord tissue with $CO_2$ laser, 1966.

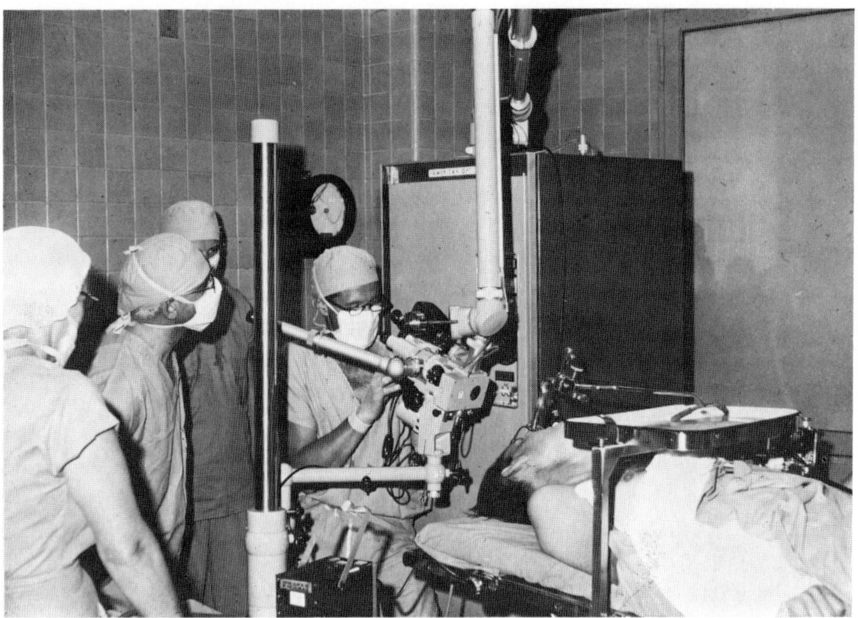

**Fig. 15.3.** First laser surgery of the larynx in a human, 1970.

vocal cord in laryngeal specimens (Fig. 15.2). The potential for laser application in human surgery was then conceived. Microscopic and endoscopic delivery systems were constructed, and in dog experiments it was shown that the focused $CO_2$ laser beam is excellent for cutting soft tissue.

In 1968, the removal of a vocal-cord nodule in a dog demonstrated the practical clinical application of this new precision surgical tool (Jako, 1972). Clinical application in humans began in 1970 at the Department of Otolaryngology of Boston University School of Medicine (Fig. 15.3). A report published by Strong and Jako in 1972 described the first clinical study, representing a new era in laryngeal surgery, which expanded into various other surgical specialties in the following years.

## Action and Absorption of Laser Energy

Electromagnetic radiation interacts with material depending on its wavelength and the atomic/molecular structure of the material. Inorganic materials like metals will absorb or reflect the energy in various degrees depending on its wavelength. If energy is absorbed by the material, heat develops. In the case of lasers, where the radiation is coherent and can be focused into a small spot, high-density localized heating results. Heat is utilized for laser machining of metals in drilling, milling, and cutting operations. Local melting of metals is used for precision welding with lasers. In these industrial applications, high-output energy is required. Therefore in most instances, continuous-wave $CO_2$ and neodymium-YAG lasers are used. These lasers are also used for other industrial applications, such as cutting fabrics and machining plastics, wood, and ceramics.

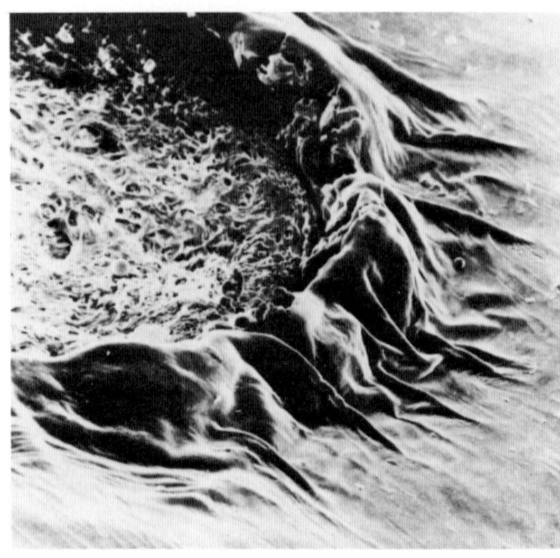

**Fig. 15.4.** Impact of $CO_2$ laser on mucosa, as seen with the scanning electron microscope.

Similarly, lasers can be used for machining biological material or living tissue. This machining of living tissue is also called surgery. Biological material contains a large amount of water: living human soft tissue, normal or pathological, is composed of approximately 80% to 95% water. Therefore, the absorption of a particular wavelength in water plays a great role in surgery. Pigmented biological materials and hemoglobin have maximum specific absorption in the visible spectrum. For this reason, lasers in the visible range can be used to create selective coagulation of blood or pigment. The high absorption of the $CO_2$ laser beam at 10.6 $\mu$m explains the localized heating in the high-water-containing soft tissues. This makes the $CO_2$ laser especially useful for cutting applications (Fig. 15.4). The neodymium-YAG laser beam at 1.06 $\mu$m is absorbed less in water; therefore, the heating effect in biological tissue is less localized, resulting in a larger area of tissue coagulation, not evaporation. In living tissue, the neodymium-YAG laser is better suited to creating a hemostatic effect.

In general, for theoretical and practical calculations of laser-beam absorption at a particular wavelength, we use data available for water. Recently, however, a sensitive method was developed by the author and coworkers for measurement of light absorption in biological material.

**In-Vitro Measurement of Absorption by Photoacoustic Spectroscopy.** The photoacoustic phenomenon was first described by Alexander Graham Bell in 1880. In his experiment, he utilized focused sunlight to heat air in a small cell (Fig. 15.5). I observed this phenomenon during laser surgery when an ac-powered $CO_2$ laser was used. In 1973, Rosencweig utilized this phenomenon for measuring absorption spectra in the visible region of solids, liquids, and blood. He called it photoacoustic spectroscopy. In the past few years, the author and coworkers at the Massachusetts Institute of Technology built an instrument to perform absorption measurements of biological material utilizing tunable lasers (Fig. 15.6). Preliminary measurements in human tissues are shown in Figure 15.7.

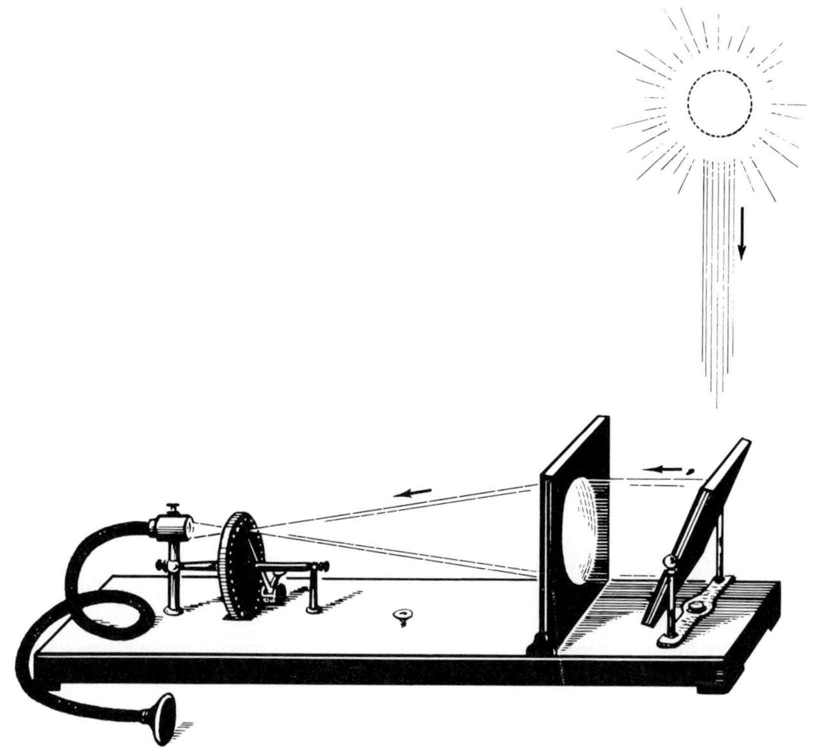

Fig. 15.5. Photophone built by Alexander Graham Bell, 1880.

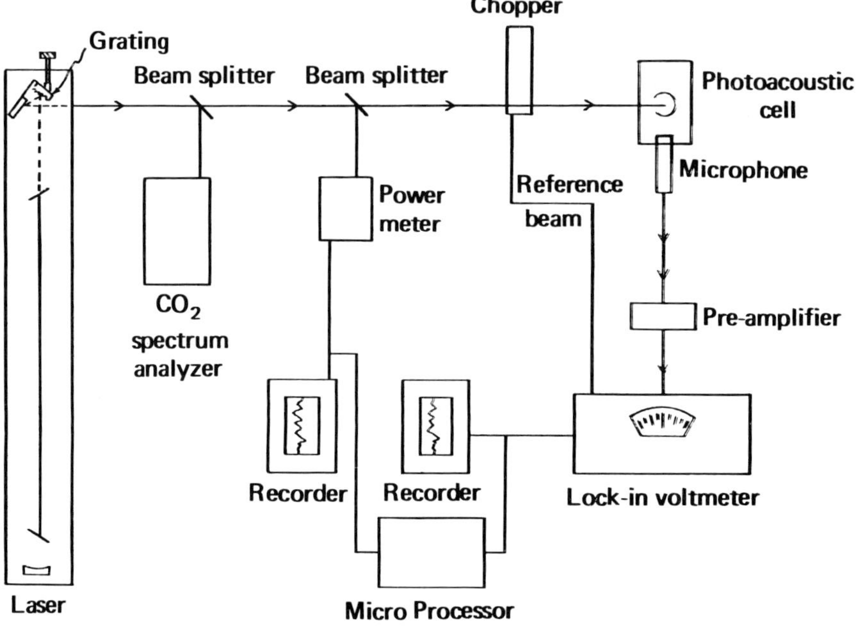


Fig. 15.6. Infrared photoacoustic spectroscope.

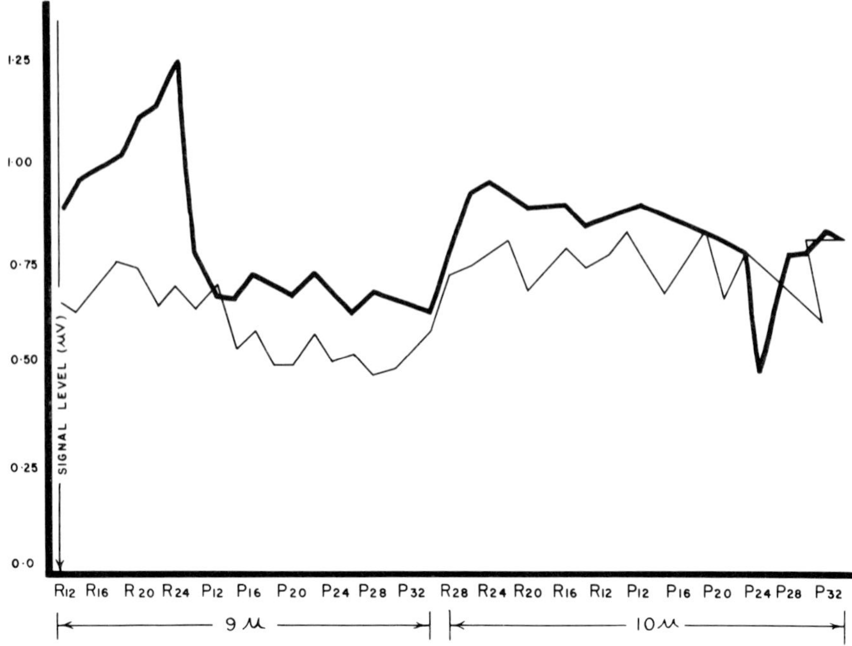


**Fig. 15.7.** Photoacoustic measurements of human tissue made with tunable $CO_2$ laser at 41.1 Hz chopping frequency. *Heavy line*, cancerous; *light line*, normal.

## Development of Endoscopic Microscope-Micromanipulator Delivery Systems

Since the coherent beam of a laser is well collimated, it can be delivered through the tube of an endoscope (Figs. 15.8 and 15.9). The delivery of the laser beam can be accomplished with mirrors or with a combination of mirrors and relay lenses (Figs. 15.10 and 15.11). Visible and short infrared wavelengths can be delivered through a quartz optical fiber. Fiber optics for the $CO_2$ wavelength are still experimental. Aluminum-tube wave guides for $CO_2$ laser delivery have also been experimented with. Polanyi and coworkers developed the first endoscopic delivery system for use in dog experiments. His team also developed a bronchoscope that was first used clinically at Boston University. Since then, various companies have built bronchoscopes and bronchoscopic attachments (Fig. 15.12). A prototype cystoscope for $CO_2$ laser was developed at Boston University and then improved by the Wolf Company in Germany.

Polanyi and coworkers developed a microscope-micromanipulator system. After initial experimentation in the dog, it became evident the $CO_2$ laser beam is very useful in microsurgery. Because a relatively small amount of tissue has to be evaporated in microsurgery, small-output lasers can be used. As for any precision work, magnification is required. This is provided by a surgical microscope. The laser beam is directed by a micromanipulator system, in which the movement of the

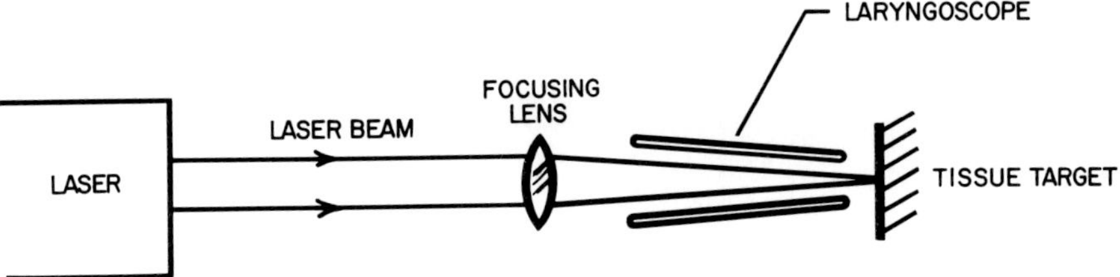


**Fig. 15.8.** Laser delivery system for laryngoscopy.

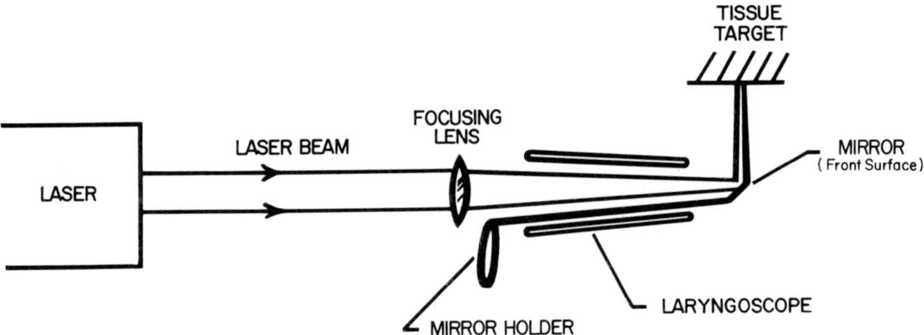


**Fig. 15.9.** Laser delivery system with mirror.

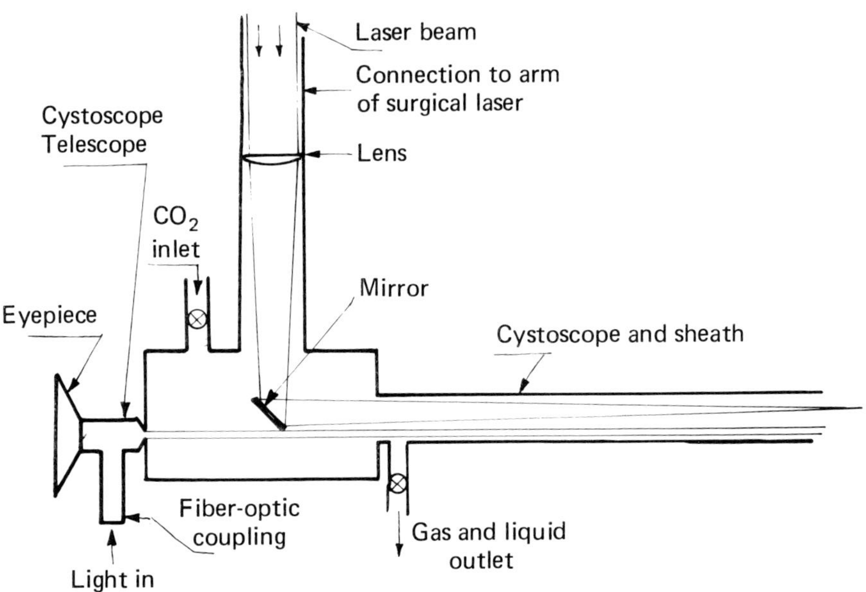


**Fig. 15.10.** Laser endoscope (bronchoscope, cystoscope) with mirror.

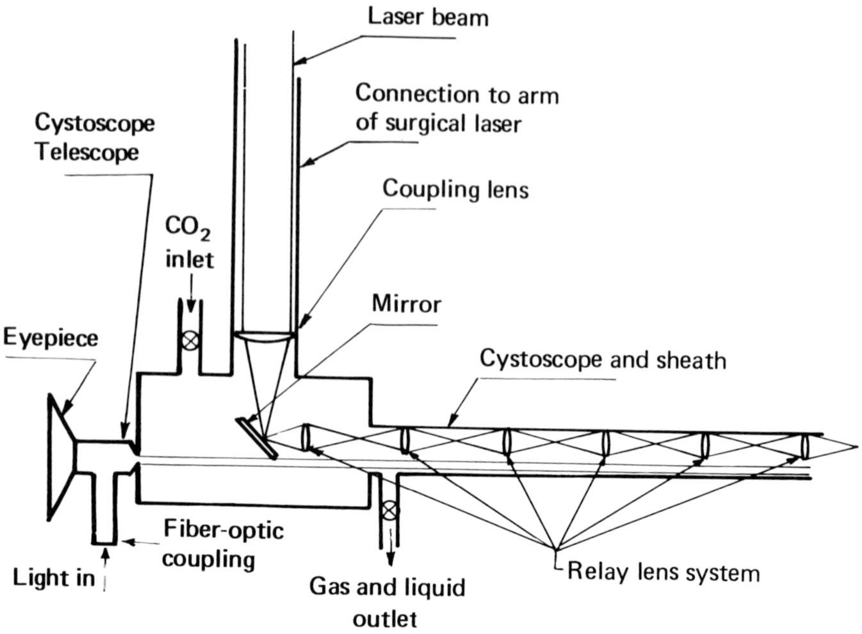


**Fig. 15.11.** Laser endoscope with infrared relay lenses.

beam is mechanically demagnified. The aiming light is a small green point seen only through the microscope. In other systems, a coaxial helium-neon beam is projected onto the target. Further advances in microscope-micromanipulator systems, including compatibility with microprocessors, are being developed.

## Microsurgery with the Carbon Dioxide Laser

Microsurgical application of the laser began in the larynx and expanded into gynecology, neurosurgery, and skin and plastic surgery. In the beginning, a relatively large 1.5–2 mm spot size appeared to be satisfactory for tissue ablation. In the flowing laser systems that were used first, higher-order-mode laser beams also appeared to be satisfactory. It was subsequently realized that for more precision cutting, lasers running in a single mode would be required. Microsurgical instrumentation improved surgical precision in general. Laser microsurgery improved that precision even further. After many years of experience with laser surgery, it now appears that its greatest significance is the precision it brought to surgery.

Laser surgical systems can be classified according to their output ranges. A small 5–10 W system is required for ear surgery, skin surgery, and minor surgery in the nose, throat, and larynx. I developed a prototype of such a small laser (Fig. 15.13). This laser has a single-mode output beam, and its spot size can be varied. A medium-range 10–25 W system is widely used in laryngology and gynecology. The original system was conceived by the author and developed by Polanyi and

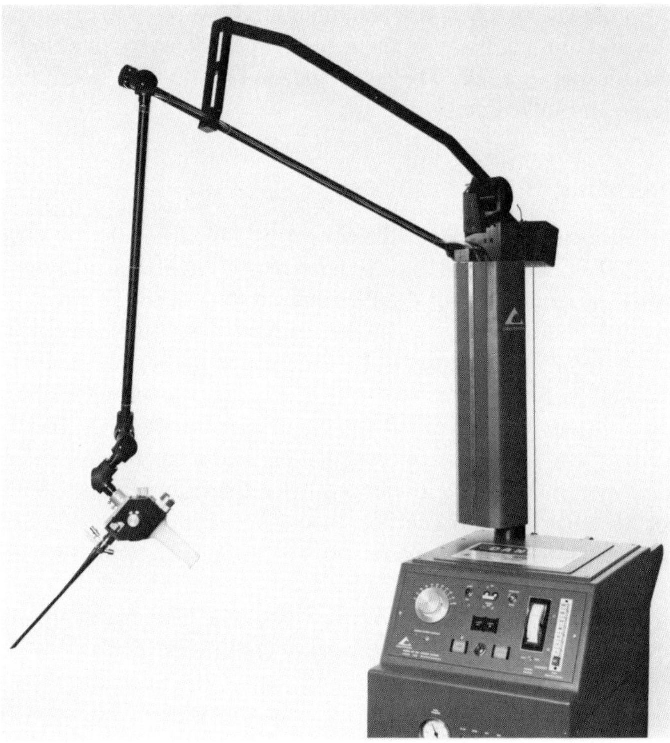

**Fig. 15.12.** Laser bronchoscope. (Courtesy of Cavitron Corp.)

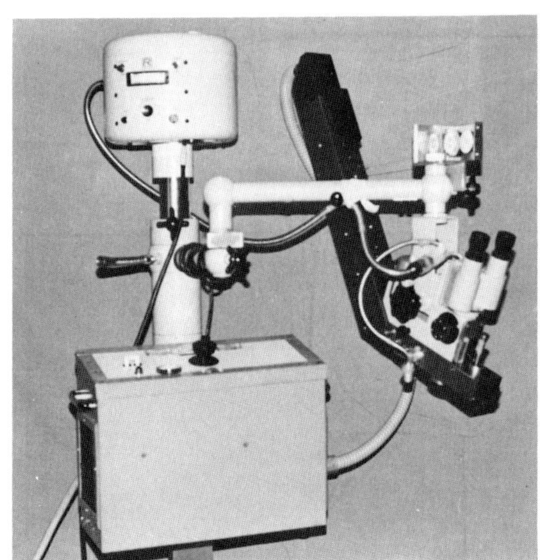

**Fig. 15.13.** Prototype small $CO_2$ laser surgical system for ear surgery. (Courtesy of Dr. G. J. Jako.)

coworkers. Modifications of it are manufactured by several companies in the United States and abroad. None of these laser systems operate in a single mode or allow for variation of spot size. These systems use flowing-type laser tubes, and are relatively large and inflexible.

## Large Operating Room Systems

The original surgical laser system developed by Polanyi and coworkers had an output up to 100 W, and the beam was delivered through an articulated arm. The instrument was large and rather cumbersome in the operating room. It could be attached to a micromanipulator. A smaller copy of this system was built by Laser Industries with up to 50 W output. In the future, a more flexible general operating room system will be needed for head and neck surgery. I am developing a prototype of such a system (Fig. 15.14). This system includes the $CO_2$ laser for cutting and the neodymium-YAG laser for coagulation, and a microscope-micromanipulator delivery system. It has a miniature color television camera built into the microscope. An articulated arm can be attached as a handpiece or for endoscopic application, and the micromanipulator can be driven with a microprocessor.

**The Argon Laser Microsurgical System.** The argon laser has been used for several years for coagulation in the eye. Its wavelength is particularly well absorbed by pigmented tissue and hemoglobin, and very minimally absorbed in water. Therefore, unnecessary damage can result when the beam or scattered beam traveling through fluid is absorbed by well-absorbing tissue elements. In using the argon laser, protective goggles must be worn to protect the eyes of the patient and attendant. Because of the lower wavelength of the argon laser, it can be focused easily to a small spot size, resulting in a relatively high power density. This wavelength can also be conducted in optical fibers (quartz) with minimal loss. Several companies have modified their eye laser systems by adding a micromanipulator delivery system for ear surgery. This system is used by Perkins for stapes surgery and vascular tumors of the ear, such as acoustic neurinoma and glomus tumor. The argon laser with fiber optics is also used for coagulation in the skin and in the nasal turbinates.

**The Neodymium-YAG Laser.** The neodymium-YAG laser was first used to coagulate bleeding esophageal varices. In this endoscopic application, the beam is delivered through a quartz optical fiber. Similar systems have also been reported for laryngeal, neurologic, gynecologic, and urologic surgery. The beam can also be delivered through an articulated arm from a high-output continuous-wave neodymium-YAG laser. This appears to be especially useful for treating cavernous hemangiomas of the head and neck. It is also used in liver surgery.

**The Carbon Monoxide Laser.** The wavelength of the carbon monoxide laser is also well absorbed in water and water-containing tissues. Experimentally, it was used for cutting tissue by Jako, Freed, and Freed. Since a high-output CO laser is relatively large in size and difficult to maintain (cooling), it does not seem to be practical for surgical use at this time.

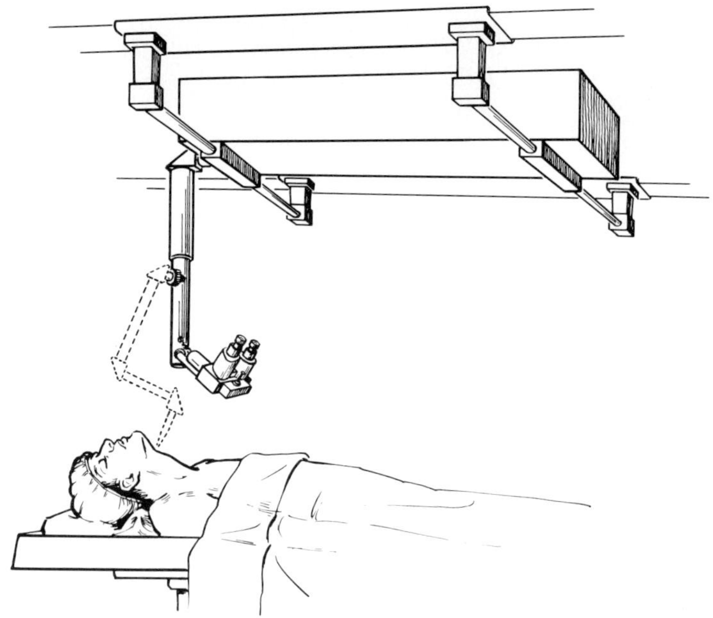

**Fig. 15.14.** Jako general operating room laser system.

**The Helium-Neon Laser.** Mester used the helium-neon laser for stimulating tissue healing experimentally as early as 1968. Since then, it is used for enhancing wound healing in routine clinical work in Hungary, Italy, China, and many other countries. In otolaryngology, this laser is used for enhancing healing of tracheostomas and in perichondritis of the auricle in China (Fig. 15.15). In China and Germany, it is also used for laser acupuncture.

**The Nitrogen Laser.** Nitrogen lasers have a pulsed output in the ultraviolet range at .337 $\mu$m. Medical experimentation and clinical work with them is being performed in China. Experiments were performed using tissue cultures of mouse melanoma. Preliminary results indicate that this wavelength has tumoricidal effects. In humans, two patients who had recurrent cancer of the maxillary sinus were reported to show tumor regression after a course of irradiation with the nitrogen laser.

## APPLICATION OF THE CARBON DIOXIDE LASER—MICROSURGERY IN OTOLARYNGOLOGY

The precision with which the laser beam can be directed by a micromanipulator through an endoscopic tube makes it especially useful for endoscopic microsurgery of the larynx. In 1962, I introduced the instrumentation and technique for microsurgery of the larynx. This technique improved the precision of endoscopic laryn-

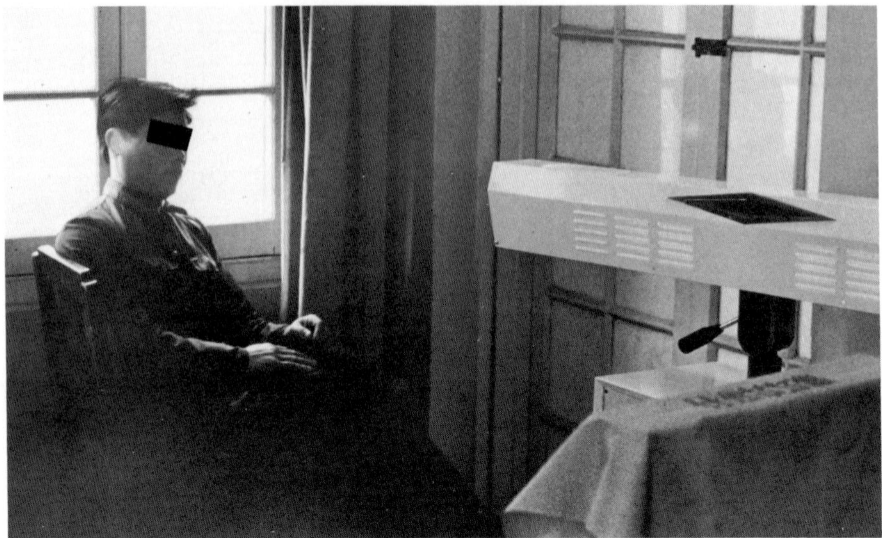

**Fig. 15.15.** Irradiation with 25-W helium-neon laser to treat perichondritis of the auricle, Shanghai.

geal surgery about one order of magnitude. Surgery is performed under general anesthesia and, in most cases, an endotracheal tube is used with oxygen. Endotracheal tubes are made of either plastic or rubber. In this oxygen environment, the plastic or rubber can ignite and burn briskly. If the tube were perforated by the laser beam, the fire could be as intense as a blowtorch. For this reason, every precaution must be taken. Understanding and cooperation between the surgeon and the anesthesiologist are very important. Reasonable protection can be achieved

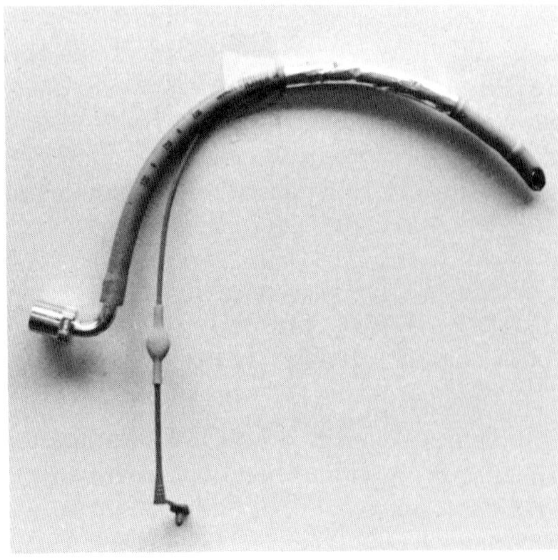

**Fig. 15.16.** Rubber endotracheal tube wrapped with adhesive aluminum foil.

using a red rubber endotracheal tube (Ruesch Co.) wrapped with an adhesive aluminum foil (Fig. 15.16). Use of an unprotected tube is negligence on the part of the surgeon and the anesthesiologist, and can result in fatal accident. Plastic endotracheal tubes, even with aluminum taping, absolutely should not be used. Other endotracheal tubes made of special silicone rubbers have also been tried. Anesthesia techniques without tubes, like Venturi jet, etc., can be used. It is most important that the surgeon and the anesthesiologist learn the importance of safety. This can be best accomplished by learning from an experienced surgical team or by attending a special course.

Special precautions must also be taken to protect the skin, mucosa, and eyes of the patient and operating personnel. This can be best accomplished with wet saline-soaked pads, which will absorb accidental short laser exposure. The soaked pads should be remoistened frequently. The surgeon's eyes are protected by the glass optics of the microscope. The operating room personnel should wear protective glasses or plastic goggles.

## CLINICAL APPLICATIONS

### Larynx

**Benign Tumors.** Precise bloodless removal of vocal-cord nodules, polyps, and cysts can be accomplished easily. If the tumor is larger, it is held by forceps and excised at its base with the laser beam. This way, a biopsy specimen is also obtained for histologic examination. With a small vocal-cord nodule, a similar technique can be used, or the nodule can be evaporated by laser. In the latter case, there is no specimen for histologic examination, and the pathology is recorded by colored photographs shot through the microscope. Papilloma of the larynx usually involves the vocal cords and other mucosal surfaces of the larynx. This tumor bleeds readily when removed with instrumentation. Laser excision provides a nearly bloodless technique (Figs. 15.17 and 15.18). For bilateral polyp or papilloma removal in the anterior commissure, care should be taken to leave the epithelial covering of one vocal cord or a small piece of papilloma on one vocal cord to prevent web formation. The laser for laryngeal surgery has a spot size of about 1.5–2 mm. This results in a cut width of approximately the same size. If the tissue is stretched with the forceps, a finer cut will result. Postoperatively, the laser wound heals fast and results in minimal edema. Occasionally, one can observe more edema during healing, which can be the result of a bad beam caused by misalignment or degradation of mirrors. Laser surgery is usually performed for lesions of the vocal cord. Part of the false vocal cords can be removed in the case of a wedge resection of the false cords for spastic disphonia.

**Malignant Tumors.** Endoscopic excision of carcinoma in situ and small $T_1$ cancers of the vocal cords can be performed with high precision. Partial or total cordectomies and other partial endoscopic laryngectomies are useful in treatment and in classifying tumor for diagnosis. Debulking of large tumors can open up the airway before radiation treatment. In cases of verrucous carcinoma of the larynx, 5-

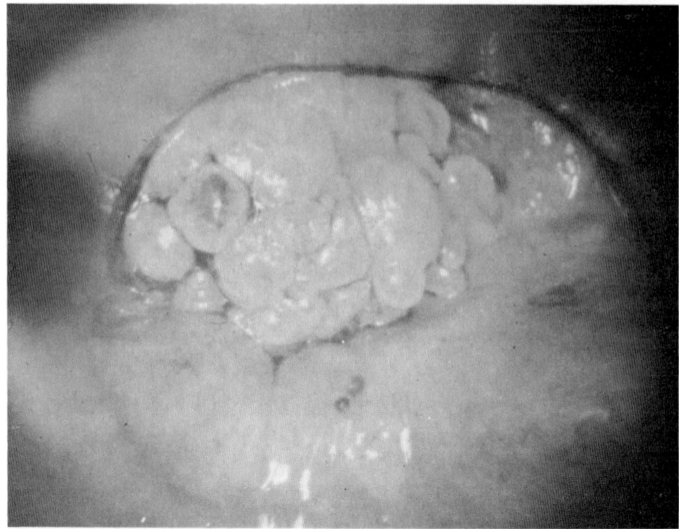

**Fig. 15.17.** Papilloma of the larynx.

year follow-up showed that these tumors responded excellently to this type of conservative surgery (Figs. 15.19–15.21). A 5-year follow-up of small localized vocal-cord tumors resulted in equal or better results than radiation treatment. Recurring cancer of the vocal cords after radiation treatment can also be removed with laser surgery.

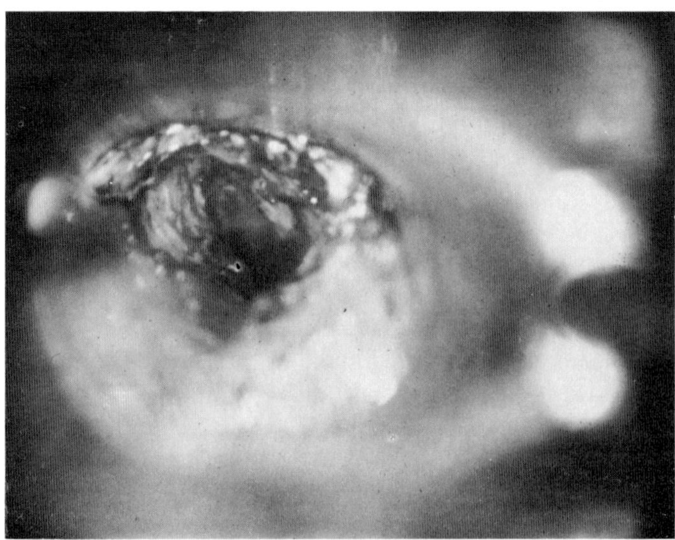

**Fig. 15.18.** Larynx from Figure 15.17 after laser surgery.

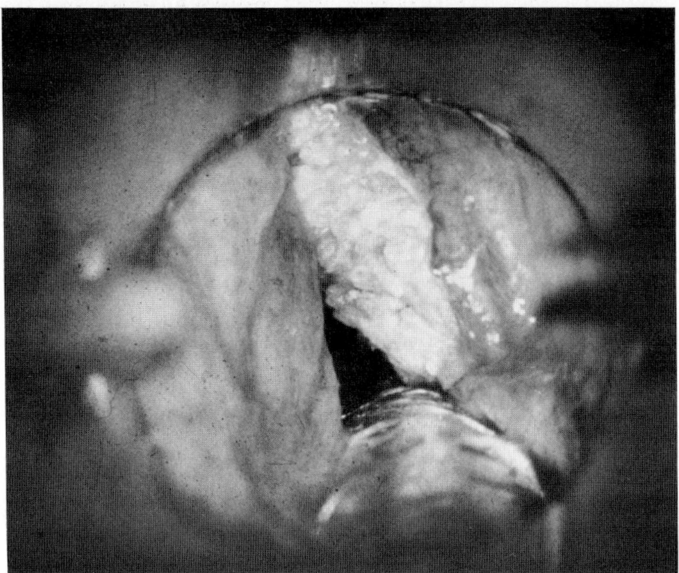

**Fig. 15.19.** Verrucous cancer of the vocal cord.

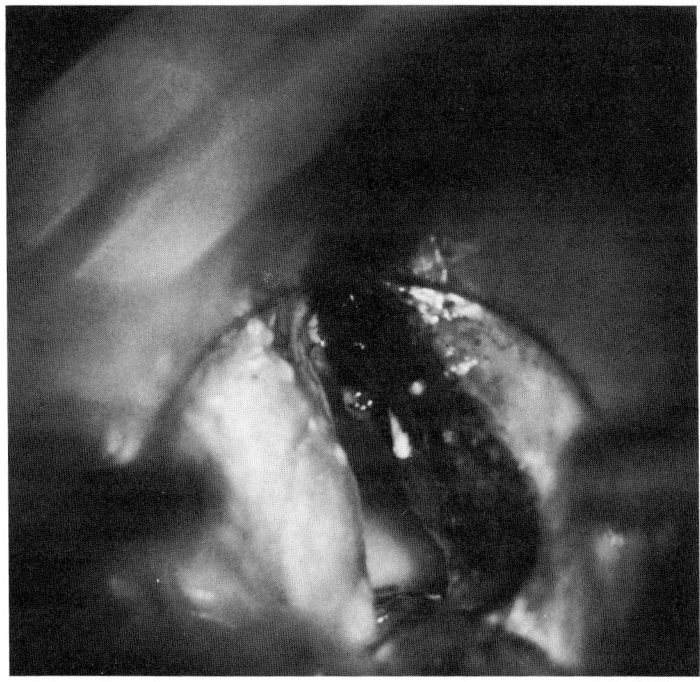

**Fig. 15.20.** Tumor and vocal cord from Figure 15.19 excised.

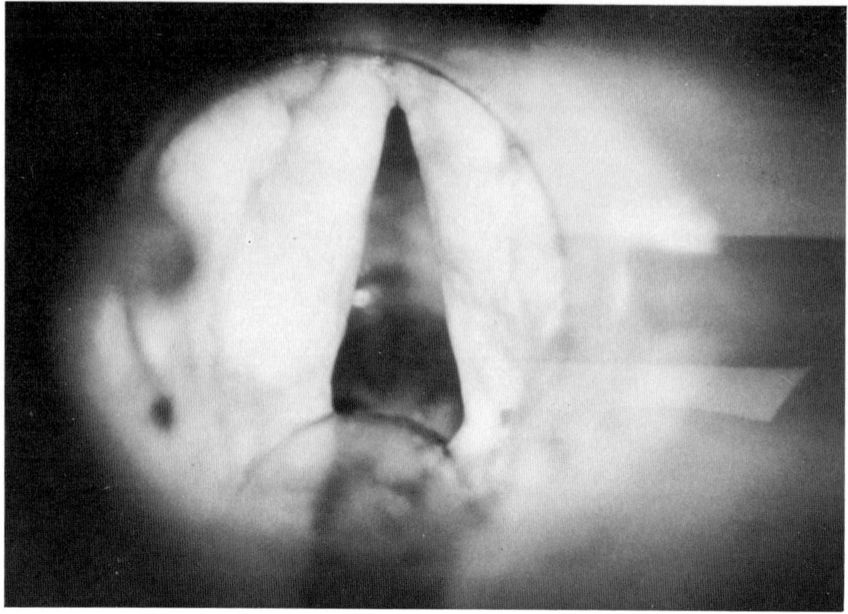

**Fig. 15.21.** Vocal cord from Figure 15.19, 2 years postoperatively.

## Trachea, Hypopharynx, and Esophagus

Papilloma and carcinoma occasionally involve the trachea. Bronchial adenoma in the main bronchus could develop airway blockage. The $CO_2$ laser bronchoscope is used routinely by laryngologists and chest surgeons to improve the airway in the treatment of these lesions. Repeated surgery can be performed to prolong the patient's life. Blocking cancer in the hypopharynx or upper esophagus can be temporarily debulked using the large Jako laryngoscope and the laser microscope.

## Oral Cavity

Small lesions of the buccal mucosa including hyperkeratosis, leukoplakia, and other small benign or malignant lesions can be biopsied and shaved off with the laser. Obstructed salivary-gland openings can be opened or marsupialized with the laser. Small $T_1$ carcinomas can be excised. Surgery on the oral mucosa or gingiva can be performed with practically no bleeding. For surgical procedures of the gingiva

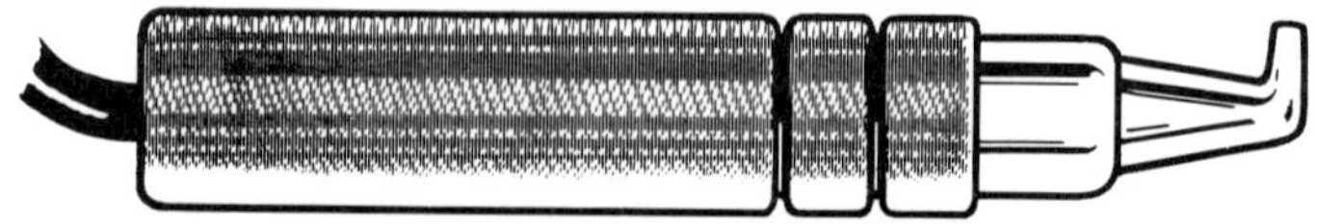

**Fig. 15.22.** Hand-held $CO_2$ dental laser for microsurgery.

and the tooth, a small dental laser was developed (Fig. 15.22). This laser is hand-held and used in connection with the dental microscope.

## Tongue

Surface lesions on the tongue can be precisely shaved off with the laser (Fig. 15.23). Biopsy specimens can also be taken. Laser procedures on surface lesions of the tongue are relatively bloodless. Small malignant lesions of the tongue tip can be excised with the laser alone or combined with electrosurgery.

## Tonsils

Removal of the tonsils with $CO_2$ laser was introduced by French in 1973. It is a relatively bloodless procedure and the postoperative pain is less than that experienced with conventional surgery. The surgery is usually performed with the microscopic delivery system. It is recommended that the laser cut be made more on the side of the tonsil to avoid encountering larger blood vessels in the tonsillar fossa. Bleeding from larger blood vessels requires the use of a hemostat. French developed a black anodized hemostat, the tip of which can be heated with the laser to coagulate the blood vessel.

Retention cysts, papillomas, and other small lesions of the tonsils can be easily excised now. In chronic tonsillitis, frequently the tonsillar crypts are covered and blocked by a thickened inflammatory anterior pillar. In these cases, excision of the

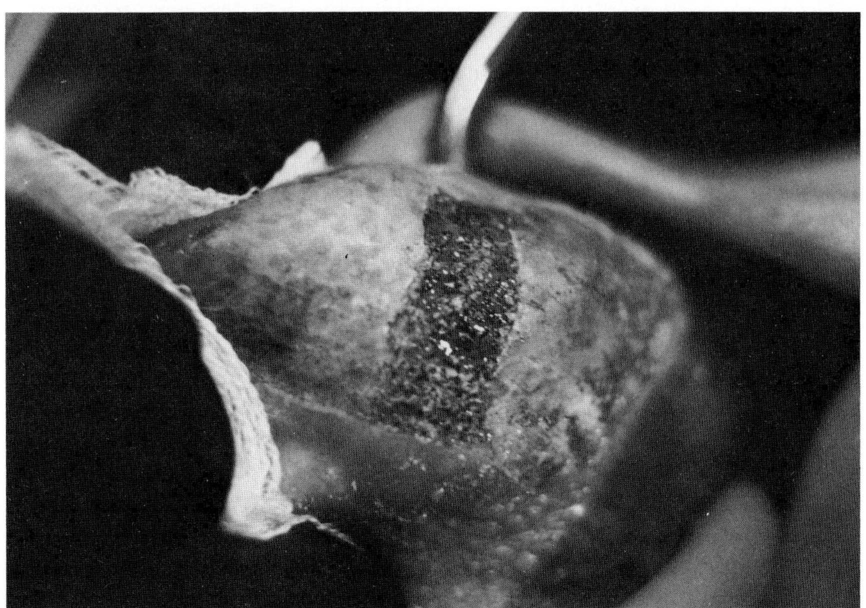

**Fig. 15.23.** Surgical shaving of the tongue with $CO_2$ laser.

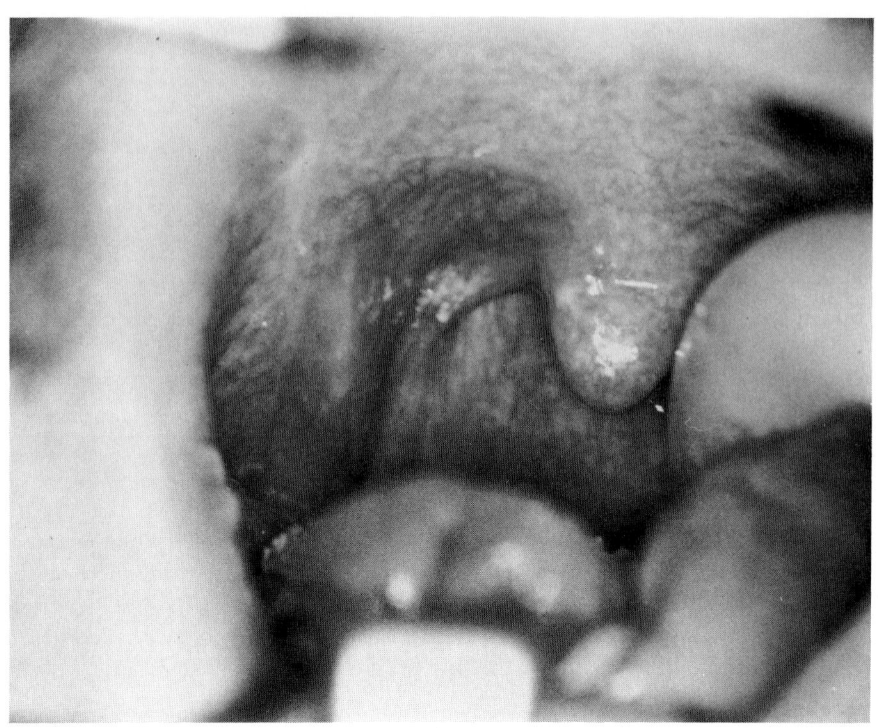

**Fig. 15.24.** Anterior pillar in chronic tonsillitis.

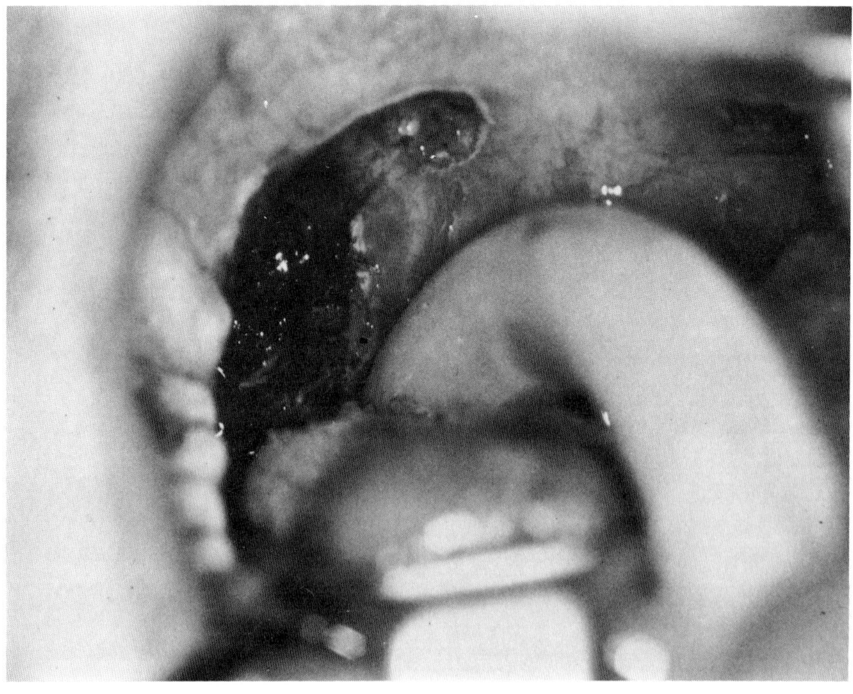

**Fig. 15.25.** Excision of anterior pillar in Figure 15.24.

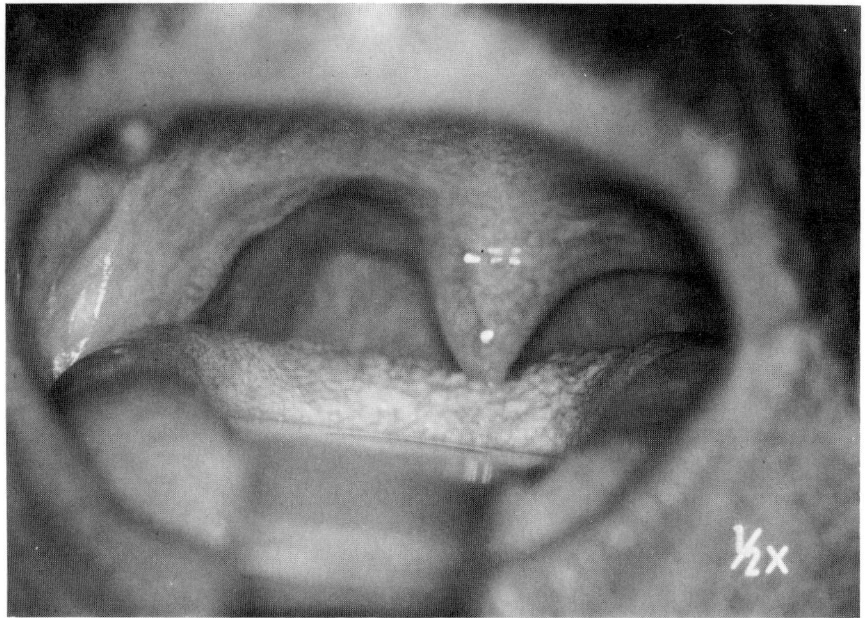


**Fig. 15.26.** Healing of patient in Figure 15.25.

anterior pillar can be easily accomplished without bleeding. This provides a new surgical treatment for certain types of chronic tonsillitis (Figs. 15.24–15.26). The postoperative course here is also relatively painless. For malignant tumors, biopsy or excision of the tumor can be accomplished with precision using the microscope.

## Nose

A low-powered, diffused $CO_2$ beam will coagulate the nasal mucosa. This can be used for cauterization of the small blood vessels in the nasal mucosa. The microscopic laser delivery system is suitable for surgery of both the nasal skin and the nasal mucosa. Small polyps inside the nose can be precisely removed in the area of the sinus openings (Fig. 15.27). Choanal atresia, the membranous type or where only a thin bony septum is present, can be excised with the aid of a special, long nasal speculum. This can also be accomplished using a front surface mirror held in the nasopharynx (Fig. 15.28). Special care should be taken that the underlining bone does not become overheated by the laser.

Surgery of the nasal turbinates, including removal of turbinate tissue and coagulation, has been reported. Argon laser coagulation in the treatment of hypertrophied nasal turbinates is preferable since it causes more scarring than the $CO_2$ laser. Excision of rhinophyma is a practical application for the $CO_2$ laser. Small areas of basal-cell or squamous cancer of the nasal skin or vestibule can also be precisely excised.

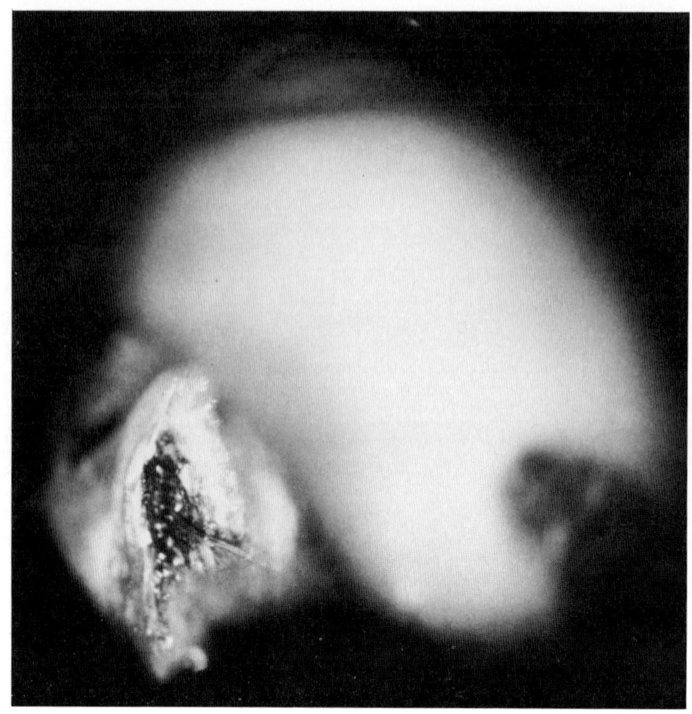

**Fig. 15.27.** Laser excision of small polyp blocking the opening of the nasofrontal duct.

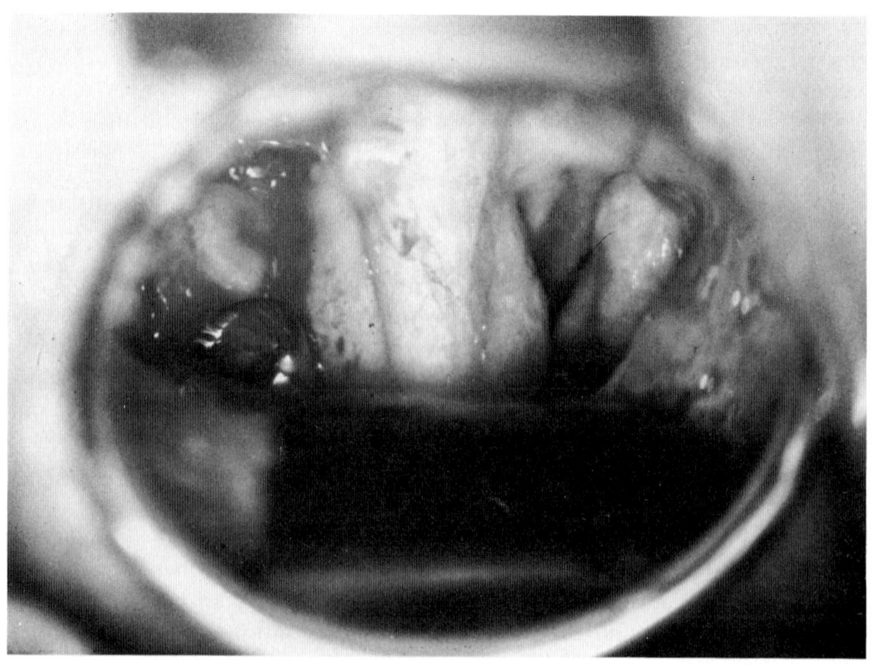

**Fig. 15.28.** Posterior choanae seen under the microscope and mirror.

## Nasopharynx

With the aid of a microscope and a front surface mirror, an excellent view of the nasopharynx can be obtained. The patient's mouth and tongue are retracted with a special self-retaining retractor. The soft palate is retracted with a self-retaining retractor or with rubber catheters inserted through the nose. For the front surface mirror, a metal mirror is not very satisfactory; a surface-coated glass mirror provides better visualization and also reflects the infrared $CO_2$ beam. The beam is moved with the micromanipulator or simply directed by the hand-held mirror. The microscope provides adequate illumination and additional light can be obtained with fiber optics. For removal of smoke and vapor, a plastic catheter is inserted through the nose.

Laser adenoidectomy is a practically bloodless but time-consuming procedure. Removal of small secondary adenoid remnants, especially around the eustachian-tube openings, can be accomplished with great precision. Angiofibroma of the nasopharynx, since it contains large blood vessels, is not suitable for $CO_2$ laser excision. However, after conventional removal, small islands of tumor left in the nasopharynx and posterior nose can be very precisely located with the microscope and removed with the $CO_2$ laser. Cancer of the nasopharynx is generally treated with radiation. Excision of early lesions, if recognized, could be attempted with the microscope and mirror.

## Ear

In 1969, I carried out experimental work in the temporal bone, including perforating the stapedial footplate, ossiculotomy, and myringotomy. In the same year, Jansen and Jako experimented with bone cutting and soft-tissue removal using fresh human temporal bones (Fig. 15.29). From these experiments, it was concluded that the $CO_2$ laser is not practical for cutting bone in the mastoid. It appeared to be useful for thin-bone cutting and especially for soft-tissue removal. Detailed experimental study in the ears of squirrel monkeys was performed by Wilpizeski (1977). I performed myringotomies in two patients in 1974. Ear surgery with $CO_2$ laser has not progressed until recently, because of the need for a small flexible $CO_2$ laser for microsurgery. I built such a laser in 1979 (Fig. 15.13).

**External Ear.** Removal of benign tumors, papilloma and granuloma, and debulking of cancer from the ear canal are practical applications for $CO_2$ laser surgery. Basal-cell carcinoma is another application where precision diagnosis and surgery can be performed under the microscope (Fig. 15.30).

**Middle Ear.** Myringotomy, removal of epithelium and fibrous parts of the tympanic membrane, can be accomplished with precision and without bleeding. Probably the most practical application in ear surgery is the removal of pathological soft tissues, polyps, and cholesteatomas. Since glomus tumor contains large blood vessels, hemostasis is not satisfactory with the $CO_2$ laser.

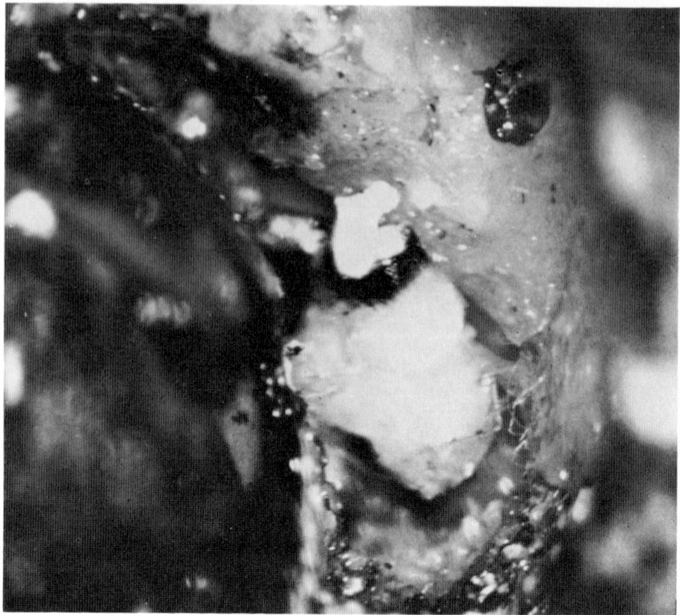

**Fig. 15.29.** Laser surgery of human temporal bone, middle ear, and mastoid, 1969.

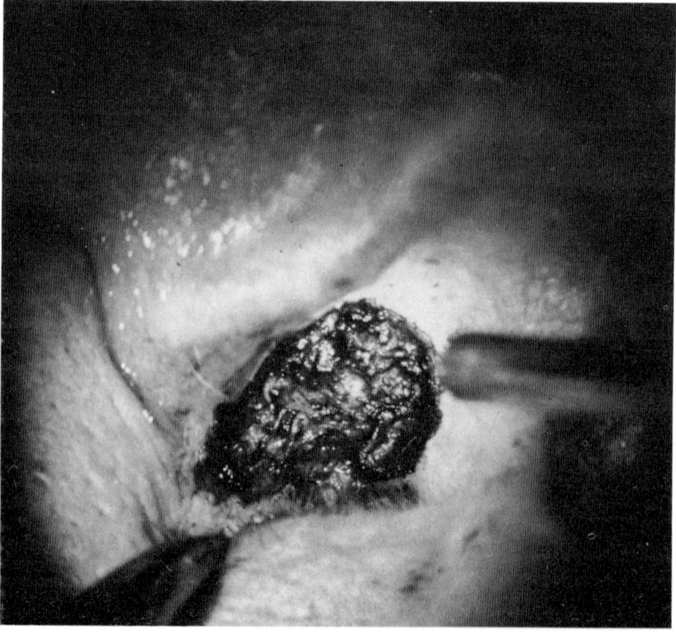

**Fig. 15.30.** Basal-cell carcinoma of the ear excised with $CO_2$ laser microsurgery.

Perkins reported the use of the argon microsurgical system for removing acoustic tumors.

## SUMMARY

After 14 years of use, it appears that the $CO_2$ laser's greatest attribute is precision cutting. The combination of a surgical microscope and the $CO_2$ laser assures great improvement in diagnosis and in microsurgery. Now, with the microscope and the $CO_2$ laser, we can achieve surgical accuracy in the range of 50–100 $\mu$m. The applications in otolaryngology which I have discussed are within the scope of presently available instrumentation. For further progress, new instruments, as suggested in this chapter, will be necessary. In head and neck surgery and in general surgery, the operating room system shown in Fig. 15.14 is a great advance. With this system, the use of the microscope will enable us to differentiate better between normal and pathologic tissues. The combination of the $CO_2$ laser for precision cutting and the neodymium-YAG laser for coagulation greatly advances our surgical capabilities. With this development, combined surgery of the larynx, endoscopic and external, can be performed. Removal of tumorous tissue in the neck can be accomplished with more precision—therefore with more conservation of tissue. The use of this system in general surgery and in other surgical specialties will contribute to medical progress because, with the microscope, smaller details can be seen better and, with the laser, surgery can be performed with greater precision.

## REFERENCES

Andrews AH Jr, Moss HW (1974) Experience with the carbon dioxide laser in the larynx. Ann Otol Rhinol Laryngol 83:462–470.

Conti A, Bergomi A (1966) Irradiazione laser del labirinto posteriore. Arch Ital Biol 77:546–567.

Jako GJ (1970) Laryngoscope for microscopic observation, surgery and photography. Arch Otolaryngol 91:196.

Jako GJ (1972) Laser surgery of the vocal cords. Laryngoscope 82:2204.

Jako GJ (1976) Microsurgery of the larynx with the $CO_2$ laser. In: English G (ed) Otolaryngology, vol. 3. Harper & Row, New York.

Jako GJ, Polanyi TG (1976) Carbon dioxide laser surgery in otolaryngology. In: Kaplan I (ed) Laser Surgery. Academic Press, Jerusalem.

Jako GJ, Wallace RA (1977) Carbon dioxide laser microsurgery and its applications in laryngology. In: Waidelich W (ed) Laser 77 Opto-Electronics: Conference Proceedings. Science and Technology Press, Schenectady, New York.

Jako GJ, Vaughan CW, Polanyi TG (1978) Surgical management of tumors of the upper aerodigestive tract with carbon laser microsurgery. J Surg Oncol 1:265.

Kelemen G, Laor Y, Klein E (1967) Laser induced ear damage. Arch Otolaryngol 86:603–609.

Kiefhaber P, Nath G, Moritz K (1977) Endoscopical control of massive gastrointestinal hemorrhage by irradiation with a high power neodymium YAG laser. Prog Surg 15:140–155.

Lenz H, et al. (1976) Biophysical considerations of laser surgery and the application in otolaryngology. Laryngol Rhinol Otol (Stuttg) 55(7):529–544.
Mester E (1971) Effect of laser rays on wound healing. Am J Surg 122: 532–535.
Mihashi S, Jako GJ, Incze J, Strong MS, Vaughan CW (1975) Laser surgery in otolaryngology: Interaction of $CO_2$ laser and soft tissues. Ann NY Acad Sci 267:263–294.
Norton ML, Strong MS, Vaughan CW, Snow JC, Kripke BJ (1976) Endotracheal intubation and Venturi (jet) ventilation for laser microsurgery of the larynx. Ann Otol Rhinol Laryngol 85:656.
Polanyi TG, Bredemeier HC, David TW Jr (1966) A $CO_2$ laser for surgical research. Med Biol Eng Comp 8:541–548.
Rosencwaig A (1975) Photoacoustic spectroscopy of solids. Physics Today 28:23–30.
Sataloff J (1967) Experimental use of laser in otosclerotic stapes. Arch Otolaryngol 85:614–616.
Snow JC, et al. (1974) Anesthesia for carbon dioxide laser microsurgery on the larynx and trachea. Anesth Analg (Cleve) 53:507.
Stahle J, Hoegberg L (1965) Laser and the labyrinth. Acta Otolaryngol 85:367–374.
Strong MS, Jako GJ (1972) Laser surgery in the larynx. Ann Otol Rhinol Laryngol 81:791.
Strong MS, Vaughan CW, Polanyi TG, Wallace RA (1974) Bronchoscopic $CO_2$ laser surgery. Ann Otol Rhinol Laryngol 83:769–776.
Willscher MK, Filoso AM, Jako GJ, Olsson CA (1978) Development of a $CO_2$ laser cystoscope. J Urol 119:202–207.
Wilpizeski CR (1977) Otological applications of lasers. In: Wolbarsht ML (ed) Laser Applications in Medicine and Biology, vol. 3. Plenum Press, New York, pp. 289–328.

# 16

# Techniques of Laser Burn Surgery

*James P. Fidler*

The two major problems in laser burn surgery are the excision or removal of thermally injured tissue and the closure of the wound with a skin graft. The excision of a thermal burn performed with conventional instruments requires major blood-volume replacement. Skin grafts placed on an excised surface must acquire new circulation in order to remain viable and survive. The ideal laser must cut or excise tissue efficiently, coagulate or close the ends of blood vessels, and permit the growth of new blood vessels into a skin graft.

## HISTORY OF LASER BURN SURGERY

Laser burn surgery began in the experimental laboratory in 1968 (Fidler et al., 1974). Standardized burns were produced in animal models and excised with the available lasers of the day. After preliminary trials, the argon laser and the carbon dioxide ($CO_2$) laser were chosen for the comparative studies with two conventionally used knives, the cold knife (scalpel) and the electric or Bovie knife. At that time, only the argon and $CO_2$ lasers met the qualifications of delivering the necessary power density through an operating arm in a continuous-wave (CW) output. Research models were developed to (1) measure blood loss, (2) study the effect of laser beams on tissue, and (3) measure operating time or speed compared to conventional instruments.

### Blood Loss

Multiple studies followed the report of Hoye and Minton (1965) that the high-powered continuous-wave laser decreased blood loss. The early studies were frequently without controls, but everyone was impressed that a small rat's liver, spleen, and even kidney could be partially excised with the $CO_2$ laser without hemorrhage. In larger animals (e.g., dogs), vessels 1–2 mm in diameter could be coagulated but frequently required additional means of hemostasis. The hemostasis was aided by temporarily lowering the blood pressure or interrupting blood flow through arteries and veins. The partial excision of a dog's liver lobe required dissection of the hepatic artery and portal vein and a vascular clamp control until the resection was completed (Fidler et al., 1975; Mullins et al., 1968). The same proved true in burn experiments. The blood vessels of the skin and subcutaneous layer in rats were controlled without difficulty, but the same vessels in humans were more easily controlled by applying a tourniquet, where applicable, to limbs or by placing traction on the eschar or devitalized tissue until spasm decreased the filling of vessels (Fidler et al., 1974).

In experimental studies on liver and skin tissues, the laser appeared statistically better than the electric knife (Fidler et al., 1975a, 1975b; Levine et al., 1975). The electric knife can incise with a cutting-mode current, coagulation-mode current, or spark-gap current. These three modes affect the coagulation of blood vessels differently and produce different amounts of heat damage. The coagulation current of the Bovie and the spark-gap technique proved as hemostatic as the $CO_2$ laser but increased the damage to the underlying recipient bed. Only the cutting mode of the electric knife compares with the tissue damage of the focused $CO_2$ laser beam. In comparison studies between the two modalities, the $CO_2$ laser had less blood loss than the cutting mode of the electric knife.

## Effect of Laser Beam on Tissues

Wound healing following laser-produced incisions or excisions were of marked interest to clinicians. In the laboratory, all the thermal knives—which include the plasma scalpel, electric knife, and lasers—were found to prolong the healing time of incisions or wounds (Glover et al., 1978; Hall et al., 1971). This was true of incisions made on the backs of rats, compared to conventionally made incisions with knives and was true of excised portions of tissue made on the backs of rats when compared to the cold-knife–excised tissue (Hishimoto et al., 1975). When a thermal knife was used, it took 40 days for incisions to gain the same tensile strength (Glover et al., 1978) as an incision made with a knife or scalpel. The contraction or epithelialization of a 2-$cm^2$-size portion of rat's back was 20% slower when made with a thermal knife at 2 weeks and required 28 days to approach 95% closure of the wound (Hishimoto et al., 1975). Despite these delays, incisions or wounds did heal. The skin graft take and survival in animal experiments are never better than those of the cold-knife controls, and when lost, the growth of new skin or the epithelialization over denuded areas is prolonged (Fidler et al., 1974). Madden et al. (1970) found the resistance of wounds to infection significantly greater in wounds made with a steel knife than in those made with the electrosurgical unit or $CO_2$ laser. They furthermore found electrosurgical wounds more resistant to infection than the laser wounds.

## Operating Time of the Laser Compared to Conventional Instruments

None of the thermal knives, including the conventional electric knife and lasers, were able to make incisions at a rate comparable to that of the cold knife. The first limitation was the laser machine itself. This was particularly true of the argon laser, the neodymium-YAG (Nd-YAG) laser, and also the early models of the $CO_2$ laser, in which laser use at full power output was slower than the scalpel.

When more powerful outputs became available, surgeons continued to work at a slower rate with the thermal knives than with the scalpel for two reasons: First, the surgeon was unable to control the unlimited power without creating a deeper injury than was prudent. Second, the increased rate of cutting decreased the heat effect on tissues and the coagulation of vessels. The burn surgeon continued to cut at a slower speed than he normally would with the scalpel, but had a drier field. Despite the wound-healing effects of lasers and slower operating speed, the pronounced decrease in blood loss encouraged the use of lasers in burn research.

## Control Knives and Sites

It is evident from the early studies that the ideal laser has to approach the cutting speed, the wound healing, and the simplicity of the cold knife, and the decreased blood loss of the relatively cheap electric knife. Comparison studies in burns require the same size burn, the same site, and the same postburn day. Therefore, one-half of the back is compared to the opposite side of the back but not to the same size burn on the chest or limbs. The burn lesion is such that each postburn day, the amount of edema fluid, and the extent of inflammatory reaction or infection changes. These changes affect the laser, the coagulation process, and the amount of blood in the vessels. Burn excisions performed after the inflammatory reaction has reached its peak from the burn (3–5 days) or after an infection bleed more. Extremity surgery bleeds more and is technically more difficult than trunk surgery unless additional surgical adjuncts, such as tourniquets, are used.

## Identification of Side Effects

In the early animal models, the investigators were concerned with any (1) deleterious tissue change, including cancer formation, wound healing, and x-ray effects; (2) air pollution carrying viable tumor cells, infection, particulate matter, or damaging chemicals; and (3) safety of lasers in both the laboratory and the clinical setting.

**Tissue Damage.** The clinical lasers in use for animal and human tissue did not contain x rays or ultraviolet rays, and to our present knowledge, did not produce cancer. All known tissue change was believed to be explained by heat.

**Air Pollution from the Steam and Vapor of the Laser Incision.** Air pollution is a constant problem. The associated odor of burned tissue is annoying. The possible transfer of bacteria or of chemicals capable of damaging the lungs of patients or operating personnel requires constant vigilance. Attempts to grow bacteria from material collected in the filters of suction machines have failed. Special suction machines were devised to keep both the amount and the odor of burned tissue to a minimum.

**Safety.** In early animal experiments, techniques were worked out to prevent the drapes from catching fire, eye damage, skin damage, and anesthesia explosions, and routines were developed to sterilize and drape the laser equipment.

## Success of the Carbon Dioxide Laser in Burn Surgery

Although imperfect, the $CO_2$ laser emerged as the laser of choice for burn surgery. The $CO_2$ is the fastest cutting laser and produces the least thermal damage to the sides of the incision. The $CO_2$ laser achieved a greater irradiance or power density ($W/cm^2$) than other lasers for three reasons: (1) greater power output, (2) a good absorption coefficient, and (3) a nonspecific absorption for tissues involved in burn surgery.

The greater power output was due to a simpler laser device for reasons beyond the scope of this report. The good absorption coefficient ($200–900^{cm^{-1}}$) meant the beam was absorbed within 200 $\mu$m of tissue and quickly reached the vaporization point of water. The nonspecificity meant the absorption coefficient remained high for all soft tissues of the body containing water.

The 10,600-nm beam approaches an absorption coefficient of $950^{cm^{-1}}$ for water. Most tissues, with the exception of bone, contain about 40%–60% of their weight in water and provide a range of absorption coefficient from $950^{cm^{-1}}$ to $200^{cm^{-1}}$. The tissue depth penetration of the $CO_2$ laser for 98% absorption can be calculated from the equation $e^{-\alpha x} = 0.02$, where $\alpha$ is equal to the absorption coefficient, and $\chi$, the tissue depth needed to absorb 98% of the incident energy. The excellent absorption coefficient of tissues for the $CO_2$ laser decreases the volume of injured tissue, in comparison to that with other lasers and is comparable to the cutting mode of the electric knife but causes less damage than that created by the plasma scalpel.

The $CO_2$ laser was the fastest cutting laser and produced less conduction thermal damage to the sides of the incision. The amount of heat damage produced correlates directly with the cutting speed or time the beam is held in one place and the absorption coefficient or amount of tissue needed to absorb the beam. Increased power allowed for faster movement of the laser beam at any given depth and therefore less heat damage.

The minimal damage to the tissue allowed for excellent skin graft take but limited the size of blood vessels that the $CO_2$ laser could control. Thermal injuries incite an inflammatory response. A marked influx of salt solution and protein (edema fluid) accumulates in the tissue as a result of dilation of all blood vessels (hyperemia) and increased loss of the fluid through the vessel walls. This hyperemic response is the cause of the massive blood loss in burns. Fortunately, most of the vessels are capillary size at the skin and subcutaneous level, and the $CO_2$ laser seals the severed ends as it cuts. Thus, the $CO_2$ laser was chosen over other lasers because of the power output it could achieve, the nonspecific absorption coefficient, and the minimal tissue damage, permitting immediate skin grafting.

## CLINICAL USE OF THE CARBON DIOXIDE LASER

### Comparative Studies

Levine et al. (1972) reported the first clinical $CO_2$ laser excision of a burn with immediate autograft closure. Within a year of their work, a comparative study was performed at the Shriner's Burns Institute in Cincinnati, consisting of 15 excisional procedures in children (Fidler et al., 1974). The study compared blood loss, operating time, and successful autograft take between the cold-knife control excision area and the $CO_2$ laser excision area. The same study was repeated in 13 excisional procedures performed on 11 children to compare blood loss, operating time, and successful autograft take between the area of control excision with the Bovie electrosurgical knife and the area excised with the $CO_2$ laser (Fidler et al., 1975). As expected, the clinical studies tended to repeat the studies in animals.

**Blood Loss in Clinical Studies.** An average of 3.9 cc of blood and a median of 3.4 cc was lost with steel scalpel excision compared with 1 cc of blood lost with $CO_2$ laser excision per unit area. An average 3.5 cc and a median of 2.3 cc of blood were lost with the electrosurgical unit for each 1 cc lost with the $CO_2$ laser per unit area. Only in 5 of 13 operations was it apparent that more blood was lost with the electrosurgical scalpel than with the $CO_2$ laser. In 2 of the 13 operations more blood was lost with the laser than with the electric knife per unit area. In the remaining 6 operations, measurement of blood loss normalized against the size of the eschar was necessary before a difference was discernible in favor of the laser. The electrosurgical-laser results are in contrast to the $CO_2$ laser steel scalpel series in which there was a grossly discernible difference in favor of the laser in all but one procedure.

**Operating Time in Clinical Studies.** Fidler et al. (1974) found both the multimode $CO_2$ laser machine, with an irradiance of 1–5 $kW/cm^2$, and the single-mode machine, with an irradiance of 5–20 $kW/cm^2$, slower than either the cold knife or the electric knife. The $CO_2$ laser averaged 1.6 min of operating time for each minute to excise a similar area with a steel scalpel and 1.2 min of operating time for each minute with the electrosurgical knife. The operating time includes the actual cutting time and the time it took to control hemorrhage with clamps and ligatures. Levine et al. (1975) performed comparison studies on adults at the Brook Army Burn Center and found the laser excisions faster than the electrosurgical unit, 1:1.37, but slower than the knife, 1:0.67. They also found the blood loss ratios for laser, electrosurgery, and steel scalpels, 1:1.7:3.3, in favor of the $CO_2$ laser.

In clinical experiments, the operating time varied with the meticulous nature of the surgeon, the difficulty of the procedure, the awkwardness of the laser for changing planes, and the uniqueness of the patient. The more meticulous the surgeon, the more slowly he moves in order to protect the tissues and to obtain better hemostasis. The operations last longer, but the blood loss is less and the skin graft take is frequently improved. Of the knives compared—the scalpel, electric knife, plasma scalpel, and $CO_2$ laser—the $CO_2$ laser was the most awkward to manipulate and handle. Extremity work in children was particularly difficult because of a constantly changing plane of incision. A good, flexible cable for conducting the $CO_2$ beam is not yet available. The $CO_2$ laser requires a straight-arm vertical pipe that interferes with the surgeon's head, his light, and his mobility. The handpiece is heavier than other cutting modalities including other lasers. Therefore, the $CO_2$ laser, although the most ideal for burn surgery, is the most awkward in the operating room environment.

## Surgical Techniques

**The Burn Patient.** The uniqueness of the patient is of great concern in burn surgery. MacMillan (1978) noted that the excision of a 10%–20% total body surface (TBS) burn may require 2000–4000 ml or 8–10 pints of blood in adults. Excision of similar size burns on different parts of the body will result in major differences in blood loss and operating time. A burn of 18% TBS of the chest and abdomen of a child or an adult will require less blood than a similar 18% TBS from the leg. The adult may lose more per unit area than the child because of the greater percentage of larger vessels although the percent of total blood volume lost is equal.

The anatomic difference in blood loss is changed by the use of a pneumatic tourniquet placed high on the extremity and, if necessary, over the burn. The excision of a burn of 18% TBS from the anterior chest and abdomen may result in more or less blood loss than the removal of a similar area of the back 3 days later. The blood loss will depend on the blood-clotting factors of the patient, the volume of edema fluid within and around the burn, and the amount of inflammation secondary to infection within the burn itself.

The large amounts of fluid given to the patient in the resuscitation period following major burns of 15% TBS or more accumulate in the burn and in the tissues adjacent to the burn and remain until mobilized and excreted some days later. The surgeon excising the burn eschar must place his excision through this fluid. Since most body fluids have an excellent absorption coefficient for the 10,600-nm $CO_2$ laser beam, excision time and the heat effect on the tissue is decreased.

Blood itself acts as a similar impediment to an incision made with the laser beam if the beam is absorbed in the blood. The laser surgeon learns to control the blood that collects in the incision site and develops techniques that decrease the amount of blood the beam must incise in order to reach the desired line of separation. In burn surgery there is marked inflammation and engorgement of vessels at the site of the burn eschar, and it is not uncommon to replace the entire blood volume of a child or adult in excising large areas of burn surfaces using a knife or steel scalpel.

Such techniques as the lowering of blood pressure, the application of tourniquets, and the use of constricting drugs at the burn site are employed in an effort to decrease the amount of blood loss.

**The Use of Traction.** Locally, the surgeon stretches the vessels by placing Kocher clamps or other similar instruments on tissues and pulling on the eschar. This places the vessels in spasm and elevates the line of incision above the remaining part of the operating field. The laser cuts more quickly through the spastic vessel since there is less blood to absorb the energy and less blood flow for convection of heat loss. The traction on the eschar also helps to identify the tissue planes. The incision, regardless of the cutting modality, is generally placed between the fat layer and the deep fascia, and only the vessels are cut. An attempt is made to protect the underlying deep fascia from heat damage to permit a better take and survival of the skin grafts.

**Comparison with the Electric Knife.** The ultimate blood loss experiments for the $CO_2$ laser are the comparison studies with the electric knife. Unfortunately, there exist many variables with the electric knife that make studies to compare one to the other difficult to interpret. The surgeon is a major variable because of his individual surgical technique. Some surgeons prefer to cut as quickly as possible with the electric knife and then to control the resultant bleeding points after the entire specimen has been removed. Other surgeons will attempt to control the blood loss and vessels as incised or prior to the incision. This alters not only the operating time but the amount of blood loss. The electric knife has a cutting mode, a coagulation mode, and a spark-gap potential. The resulting tissue damage changes markedly with the type mode being used by the electric knife. The so-called cutting mode using a radio frequency results in heat damage on histologic examination identical to that caused by the $CO_2$ laser. The pathologist cannot determine with routine hematoxylin and eosin staining methods whether an incision has been made with the focused $CO_2$ laser beam or the cutting mode of the Bovie knife, even though the $CO_2$ laser is more hemostatic. The difference may be due partly to the slower use of the laser than the electric knife, thereby producing the drier field.

The coagulation mode, a blend of the coagulation and cutting modes, or the spark-gap method are all more hemostatic than the cutting mode alone but cause more heat damage than either the $CO_2$ laser or the cutting mode. We reserve their use for very edematous tissues.

**Skin Graft Take and Survival.** We have been unable to ascertain any short-term difference in skin graft take or survival among patients who have undergone excision by the $CO_2$ laser, those on whom the electric knife was used, or those whose excision was by cold knife. Although a carefully controlled experiment in the laboratory might show a difference, our attempts to find a model to measure the tensile holding ability of the grafts have not led to reproducible results.

**Suctioning the Laser Plume.** The $CO_2$ laser causes vaporization of extracellular and intracellular water at the incision site and produces a great deal of steam or smoke, called the laser plume. The steam is suctioned from the operating site. We have failed to grow bacteria or fungi from the filtered vacuum hose despite almost uniform contamination of burn wounds and granulating tissues with these organisms. The pollution of the air with the steam and smoke contents is unpleasant to operating room personnel. We have used a commercial vacuum built to clean hospital floors and attached it to a hose wrapped in a gas-sterilized plastic drape. A sterile trouble light (Fig. 16.1) is placed on the end of the hose to prevent the suction of sponges into the vacuum.

**Incidence of Cancer.** There is interest in whether an increased incidence of cancer can be expected from laser-beam burns, particularly when imposed on a lesion associated with Marjolin's ulcers. A Marjolin ulcer is a malignant change in an indolent ulcer or scar secondary to an old burn or roentgen-ray treatment. Despite watching for these lesions, we are not aware of their presence in either sheet grafts or expanded grafts (which have more scarring).

## Safety Techniques in the Operating Room

*Eyes.* All operating personnel use either their own personal glasses or safety glasses to protect the eyes from possible reflected or direct beams of laser light. The lesion produced in the eye depends on whether the beam is absorbed in the superficial layers of the eye (e.g., $CO_2$ laser in the conjunctiva) or in the pigmented layers (e.g., the selective lasers, ruby and argon, for the retina). The visible-light lasers require special glasses to absorb their respective frequency. This, unfortunately, makes the beams invisible like the $CO_2$ laser beam. Regular glass protects the eye from the $CO_2$ laser beam, but contact lenses alone are not adequate protection. My preference is visors with low magnification for protection as well as for visualizing blood vessels during the operative procedure.

*Skin Protection.* Surgical gowns and gloves protect the surgeon from most non-focused reflected beams unless the energy is such that a fire can be created. Direct focusing of the beam will burn a hole directly through the cloth or rubber gloves of the surgeon. Care must be used around the drapes and towels near the operating wound. This is particularly true of paper drapes, gauze sponges, or laparotomy tapes that may be in the operating field. A wet saline-soaked laparotomy tape or towel is usually sufficient to protect the edges of the wound or underlying drapes from incidental or direct laser-beam injury or fire. A directly focused beam will penetrate gown, gloves, and thin-glass materials, and is a potential hazard to the operating personnel and patient.

Accidents are most likely to occur on terminating an incision when the surgeon completely severs a fragment of tissue. The beam continues in a straight line until

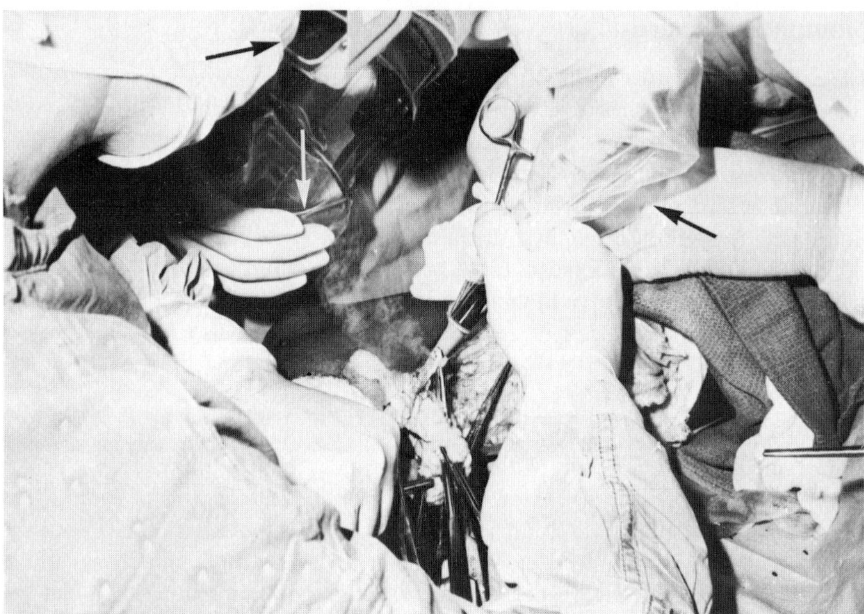

**Fig. 16.1.** Sharplan $CO_2$ laser operating arm wrapped in sterile plastic in the surgeon's hand *(right arrow).* Note protective glasses *(left arrow).* A trouble light *(white arrow)* seen in the operating field is attached to strong suction to remove steam and smoke.

absorbed, reflected, or scattered, whether the object in its path be the surgeon's or assistant's operating hand or a wet sponge.

This is a particular problem for novices who are becoming acquainted with the laser. There is a tendency to forget that the beam continues until absorbed by some structure or turned off. This is not true of any other knife (Bovie, plasma scalpel, heated knife, or cold-steel scalpel) that the surgeon leaves in an "on" position. The surgeon must learn always to aim the laser beam at a safe structure. In contrast to the laser, almost all other foot-driven instruments used in the operating room, such as the electric knife, dermatomes, etc., terminate their action once the instrument is lifted from the patient. Neither the surgeon nor the assistants easily forget a laser impact on their operating hands. The sensation is similar to that of the burn suffered with the electric knife when a hole occurs in the surgeon's glove. Even when the burn is less than a millimeter in diameter or point size, it is painful for several days.

Only nonexplosive anesthetic agents are used in the room with the laser. This is also true when all other thermal knives are used.

The electric knife is the only thermal scalpel that is currently competitive with the $CO_2$ laser in the operating room. At the time of this writing, the plasma scalpel and other experimental thermal knives are not considered conventional instruments.

## Competing Thermal Knives in Burn Surgery

**Electrosurgical Unit.** The most frequently used thermal knife in burn surgery is the electric knife. It is relatively cheap, easy to operate, available, requires no special eye protection, allows physical contact of the knife with tissue, and may be used in a variety of modes. No special permits are needed for its use. It has the potential hazard of electrocuting both the patient and the operating personnel unless care is taken in grounding the patient. Most operating room floors are conductive and place the operating room personnel at risk if their gloves acquire a hole during the procedure. Monitoring devices, e.g., an electroencephalograph, may offer a low impedance path for the current to complete its circuit, and serious burns can result unless protective circuitry is built into the machine.

**Plasma Scalpel.** The plasma scalpel, as developed by Glover et al. (1978), cuts and cauterizes simultaneously with a hot plasma-gas jet. The plasma gas is generated by passing a noble gas (argon, helium) through a direct-current electric arc. The temperature of the gas approaches 6000°C and is partially ionized until the gas cools. When a free electron recombines with an atom, a photon of light is released. Hazards include deeper thermal damage than that caused by either the focused $CO_2$ laser or cutting mode of the electrosurgical unit. Although this heat produces a drier operating field, theoretically it makes grafting more hazardous. However, animal skin grafts take well in excised burn surfaces in the pig. The initial animal experiments show that for each milliliter of blood lost with the plasma scalpel, 2.5 ml and 5.5 ml were lost with the electrosurgery scalpel and steel scalpel, respectively. Studies on patients are not complete. A second hazard involves argon-gas embolism. Liver excisions in rhesus monkeys resulted in lethal injuries in the experiments of Hishimoto et al. (1975). This hazard has supposedly been corrected in the recent plasma scalpel models and experiments on dog liver in the laboratory studies by Glover et al. (1978).

**Argon, Neodymium-YAG, and Ruby Lasers.** There was early failure of the argon, neodymium-YAG (Nd-YAG), and ruby lasers in burn surgery despite the fact that photocoagulation of blood vessels or the control of a bleeding surface was easier to achieve in pigmented surfaces with these lasers than with the $CO_2$ laser. However, the ruby laser was available only as a pulsed laser and could not incise or compete with the CW lasers. As noted by Goldman and Rockwell (1971a), the argon laser was hindered by three factors: (1) poor output; (2) a fair, $37^{cm^{-1}}$ absorption coefficient for pigmented tissue; and (3) marked specificity or absorption of the beam. A large part of the 488-nm argon beam is reflected (35%) from human skin, and although absorption increases with the amount of pigmentation, incision of lightly colored fat is almost impossible and ruled out the argon laser for burn excision. Similar arguments were made against the Nd-YAG laser. The output was greater than that of the argon laser, but the absorption coefficient for excisional purposes was poor and grafting over the excised surfaces was therefore at high risk of failure. New machines constructed in the late 1970s have high-output energy in both the argon or Nd-YAG frequencies and make incision with these instruments possible, but they result in greater depth of injury than does the $CO_2$ laser. An adaptation of the argon laser, in which the optical radiation is coupled with a transparent blade that mechanically cuts and photocoagulates, is now being introduced by Auth (1979).

**Heated Mechanical Blades.** The heated knife, popularized by Shaw and described by Levenson (1979), and the argon-coagulation knife of Auth (1979) both use a mechanical blade to incise tissue and control bleeding by heating a steel blade, in the first instance, or argon photocoagulation, in the second instance. Animal laboratory trials are currently being replaced by human studies. The advantage of these instruments may lie in their ability to incise in layers or to shave tangentially the necrotic burn tissue until pinpoint bleeding and a viable base capable of supporting a graft is achieved. The cosmetic and functional results of the current tangential method of Janzkovič (1976) is superb compared to the fascial plane at which the $CO_2$ laser excision is usually performed. The tangential method currently is limited to burns of 20% TBS by most surgeons (or one total blood volume of the patient) because of the severe blood loss. If these knives prove capable of tangential excisions, they will have a distinct advantage over the $CO_2$ laser, the electrosurgical unit, or the plasma scalpel, as these instruments are currently used.

**Carbon Dioxide Laser.** The $CO_2$ laser is currently the laser of choice in burn work. It has proved in both animal and clinical trials to be dependable and more hemostatic than the electrosurgical knife. Any size burn can be excised but usually in 15%–20% TBS stages and grafted immediately. The $CO_2$ laser's main disadvantages lie in its awkwardness and the inability to perform tangential excisions. The latter problem could theoretically be overcome by using a $CO_2$ laser dermatome with unlimited power but incising a measured segment of tissue.

**Topical Enzymes.** Topical enzymes and chemical agents also have the potential of competing with the thermal knives in the debridement of burns. Their widespread use is hampered by a slow (5- to 7-day) debridement period, uneven debridement when necrotic fat is present, and an increase of invasive infections. All of the foregoing problems are currently being investigated in the laboratory and may prove correctable. If perfected, topical debridement would avoid any mechanical excision and blood loss.

## Specifications for Placing the Laser in the Operating Room

**Electrical Codes.** Operating room (OR) electrical codes make it difficult to place some lasers in the OR. This is particularly true of the argon laser, which requires special wiring. Conductive floors and regulations introduced at the height of the use of combustible anesthetic agents are partly to blame for the severe restrictions of the electrical codes. These codes are beyond the scope of this chapter and should be reviewed by any manufacturer wishing to produce instruments for clinical use.

The more current required by the laser, the greater the necessity for the physical exclusion of these machines from the operating room itself and for bringing the laser beam through conduits into the room. Even the $CO_2$ laser, which is plugged into standard electric wall sockets, may set off alarm systems unless specially wired.

**Safety Measures.** Most safety measures needed for the protection of OR personnel and patients relate to the reflections of nonfocused beams off glazed or polished surfaces and were discussed earlier under the section Surgical Techniques. We have made no special effort to change the type of commercial drapes used in most ORs. However, the less fire-resistant the drapes are, the more serious the problem is for the laser surgeon. The light-visible lasers ideally should be used only when deeply pigmented drapes have been supplied to absorb the nonfocused reflected beams. Laser surgeons who are using their machines on a daily basis have found it helpful to use non-chrome-plated instruments to decrease the reflection and scatter of laser light around the OR. The marked amount of steam and vapor produced by the laser incisions or impacts has required a suction apparatus more powerful than the usual wall type in burn surgery and was described earlier under Surgical Techniques. The apparatus decreases the odor and the amount of debris inhaled by the OR personnel. It is practical and important to have tubing that is easily cleaned and to have the filters inspected, cleaned, and changed on a regular basis. The exhausts of these suction machines must be carefully planned so they will not contaminate other parts of the hospital, and the outdoor vents should be placed away from the intake of air conditioners or open hospital windows.

**Space Requirements.** The space requirements for the laser are a constant irritation to the operating personnel. When in use, the laser, with its electrical wiring, foot-pedal lines, two water hoses, and suction hose, must be placed so that the foot traffic does not become entangled in the lines. This is particularly true when the surgeons are walking blindly while wearing their protective eyepieces or magnifying glasses and the loosely fitting shoecovers make it easy to trip over these unseen obstacles. Since it is cheaper to buy the necessary gas ($CO_2$, helium, $H_2$) in large amounts, the gas tanks may also be separated from the machine and add to the confusion of what to move when the laser machine is shifted around the OR. The operating arms, particularly of the $CO_2$ laser, are constantly in competition for our head space with the OR lights, intravenous poles and lines, and block the vision of the surgical assistants and the OR television cameras and photographers. The surgeon's head may make contact with the delivery arm, not only contaminating the drapes, but causing lint to fall into the operating field. Conduction fibers used with the light-visible lasers decrease this problem.

**Sterilization.** Part of the operating armpieces of the $CO_2$ laser may be sterilized by steam sterilization, a technique performed daily by operating personnel and one that is relatively cheap. The sterilization procedures mean that the materials used are capable of enduring steam heat, 260°F, 27–39 lb pressure for 10 min. Special plastic coverings for the operating arm of the $CO_2$ laser require ethylene oxide gas sterilization for 8 h at 115°–130°F, usually performed only once or twice a week in most OR suites. This requires some planning but is worth the additional trouble, as the plastic covers are waterproof and are not contaminated by blood or other wetting agents. The use of these transparent plastic coverings decreases the number of layers that must be placed around the operating arm, reducing its bulkiness.

## Laser Incision and Excision of Tissues and Control of Hemorrhage

Incision with the focused $CO_2$ laser is produced when skin temperatures exceed a temperature of 100° and the intracellular and extracellular water begin to evaporate. Although protein is denatured at 60°C, a temperature of 100°–600°C is required to achieve pyrolysis with changes in the bonding of the molecules. Both the width and the depth of the incision can be affected by the surgeon.

**Width of the Incision.** The width of the incision is determined by the spot size of the focused beam. The spot size or diameter is given by the equation $d = f\theta$, in which $d$ is spot diameter in centimeters; $f$ is focal length of lens in centimeters; and $\theta$ is beam spread in radians. The area of a spot size (A) is given by the equation

$$A = \frac{\pi f^2 \theta^2}{4}$$

As the spot diameter approaches the order of magnitude of the wavelength of light, the spot size becomes diffraction-limited (Goldman and Rockwell, 1971b). In a highly coherent single-mode ($TEM_{00}$) gas laser, about 80% of the beam energy is contained in a diameter

$$^{d}TEM_{00} = \frac{2.44 f\lambda}{D}$$

where $\lambda$ is wavelength of light; $D$ is diameter of the beam; $f$ is focal length of lens.

Therefore, the smallest possible spot size of a focused beam ($f/D = 1$) is never smaller than the wavelength of light. The power density (power per unit area) varies inversely with the square of the focal length of the lens or the square of the beam divergence angle ($\theta$). Once the surgeon has chosen a laser, the mode or divergence is usually fixed, and the only variable is the lens or focal length that he places between the beam and the patient. At any given power output, the shorter the focal length, the smaller the spot size and the greater the radiance per unit area of the spot size. A smaller focal length decreases the width of tissue damage in the incision. However, the surgeon's limitations in directing a hand-held laser beam in the line of a proposed incision or to deepen an existing incision are made more difficult with a small spot size. A range of 0.2–1 mm for cutting is acceptable to most surgeons. When the spot size is small, surgeons will often hold the laser beyond the focal length of the lens to increase the spot size, to slow down the cutting speed, or to decrease blood loss by allowing more time for the beam to act thermally on the wound edges through conduction. Coagulation without vaporization begins to occur at a beam irradiance of 6–12 $W/cm^2$ with the $CO_2$ laser. This irradiance is achieved by the surgeon by controlling the power of a focused beam or defocusing the more powerful output and increasing the spot size. Cutting is achieved at 1–20 $kW/cm^2$.

**Depth of the Incision.** The depth of the $CO_2$ laser incision depends on the following:

1. The time the beam is held at one point, or rate of cutting
2. Absorption depth
3. Beam irradiance and focused spot size
4. Dryness of field and tissue tension

*Rate of Cutting.* There is an inverse relationship between the depth of the incision and the rate of cutting. The depth of the incision is increased by slowing the rate of movement of the laser beam.

*Absorption Depth.* The absorption coefficient of the beam is the depth of tissue that is required to absorb a laser beam before thermal injury. The greater the absorption coefficient, the smaller the amount of tissue needed to absorb the beam and the shallower the depth of incision.

*Beam Irradiance and Focused Spot Size.* The greater the power output and the smaller the spot size, the greater the irradiance. The depth of the incision varies directly with the irradiance or power density of the focused beam.

*Dryness of the Field and Tissue Tension.* The depth or rate of an incision can be affected by how dry the surgeon keeps the wound and the tension the surgeon places on the sides of the wound. Since most tissues are poor conductors of heat and there is minimal convection of heat through circulation, the major tissue variable is the amount of edema fluid or blood that is allowed to accumulate in the path of the incision.

Tension or traction on the burn eschar is used to decrease the edema fluid and blood at the incision or excision site. Traction is increased until the dead eschar is almost avulsed from underlying structures. The tension facilitates visibility of the tissue planes between the deep fascia overlying the musculature and the fat layer. The perforating vessels between the muscle and fat are placed on stretch and incised.

The use of tension is of great importance with any thermal knife. The incision will collect carbon on its sides that not only changes the absorption coefficient and slows the incision rate, but also causes marked damage to the tissue itself. Ideally, there is no visible carbon on the edges if adequate tension is applied.

**Rate of Incision.** The rate of incision varies mainly with changes in the power output of the laser, but is further increased by decreasing the spot size, selecting a laser with a high absorption coefficient for the structure to be incised, and maintaining a dry field and tissue tension.

**Control of Hemorrhage.** Control of hemorrhage is the main reason for using the laser in burn surgery. The size of vessel that is controlled depends on the techniques available to the surgeon. Bleeding from a vessel is changed by placing a tourniquet proximal to the incision, placing the vessel on stretch, or applying pressure over the vessel to occlude its lumen or opening. All these techniques are generally used in any given operation to help make the laser more effective. If the vessel is too large to seal by coagulation of the ends, a hemostat is applied and later replaced by a ligature. Some surgeons will coagulate the clamped vessel wall with a defocused laser beam, but highly polished chrome-covered instruments will reflect or scatter the laser rays. When it is possible to dislodge blood from the lumen of a large vein, the vessel may be "painted" with the nonfocused laser beam. Coagulation of the intact vessel for a 5–10 mm length is achieved prior to incising it. This will permit the control of the vessel that normally would bleed if incised when engorged. The electrosurgical unit or Bovie knife can be used to coagulate a vessel after control with a hemostat or other surgical instrument or to paint the vessel prior to incising it. There is no reason that other modalities, such as the electric knife, or clamping then incising the vessel with a scalpel, cannot be used as an adjunct to laser surgery. Tension, a dry operative field, and adequate exposure of vessels are important in the control of hemorrhage in any procedure. A tourniquet permits the $CO_2$ laser to seal blood vessel lumens that normally would not be controlled with a thermal knife. The vessels are partially emptied by gravity drainage, and the blood flow and pressure are decreased to a point that the cutting time is also decreased. Therefore, the tourniquet and other techniques used to slow blood flow to a given area not only decrease blood loss but speed up the operation.

## Closing the Laser Burn Wound

The $CO_2$ laser–excised burn wound may be closed by primary suture or with a permanent or temporary skin graft.

**Primary Closure.** Primary closure of the wound edges is possible in small burns that are not markedly contaminated with bacterial organisms. The skin edges must be capable of approximation. Proline or other monofilament stay sutures are used to minimize tension on the skin edges, and the skin edges are loosely closed. The wound must be examined frequently and, if infected, either drained or opened widely.

### Grafting the Wound Defect

*Permanent versus Temporary Graft.* An autograph, i.e., skin taken from a donor site on the patient, is the ultimate or definitive procedure in large burns. This permanent skin graft protects the patient from infection, stops the loss of body fluids, and decreases the number of calories required by the patient. When donor sites are not available, when the patient's general condition does not permit, or when the appearance of the recipient bed is incapable of supporting an autograft, temporary allograft cadaver skin or xenograft pigskin is applied.

*Expanded versus Sheet Grafts.* Skin that is passed through a cutting device (Meshgraft or Drapier Expanders) and stretched to 1.5:1, 2:1, 3:1, 4:1, and 6:1 of the original size is known as an expanded graft. The interstices of the expanded grafts permit body fluids (serum and blood) to drain through the graft. Any foreign material, whether it is air, blood, serum, suture material, or devitalized tissue, may complicate the growth of capillaries into the graft and threaten its survival. Sheet grafts, however, are more cosmetic, particularly for the face or neck, and provide better protection when placed over joints and hands. The grafts need to be secured to the underlying recipient beds with sutures, staples, or a secure dressing unless the patient is cooperative and the grafts are placed on a unilateral surface. We prefer to dress all wounds initially with a pressure dressing that is thick enough to absorb secretions from the burn wound, supply antibiotic protection to the contaminated wound, and protect the graft from movement or tearing of the new capillary vessels growing into the graft.

*Dressing.* The dressing includes, from graft to outer cover, a single layer of coarse mesh gauze, a single layer of fine mesh gauze impregnated with an antibiotic cream or ointment, fluffs or bunched gauze, and a prepackaged absorbent cotton cover fastened by hog rings and capable of reaching circumferentially around an extremity. Trunk burns are covered with two of these large cotton packs, and the anterior pack is fastened to the back pack with the metal hog rings.

## Pre- and Postoperative Care Necessary for Large Burns

The use of the $CO_2$ laser does not replace good burn care. Nutritional support, sepsis control, and the prevention of burn complications—including hypertension, gastrointestinal bleeding, and contraction formation—continue to be important.

**Nutrition.** Unless the entire burn is excised and covered within the first postburn week, critical attention of the intake of calories is required to maintain nitrogen balance. The estimate of 25 kcal/kg body weight plus 40 kcal for each percentage of TBS burn will approximate the caloric needs of most adult patients and keep them in positive nitrogen balance. This need is particularly true of large burns where only 10%–20% TBS is excised on any one day. The staging of the burn excisions may require 6–8 weeks to completely cover the patient's wounds with skin grafts. During this period of time, the patient becomes one in a group of patients who suffer the largest loss of calories known from a traumatic injury, whether treated with the laser or conventional therapy.

**Sepsis Control.** Sepsis control and the monitoring of bacteria sensitivity to topical therapy is important to establish before excision to prevent invasive infections and to keep the eschar from softening. Once the bacteria have accumulated in quantities sufficient to invade the tissues adjacent to the burn, skin grafts may be threatened in their take and survival, and the patient's life may be threatened by septicemia. Excellent monitoring can keep bacterial contamination to $10^5$–$10^4$ organisms and permit excision of the burn, so long as traction can be applied without pulling the burn tissue apart.

**Other Complications.** Other complications that occur in burn closure are similar to those that have been mentioned can be reviewed in detail in MacMillan's report (1978).

## Why the Laser Is Not Widely Used

The laser is not widely used in burn surgery although both the surgeons whose work is at the academic level and those engaged in private practice are interested in contrasting the laser's use to that of other thermal knives. The former regard lasers as a semi-experimental tool that decreases blood loss but may increase operating time or affect wound healing. The latter are curious enough to use the laser for difficult procedures. Inherent problems in the instrument, the learning of new surgical techniques, the specificity of use of lasers, and the surgeon's personal idiosyncrasies all tend to inhibit wide usage.

**Instrument Problems.** Instrument problems consisting of cost, awkwardness, and medicolegal aspects deter the use of this cutting modality.

*Cost.* The cost of a $CO_2$ laser with an operating arm capable of focusing a 50-W single-mode beam ranges upwards from $50,000 to $80,000. Special attachments such as guide lights and microscopes, may increase the price. The upkeep of the laser requires an annual inspection to calibrate the instrument panel and align the laser to its lens. The cost of the machine is cheaper when the laser is used for photocoagulation alone and cutting is not necessary. The cost alone has prohibited widespread distribution of the instrument. Special arrangements with insurance companies to recoup these costs are possible in some parts of the country.

*Awkwardness of the Carbon Dioxide Laser.* The $CO_2$ laser remains an awkward instrument compared to other lasers using a flexible fiber, and a pipe is required to contain the beam. Although the pipe is lightweight, it must compete for space above the operating table and with the foot-control pedals below the table. The new fiber optics for the $CO_2$ laser will make the limit more flexible. Water hoses to cool the machine must be attached to the OR plumbing and gas-tank supply, and storage must be convenient. Special suction machines to keep the OR free of steam, smoke, and odors must be vented to a safe exhaust system. Eye protection and other safety measures need chronic policing.

*Medicolegal Aspects.* The medicolegal aspects of introducing a new machine or instrument into the operating room are annoying and make comparison studies frustrating. Special informed-consent forms for the patient, federal regulations, human research committees, and OR safety procedures require patience and persistence on the surgeon's part. Malpractice insurance coverage thus far is not a deterrent to the use of the $CO_2$ laser, partly because most surgeons make the effort beforehand to explain both the advantages of the laser and its risks.

**Surgical Techniques.** New techniques must be learned to use the laser. Instead of changing mechanical pressure to control the depth of cutting, the surgeon must learn to use an invisible beam and to change power output, spot size, absorption coefficient, tension, or blood supply to the operating field.

**Specificity of Use.** The specificity of the $CO_2$ laser for use in burns is not present, as it is in vocal cord tumor excisions, for example. It is unlikely that unless an institution already owns a $CO_2$ laser for other purposes that one will be purchased for burn work. None of the thermal knives in clinical use are able to compete with the knife in performing tangential burn excision. The latter form of excision removes only the necrotic tissue until pinpoint bleeding is observed and the recipient tissue bed can support circulation to a graft. The use of thermal knives generally requires that a safe plane be reached, and most of the subcutaneous tissue is sacrificed, whether damaged or not. Many burn surgeons prefer the knife for tangential excision to preserve the subcutaneous fat layer and achieve better cosmetic and functional results despite the almost prohibitive blood loss. A laser knife capable of tangential excision with primary grafting would markedly increase the specificity of lasers in burn surgery.

**The Surgeon.** Surgeons are loath to accept new types of operations or techniques if present ones are satisfactory. The use of the laser for most surgeons requires additional training. Older, well-established surgeons with good referral systems find it hard to interrupt their routines to gamble on something new that has not been proved to be a necessity.

## FUTURE OF LASER BURN SURGERY

Ideally, the burn surgeon needs to be able to perform a tangential resection with the laser. This is not likely to happen with a hand-held instrument unless it is incorporated into a dermatome or associated with a mechanical blade. A laser dermatome would theoretically permit a known depth of cut, unlimited energy output, and minimal tissue damage. If skin grafts could be applied following the use of such an instrument, the ideal laser would exist. The unlimited power would result in a fast and efficient cutting edge. The dermatome would absorb laser rays not absorbed in the incision. The current prohibitive blood loss from hyperemic subcutaneous capillaries could be overcome, as these vessels are the best size for laser control. A short-focal-length lens or small spot size could be utilized. This would increase the power density, shorten the width of the incision, and decrease the operating time and heat damage. Better functional and cosmetic results would result than are now achieved if the grafts were placed on the fat layer.

Until such an instrument is developed, laser burn surgery will depend on the availability of lasers in the hospital, which were obtained for other purposes and used by a surgeon who found they served as well as or better than the electric knife. The new heated knives and the lighted mechanical blade (argon laser) may be additional ways of achieving these ends, but as yet they have not clinically proven themselves.

## REFERENCES

Auth DC (1979) Techniques for burn wound debridement. J Trauma 11 (Suppl): 926.

Curreri PW, Richmond D, Marvin JA, Baster CR (1974) Dietary requirements of patients with major burns. J Dietet Assoc 65:415–417.

Fidler JP, Hoeffer RW, Polanyi TG, Bredemeier HC, Siler VE, Altemeier WA (1975a) Laser surgery in exsanguinating liver injury. Ann Surg 181:74–80.

Fidler JP, Law E, MacMillan BG, Fox SG, Rockwell RJ (1975b) Comparison of carbon dioxide laser excision of burns with other thermal knives. Ann NY Acad Sci 267:254–262.

Fidler JP, Law E, Rockwell RJ, MacMillan BG (1974a) Carbon dioxide laser excision of acute burns with immediate autografting. J Surg Res 17:1–11.

Fidler JP, Rockwell RJ, Siler VE, MacMillan BG, Altemeier WA (1974b) Early laser excision of thermal burns in the white rate and miniature pig. Burns 1:5–12.

Glover JL, Bendick PJ, Link WJ (1978) The use of thermal knives in surgery; electrosurgery, lasers, plasma scalpel. Curr Probl Surg 15:1–78.

Goldman L, Rockwell RJ Jr (1971) Lasers in Medicine. Gordon and Breach, Science Publishers, New York, London, Paris, pp. 163–209 (1971a), pp. 83–107 (1971b).

Hall RR, Beach AD, Baker E, Morrison PCA (1971) Incision of tissue by carbon dioxide laser. Nature (Lond) 232:131–132.

Hishimoto K, Rockwell RJ Jr, Epstein RA, Yunis NG, Fidler JP (1975) Plasma scalpel surgery: Report of some experimental evaluations and incidence of gas emboli. Burns 1:128–134.

Hoye RC, Minton JP (1965) The noble gas laser as a light-knife. Surg Forum 16:93.

Janzkovič Z (1976) A new concept in the early excision and immediate grafting of burns. J Trauma 10:1103–1108.

Levenson S (1979) Supportive therapy in burn care. Debriding agents. J Trauma 11(Suppl):928–930.

Levine NS, Salisbury RE, Paterson HD, Pruitt BA (1975) Clinical evaluation of the carbon dioxide laser for burn wound excisions: A comparison of the laser, scalpel and electrocautery. J Trauma 15:800–807.

Levine N, Seifter E, Ger R, Stellar S, Levenson SM (1972) Use of Carbon-Dioxide Laser for the Debridement of Third Degree Burns. Abstract Book, Fourth Annual Meeting, American Burn Association, San Francisco, 1972.

MacMillan BG (1978) Closing the burn wound. Surg Clin NA 58:1205–1231.

Madden JE, Edlich RF, Cuater JR, Rauck PH, Therl J, Wagensteen OH (1970) Studies in the management of the contaminated wound. IV. Resistance to infection of surgical wounds made by knife, electrosurgery, and laser. Am J Surg 119:222–224.

Mullins F, Jennings B, McClusky L (1968) Liver resection with continuous wave carbon dioxide laser: Some experimental observations. Am Surg 34:717–722.

# 17

# Neurosurgical Laser Techniques

*P. W. Ascher*
*F. Heppner*

Neurosurgery is one of the youngest of the surgical specialties, despite the fact that neurosurgical procedures might well have been carried out in prehistoric times. Certainly, according to the Ebers papyrus, specific neurosurgical operations occurred in ancient Egypt. The beginnings of modern neurosurgery date back to the 1880s, following which this specialty developed with breathtaking speed. Under the guidance of a few outstanding workers, the range of indications for neurosurgical interventions increased with great rapidity, even given the old-fashioned instruments then available. The first true innovation was the introduction of the Bovie knife; subsequently, the bipolar forceps and then, more recently, the operating microscope came into use. For this reason, even some of the more impressive successes were attributable more to improvements in diagnostic methods and anesthetic techniques than to the skill of the surgeon. Thus it was that the industrial production of lasers stimulated great interest in the medical world: The introduction of an "immaterial" knife meant that a true "nontouch technique" was available for the very first time in surgery.

One might think that neurosurgery in particular would profit at an early stage from these possibilities. This, however, was not the case. Early attempts were made to use the laser in neurosurgery by Rosomoff (1965) and Stellar et al. (1974), but these were the only ones. The reasons were perhaps the following: (1) The lack of a practical, usable laser for neurosurgeons. This seems to us an essential precondition for success, particularly as neurosurgical techniques are completely different from techniques used in general surgery. (2) Misconceptions surrounding the use of this new cutting tool in the treatment of large malignant tumors. These attempts were doomed to failure. For these reasons, the use of the laser in neurosurgery was formally rejected by Stellar et al. (1974) as unsuitable.

On the other hand, this rejection led one of us (Ascher) to attempt to expose as untenable, statements such as "That's impossible" or, as is so often heard, "There are no neurosurgical indications for lasers; they are rather dangerous for both patient and surgeon."

The second strange motivation was naturally the concept of contact-free penetration with a beam of light into that most sensitive of organs, the human brain. A year passed between the inception of this dream in 1975 and its realization. During this year, Laser Industries Ltd. succeeded in adapting a commercial surgical carbon dioxide laser in such a way that its use for neurosurgical experiments became a real possibility.

## THE DEVELOPMENT OF A NEUROSURGICAL CARBON DIOXIDE LASER

A modified surgical $CO_2$ laser (Sharplan 791 He) was used at the University Clinic for Neurosurgery in Graz, Austria (Ascher, 1976). Two principal modifications were made during the first stage of development: (1) Replacement of iron focusing devices by a pilot laser (only this made a "contact-free" technique, as first envisaged, feasible); (2) The addition of a microadapter in accordance with the increasing proportion of microsurgical procedures in neurosurgery.

Practical considerations have been amply confirmed since then by experience, leading to the adaption of an electromechanical guiding device for the ray under the microscope. Experimental work began in late spring 1976 with this apparatus. This was rapidly followed by the first successful laser operation on a patient (by Heppner, June 28, 1976). Over 300 laser operations to date have, with increasing experience, led to these results: (1) continuing improvements in laser equipment as well as increasing interest on the part of industry; (2) the development of three different, specific surgical techniques using the laser; and (3) the discovery of fresh indications for the use of lasers and, on the other hand, their limitations.

This chapter is devoted to the continuing improvements and alterations in equipment and stresses the lines along which surgeons would like to see technology develop. The improvements and innovations have affected not only the microequipment but also the whole laser aggregate. The decisive innovation for the laser aggregate was the introduction of the pilot laser.

The limitations of the $CO_2$ laser as a cutting implement were soon recognized, and surgeons learned to content themselves with a smaller output of energy. We see no advantage in cutting skin, galea, bone, and dura with the laser. In such cases, our established instrumentarium is still preferable to laser. Nor do we believe that this situation will change in the foreseeable future.

Provided one does not regard the laser as an "instrument for all seasons" but introduces it only where there are real advantages to be gained, e.g., in nervous tissue or in the neighborhood of sensitive and well-defined organ systems, 25 W, at the most, is enough.

Narrowing the field in this way made it possible to reduce the size of the previously unwieldy laser apparatus significantly and to make it more easily manipulated, with the pleasant corollary that the cost of the machine fell by 50%. The result of these efforts is the commercially available Sharplan 733, with an integrated cooling system and hydraulic fully mobile laser head. These features have increased the laser's attractiveness among even the less enthusiastic.

A further improvement, still to be realized, is the inclusion of a microscope in the laser head. The future introduction of a fiber-optic system for $CO_2$ lasers will have a similar simplifying effect.

One particular disadvantage of our old HeNe pilot laser is the poor visibility of its red light in red tissue—e.g., blood; this problem could surely be solved with great ease. On the other hand, one important consideration in terms of the cutting $CO_2$ laser was always the need to achieve better coagulation. Both problems could be solved by the use of a green argon laser as a pilot laser in the range of some milliwatts and as a coagulation tool with 2–4 W. As we understand it, the solution to this problem is simple from the optical, but not from the economical or engineering, point of view. Certainly, recent technologic developments offer good grounds for optimism.

In contrast, the innovations and alterations in the microadapter were more numerous and difficult. In this case, also, reduction in the size of the adapter was an important basic requirement, which industry fulfilled step by step (Figs. 17.1–17.3). Even more important was the ability to defocus under the microscope. This makes it possible to achieve satisfactory hemostasis in almost all microsurgical situations. Our present microadapter possesses three lenses with focal lengths of 200,

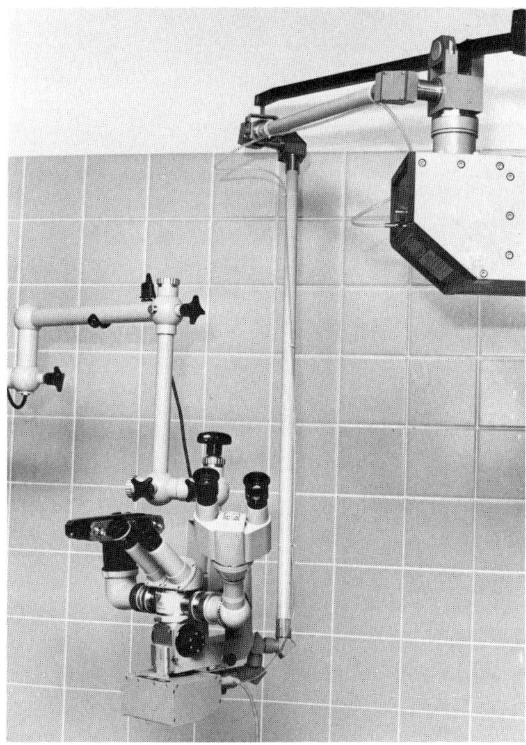

**Fig. 17.1.** Microadapter prototype II, connected to operating microscope OpMi 1 (Zeiss).

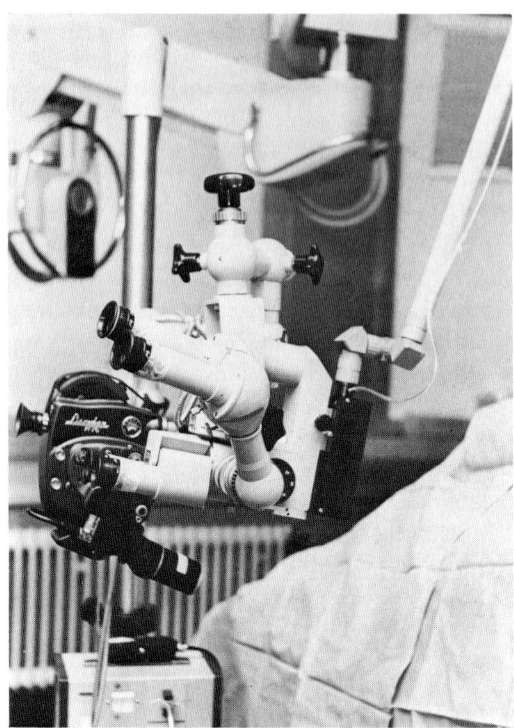

Fig. 17.2. Microadapter prototype III, connected to operating microscope.

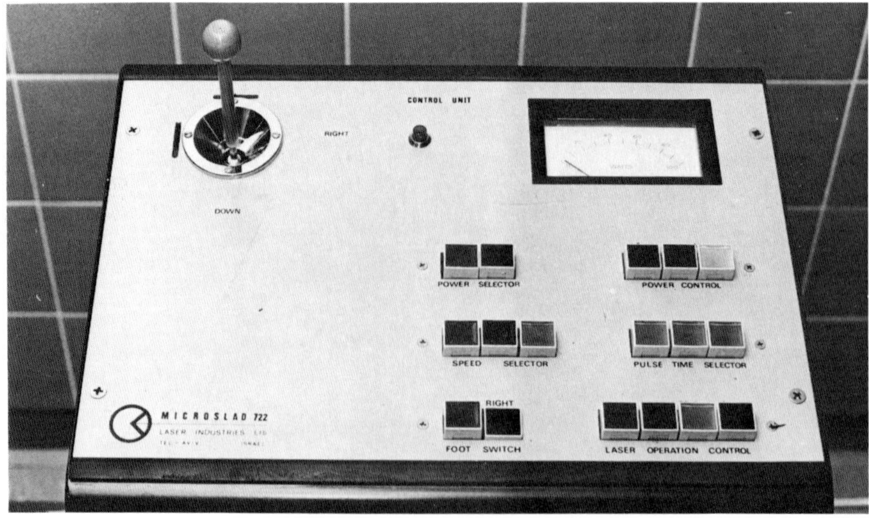


Fig. 17.3. Manipulating table, second generation.

300, and 400 mm. Of equal if not greater importance was the reduction in size of the focal spot for these extremely long lenses. This requirement was initially rejected in engineering circles as unattainable, but ultimately it was fully realized. Presently our 200-mm lens has a spot size of 0.13–0.2 mm, and this was the result of a forced compromise with respect to the volume of the adapter box required to house a lens of this size. Of thoroughly practical significance were the alterations in the manipulating table, which simplified sterile containment and utilization.

In addition, we have been pressing for the development of smaller handpieces to facilitate the freehand use of the laser under the microscope. We regard the bayonet-shaped handpiece designed by Bartal, with a working distance of 2–4 cm, as particularly important.

## SPECIFIC LASER SURGICAL TECHNIQUES

We use the $CO_2$ laser in three distinct ways: freehand; freehand under the microscope; and electromechanically controlled under the microscope.

### Freehand Surgery

The freehand technique comes closest to established surgical methods except for the replacement of the knife by an invisible light beam. Depth of penetration is therefore determined by the duration of application of the laser beam rather than the pressure of the knife. Obviously, other influencing factors are the preselected energy output of the apparatus and the energy density administered in terms of the focal distance. This implies that the more narrowly the beam is focused, the deeper and sharper is the lesion produced. Furthermore, the spot size can be preselected through the choice of lens, with the proviso that this also alters the working distance.

For normal freehand use, we have found a compromise that is in full accordance with neurosurgical demands in the shape of the 125-mm lens.

Apart from its use as a cutting instrument, the laser has proved itself highly useful in the technique of vaporization. This involves treating a larger surface area with a lower energy density (defocused beam) and vaporizing the most superficial layers (roughly 3–5 $\mu$m). A more focused beam of higher energy can also destroy a hard tumor within its capsule.

Although this technique is in many respects comparable to established surgical procedures, indications do exist which were regarded as formerly inoperable—such as hard central tumors (corpus callosum lipomas, etc.), bony roots of basal meningiomas, poorly accessible meningiomas, broadly based tumors of the floor of the fourth ventricle, and many others.

The explanation as to how this was made possible has been proved to our satisfaction in countless histologic examinations.

It is particularly important to avoid any mechanical or electrical interference in the neighborhood of sensitive systems. Even the most careful work may result in a usually fatal edema of such regions (midbrain, brain stem, spinal cord, etc.).

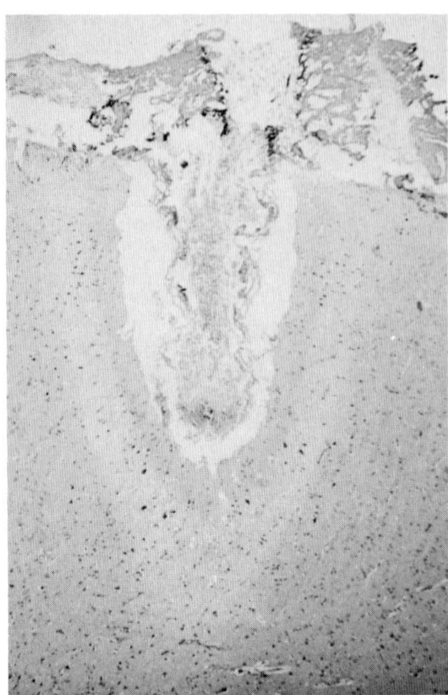

**Fig. 17.4.** Laser crater (30 W, 1 s, continuous wave) in normal brain tissue (depth 1.2 mm, width 0.3 mm) with coagulation and edema zone. H&E, ×60.

Obviously, neither mechanical nor electrical interference occurs when an "immaterial" light beam is used to replace the suction tube, the Bovie knife, or bipolar forceps. Thermal damage is limited to fractions of a millimeter, as can be seen from histologic preparations subsequent to the procedure.

## Freehand Surgery under the Microscope

Freehand surgery under the microscope has as yet been confined to theory, as industry has been unable to provide suitable handpieces (although we have great expectations of the bayonet-shaped microhandpiece) (Figs. 17.4–17.6). Experimental studies suggest that this technique can widen the range of operative procedures, particularly in concert with the use of metallic mirrors, facilitating operation around corners and in achieving coagulation in the microanatomic range. This has been developed by us and will shortly be commercially available. Possible indications for the use of this technique would be tumors of the pontine angle and microvascular surgery.

## Electromechanically Controlled Surgery under the Microscope

Hitherto unexplored territory was opened up by the introduction of the electromechanically controlled laser under the microscope. It is with this type of laser that we feel future innovations lie. Almost every operation seems to widen the boundaries of established operability.

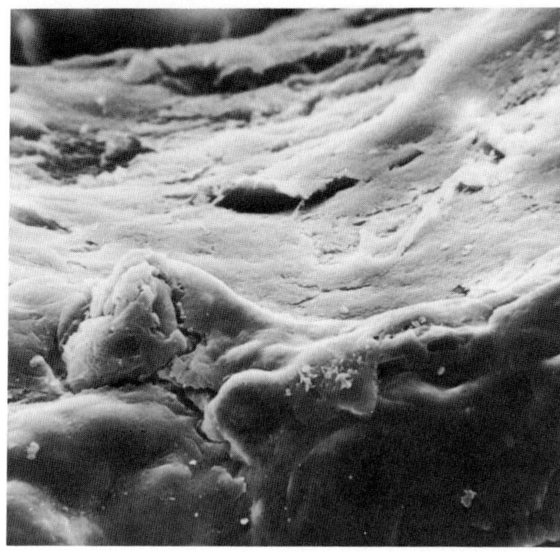

**Fig. 17.5.** Wall of laser crater in normal brain tissue. Scanning electron microscope, ×200.

**Method.** The new prototype of microadapter is fixed onto the objective lens of the operating microscope (Zeiss $O_pM_i$ 1–6) connected to the laser arm and covered with sterile drapes. The mirror in the microadapter is moved electromechanically from the manipulating table with the left hand, and the beam can be smoothly operated in any direction. Furthermore, it is possible to operate with the laser up to 5 mm over and under the focal plane without losing a significant amount of energy.

It is necessary, of course, for the purpose of coagulation, to reduce the energy density. This can be accomplished as follows:

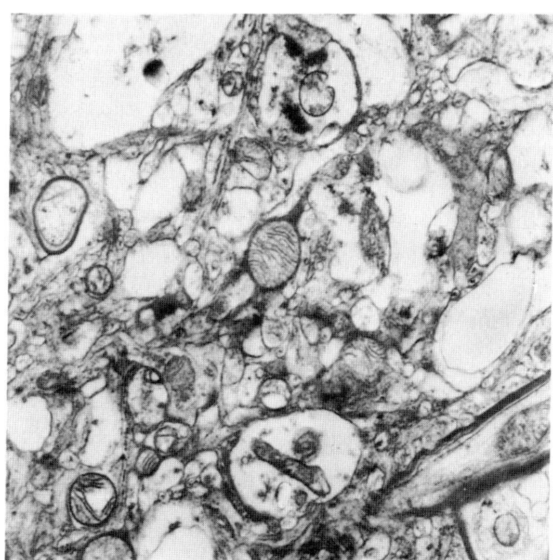

**Fig. 17.6.** Ultrastructural findings, 0.6 mm to laser lesion. Normal mitochondria. Electron microscope, ×30,000.

1. By changing the laser objective lens
2. By shortening the radiation time, which can be selected de novo, 0.1, 0.05, 0.01 s
3. By reducing the output energy (5–50 W)

There are three variations in the speed of the movement of the laser beam, which can be preselected. A rough estimate of the depth of penetration is achieved thereby. For particularly delicate membranes, it has been useful to cut, not continuously, but with interrupted single shots in series. The design of the latest models makes this possible.

Apart from cutting and coagulating, a third possibility under the microscope is the vaporization of diseased tissue. This technique has been found to be the least traumatic of all as applied to tumors of limited size (3–5 $cm^3$). Unfortunately this method cannot be applied to large and highly vascular tumors, as high-energy equipment is necessary to accomplish such a procedure in a tolerable time span. Quite apart from all the other disadvantages—e.g., size, cost, etc.—that such a machine would entail, its depth of penetration and destructiveness would make it too dangerous to be used in such sensitive areas as the brain. As the $CO_2$ laser beam has no specific affinity for pathologic tissue—i.e., increased absorption—there remains the problem of dissecting out the boundaries of a tumor. This demands all the fine skill of the surgeon and has no parallel in past experience.

Early intraoperative experiments involving fluid injections into the tumor tissue have now shown that the absorption coefficient of abnormal tissue can be changed in this way. This brings accurate dissection within the bounds of possibility. Finding tumor dyes and vaporizing the tumor and only the tumor with color-specific lasers seems to be a promising project for the future. Our present studies represent an initial step in this direction. It was a pleasant surprise to find that it was possible to produce extensive vasoconstriction with synthetic, locally active adrenalin homologues and thus largely to eliminate disruptive intraoperative bleeding.

## INDICATIONS FOR THE USE OF LASER IN NEUROSURGERY

It can be said that all disease processes that were previously regarded as inoperable, by virtue of their localization, must now be reconsidered in terms of their operability. As a rule, this applies to benign, hard, expansive lesions at the base of the skull, in relation to the midbrain, brain stem or spinal cord.

In the spinal cord, a prominent group is the intramedullary lesions, with greatly improved postoperative results. In individual cases—e.g., spongioblastoma of the brain stem—it has been possible to split the brain stem without harm to the patient.

Tumors with adhesions in the floor of the fourth ventricle can be vaporized, layer by layer, without thermal damage to important structures.

In contrast, it has been clear to us from the very beginning that the laser finds no true place in opening the cranium. In the meantime we have learned that surgical treatment of malignant brain tumors by means of the laser has resulted in no significant improvement in survival time. All the same, we observed in many cases that the patient suffered less from postoperative edema and its consequences when we used the laser. Certainly, we were able to operate more radically than previously.

In terms of peripheral nerve surgery, we were both pleasantly and unpleasantly surprised. The assumption that nerve grafting would be made easier by the unique cutting abilities of the laser had to be reconsidered after experimental studies.

Following the use of laser, we could show no growth of the proximal nerve stump 4 months after the primary grafting. On the other hand, a new indication has arisen—the neuroma—which can be successfully amputated with the laser. In all the cases we operated on there were no relapses. The first procedures of this kind were carried out in 1976.

## REFLECTIONS

After more than 2 years of clinical experience, we believe that the role of laser has become more and more important, particularly in all neurosurgical border areas. Even today, it seems to be irreplaceable in special cases. Furthermore, we found that with increasing experience there were not only new indications for use, but also new advantages in this innovation.

It should be emphasized strongly that this new method will require a rethinking and that the surgeon, who will benefit most from it, must undergo special training. So far as we can see from our own experience, we think that at least 2 or 3 years are necessary to master this new technique with all its fine points.

Last, but not least, we point out that the laser should not be a replacement for successful traditional surgery. It is, in our opinion, an additional technique, with new areas of application.

## SUMMARY

The application of the laser beam to clinical neurosurgery provides, for the first time, an opportunity to operate in the CNS without physically touching the tissue. For this reason, new horizons of neurosurgery have been opened.

## REFERENCES

Ascher PW (1976) Der $CO_2$ Laser in der Neurochirurgie. Molden, Vienna.

Rosomoff HL (1965) In: Proceedings of the 1st Annual Biomedical Laser Convention, Boston.

Stellar S, Polanyi TG, Bredemeier HC (1974) In: Laser Applications in Medicine and Biology, vol. II. Plenum Press, New York, pp. 241–293.

# 18

# Laser Instrumentation in Dermatology: Diagnosis and Treatment

*Leon Goldman*

As the subject of greatest interest in research and development of the laser for biology and medicine, the skin is second only to the eye. The availability of skin, its optical properties, normal structure and function, and its endless pathology all continue to make it an ideal test model for many phases of laser biology and for laser medicine. The first tests of the effect of the nitrogen laser (337.1 nm) on humans were done on the skin by Parrish and his associates. Parrish has continued to do extensive studies in laser dermatology.

## DIAGNOSIS

Throughout this book, many of the diagnostic instruments are mentioned. There will be brief references to many of them again for their specific applications in dermatology. The laser microprobe—that is, laser microemission spectroscopy—can be used directly on the skin to analyze for cations. This technique has been used in dermatology to detect calcium (Wilson et al., 1967), silver (argyria), gold, and arsenic in living skin, in skin samples, and in frozen sections. For control purposes, skin that has been studied for calcium by this method has also had subsequent staining with the Von Kossa stain. The laser microprobe has been used directly on the skin on tattoos for cation analyses. The same microprobe technique can be adapted to check the hair for the presence of arsenic and to record levels of some of the heavy metals, especially lead. In the child, there may be a correlation of the quantitative analyses of lead intoxication with the growth patterns of the hair, possibly supplying some clue as to the time of exposure to lead.

To obtain such microprobe laser analyses, the target area must be exposed; the laser, usually the pulsed type, must be set up with a spectrograph so that direct analysis can be performed.

Laser microscopy has been used to seek out trace metals in dried fungi. These metals are necessary for enzyme reactions.

The new laser microprobe mass analyzer (Kaufman et al., 1979) has not been used as yet for trace metal analyses of the skin in so-called nondisintegrated, freeze-dried, plastic-embedded ultramicrotome sections of skin specimens. This probe is of potential value, especially for more precise quantitative analyses and much more sensitivity than the previous laser microprobe.

## Acoustic Microscopy

The acoustic microscope, also described previously, has been suggested for examination of skin exposed to ionizing and nonionizing radiation, for trauma, for the development and progress of primary and secondary skin lesions, and for the migration patterns of parasites invading living skin. As yet, all these fascinating possibilities exist only in the planning, protocol phase.

Studies by means of photoacoustic spectroscopy were initiated, but not completed, for psoriasis cells in therapy using psoralen plus ultraviolet light (PUVA) in an attempt to examine the psoralen compounds in the cells.

## Laser Velocimetry

Dynamic studies by laser velocimetry of skin circulation have been done, especially by Holloway and Allen (1980). The new techniques of Cong and Zweibach (1979) have extended such studies into the microvascular area.

## Dermatologic Immunology

Studies of immunofluorescence are important for modern immunology. The laser nephelometer, discussed in other chapters by John Goldman, may be used as well in patients with skin diseases. When fluorescence techniques are used for immunoglobulins and complement, the dye laser may scan these under the microscope. Ueki et al. (1979) have evaluated microfluoremetry for intensity of fluorescence on antinuclear antibody serum from patients with systemic lupus erythematosus. The studies on laser fluorescence by Andreoni, Longoni, Sacchi, and Svelto in Chapter 7 should facilitate the use of lasers for this technique.

## Transillumination

In Greenberg and Tribbe's discussion of fluorescent laser transillumination (Chapter 22), the passage of laser beams through tissue is described. This technique has been used in dermatology to detect foreign bodies in the skin, including tattoo pigment masses, hemorrhage, fibrosis, leukoplakia, skin tumors, etc. Controls used were flashlight transillumination and, for certain areas, xerography.

Of particular importance in transillumination are the clear zones of invading basal-cell cancer, visible through better transmission, with less dispersion and reflection of photons. Similarly, the so-called mucinous pseudocysts of the fingers were differentiated from solid tumors (Goldman et al., 1977). For new studies of transillumination by Nath (personal communications, 1978, 1979), controls with incoherent infrared probes are to be used with low-output Nd laser with image converter.

Laser-induced fluorescence is now used for localization of early cancer of the lung and also, incidentally, for the photodynamic therapy of tumors. Laser-induced fluorescence could be adopted in dermatology for the identification of fungi and for monitoring the movements of the filariform larvae of *Ancylostoma braziliense*. We had done this previously with tetracycline and ultraviolet light.

### Computer Programming and Video Disks

In computer programs, data storage of dermatologic lesions, color, and mass size is a challenge for data image processing. So, a digital image processor with a detailed color output format will have great value for skin lesions. When research and development of programs of this type are applied to biology and medicine as thoroughly as they have been to information handling in the military, industry, and communications, laser technology will help considerably in medical record keeping. Also, when the rapidly developing program of laser video disks can be brought into biology and medicine, especially for teaching and for communications, these player units (Magnavox Division of North America, Phillips Corporation; and Pioneer Laser Disks of New York) will be of great value for information handling in these fields.

## TREATMENT

### The Skin as Test Model

In the PUVA program, important in the treatment of psoriasis, mycosis fungoides, and other nonrelated dermatoses, experiments are now underway to test model systems using laser UV-A instead of incoherent UVA (Anders and Aufmuth, 1979). Portable laser units, with controls of Nath's Superlites (UV-A and UVA + UVB) may be investigated in localized lesions in man. Ultraviolet radiation is subdivided into UV-A, 315–400 nm; UV-B, 280–315 nm; and UV-C, 200–280 nm.

### Laser Dermatologic Surgery

Lasers used for skin surgery may result in mass destruction of tissue by photocoagulation necrosis or excision. Some lasers may do both, depending on mode, whether they are CW or pulsed, their energy and power densities, beam diameters, speed, etc. These factors have been mentioned in the basic fundamentals of the effect of lasers on human tissue. The skin served as an excellent model for the first use of lasers on human tissue after the initial experiments on laser surgery of the eye.

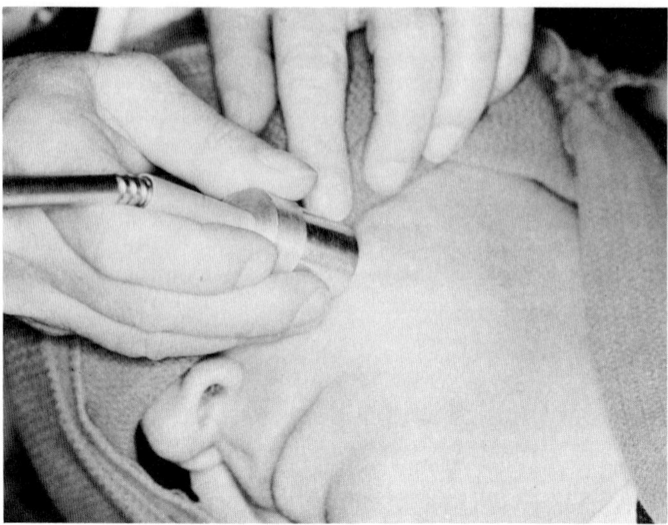

**Fig. 18.1.** Effective argon laser treatment of incurable port-wine mark of the face. Argon laser with transmission fiber and diffusing lens for areas requiring larger impacts.

With the pigmented lesions of the skin, the lasers in the visible light range—the ruby and the argon—may be used for greater intensity of reaction through greater absorption (Figs. 18.1–18.7). The first cancer treated with the laser was melanoma, identified by its intense black color (Goldman, 1979b). Similarly, the pigmented basal-cell cancer and the small spotted lesions of angiosarcoma and angiokeratomas are other examples of colored tissue responding well to laser treatments (Fig. 18.8).

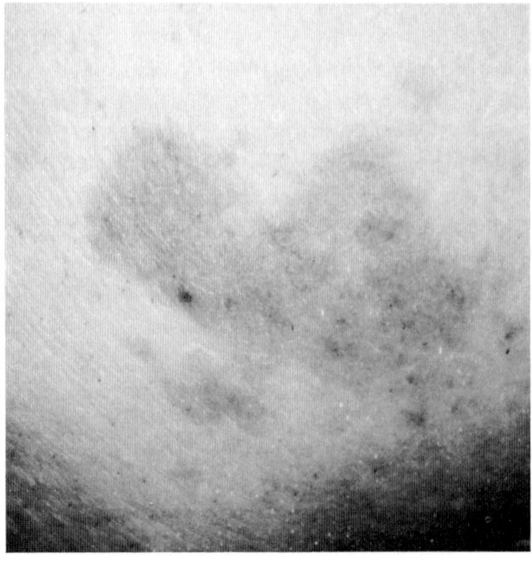

**Fig. 18.2.** Linear port-wine mark of cheek.

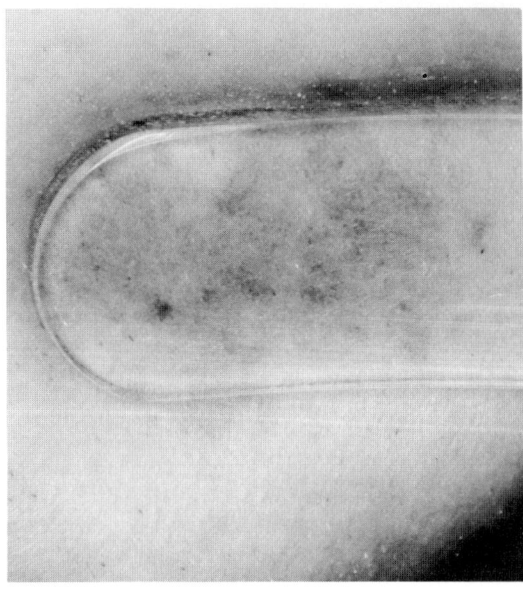

**Fig. 18.3.** Pressure of curved plastic rod (diascope) showing failure of color change after deep pressure. This indicates roughly a deep spot.

For melanoma, especially of the lentigo maligna and the peripherally spreading types, the laser may be very effective. The complete spot must be exposed. The energy densities of the laser must be adequate. For the pulsed ruby laser, up to 20,000 $J/cm^2$ may be necessary to provide adequate necrosis, especially for invasive tissue. Scarring will develop.

**Fig. 18.4.** Results after argon laser treatment.

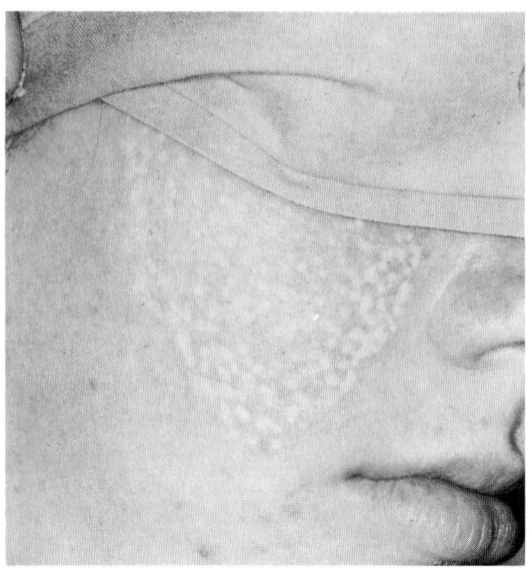

**Fig. 18.5.** Multiple impacts of argon laser on cheek, showing small, spotted character of impacts. The banding technique of Apfelberg produces a more effective, diffuse result.

It is not possible as yet to reach melanoma tumor metastases that may be underneath the skin. To do that, an incision must be made first and the tumor exposed, then the laser beam acts directly on the nodular pigmented masses. Some research is underway by Nath (personal communications, 1978, 1979) to use infrared radiation to reach tissue under the skin. The laser may be used as an adjunct to topical retinoic acid for metastatic melanoma, especially if the masses are large. In non-

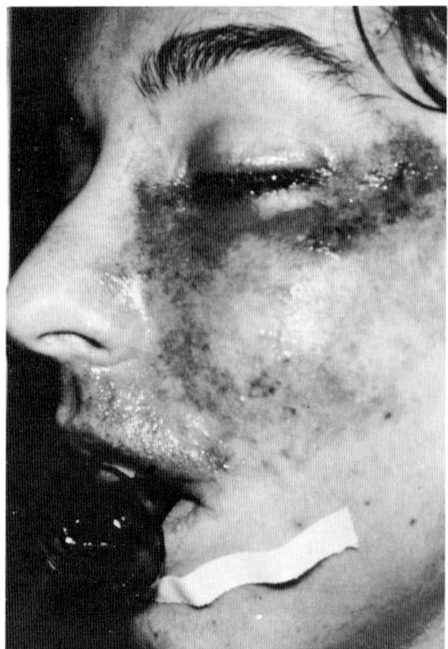

**Fig. 18.6.** Argon laser treatment given under general anesthesia after test showed good results. In this operation, the remaining spots were treated. Eye was protected with a silvered shield placed under the eyelids.

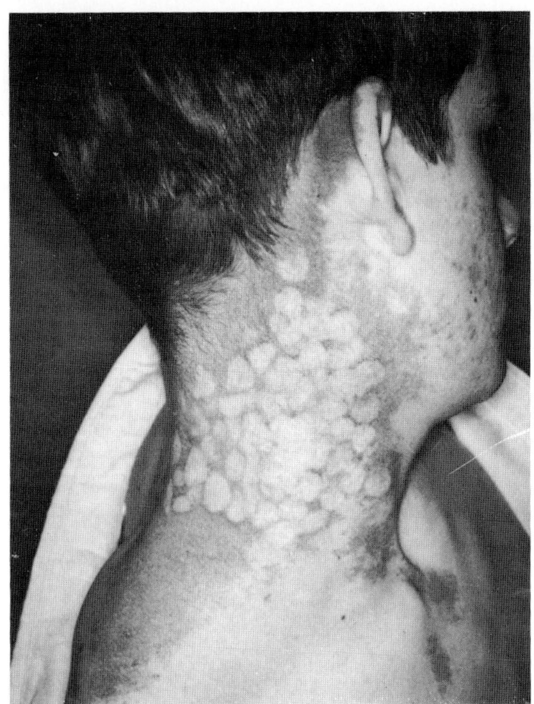

**Fig. 18.7.** Pulsed ruby laser treatment of large port-wine mark on neck showing large spotted area (50–60 cm$^2$; 2.5 cm$^2$ target area).

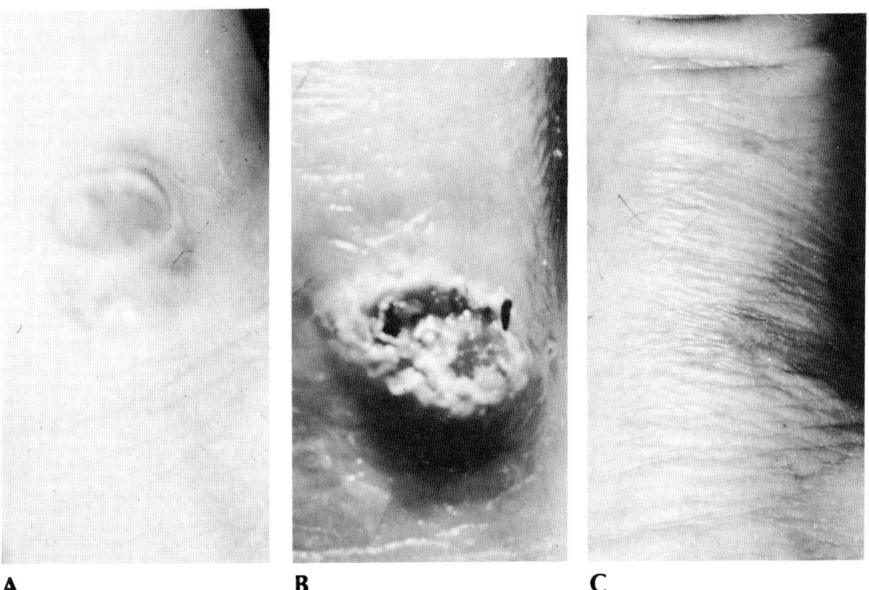


**Fig. 18.8. A.** Vascular type of cancer of finger, angiosarcoma. Upper rim (25% of lesion) served as control area for high-frequency electrosurgery; $CO_2$ laser was used to treat remaining 75%. **B.** Angiosarcoma after treatment with $CO_2$ laser and electrosurgery. A good biopsy was taken also with $CO_2$ laser. **C.** Finger is now free of any recurrence after 8 years.

pigmented tumors, lasers in the visible-light range may be used with injection of iron pigments followed by microwave radiation and the laser (Goldman, 1977, 1978).

## Treatment of Tattoos and Vascular Lesions

**Tattoos.** Tattoos may be removed by laser treatment. Ruby, $CO_2$, and argon lasers have all been used. Scarring results because of the deep-tissue necrosis. Initial experiments with Q-switched ruby lasers showed better cosmetic results than those with the normal-mode pulsed ruby laser. However, the treatment spots were small. To reduce scarring, Bailin (personal communication, 1980) and Ratz (personal communication, 1980) have used moderate magnification to localize residual pigment masses. With the $CO_2$ laser, there is initial "dermabrasion" by the laser, then selective necrosis of the individual pigment masses under microscopy. Repeat treatments may be necessary.

Laser treatments are more suitable for the small, so-called "gang-style" tattoo, than for the brilliant portraits and paintings that tattoo artists have done. The lesions of nonpigmented skin cancers may be tattooed and then treated with the laser. The iron compounds mentioned previously are an example.

**Port-Wine Marks.** A popular phase of laser treatment now is the argon laser treatment of port-wine marks (Fig. 18.1). Because of the absorption spectra of hemoglobin, use of the argon laser is more logical than the ruby laser which was used initially (Fig. 18.7). The best animal test-model system is the comb of the chicken, rather than tattooed skin of the miniature pig. The argon laser's disadvantage is that, at present, the laser's low output makes it possible to treat only small areas with each impact. It is hoped that diffusing lenses will soon be available for the operating probe of the argon laser, so that adequate and uniform energy densities may be obtained to eliminate or to lighten large areas of bluish-red marks on the skin. The banding technique of Apfelberg et al. (1978), who have had extensive experience with the laser treatment of port-wine marks, now makes it possible to treat broad areas of large facial port-wine marks. Plastic surgeons, especially, have treated a large number of patients with port-wine marks (Goldman et al., 1976; Goldman, 1980).

**Other Vascular Lesions.** The target area must be well exposed to the laser beam. The treatment of vascular lesions such as angiomas, glomangiomas, angiosarcomas, granuloma pyogenicum, etc. does not require actual contact of the instrument with the blood vessel. This is a distinct advantage in the treatment of these lesions.

The mechanism of the reaction in the blood vessels is absorption of the laser energy by hemoglobin reflection of the heat-induced energy, and absorption of necrosis of adjacent structures so that thrombi and fibrosis can develop by heat transmission from these structures about the blood vessels. Investigation must continue to determine whether thrombosis is complete without embolization and whether lymphatic vessels are sealed off in areas treated for cancer.

Surgery with the $CO_2$ laser has become popular. In dermatology, this laser can be used to excise melanomas and to destroy inoperable masses. Angiomas may also be excised by the $CO_2$ laser, as shown by the operations on the angiomas of the blue rubber bleb nevus. Moreover, in Japan, $CO_2$ lasers have been used for excision of massive cavernous angiomas by Oshiro (1980), and warts have also been treated with the ruby, Nd, and $CO_2$ lasers. Mester and his associates (1980) have studied the use of HeNe lasers in the treatment of chronic ulcers. In our laboratory, we have treated not only for stasis ulcers, but also for the necrotizing vasculitis of lupus erythematosus. Here too, controls must be used. Of interest to dermatologists are the current studies of Ginsbach et al. (1977) on the argon laser treatment of hypertrophic scars. It will be interesting to compare the argon and the Nd-YAG laser treatments of such scars.

## Controls for Laser Surgery

The controls available in laser surgical treatment are the conventional operating instruments and techniques, such as the scalpel, cryosurgery, high-frequency electrosurgery, and the infrared coagulation instruments of Nath. For investigative studies, the plasma scalpel also has been used. As always, the rule must be: *If you don't need the laser, don't use it.*

It is obvious then that progress in the research and development of laser diagnosis and laser treatment must continue. As yet, there is no single instrument for diagnosis, nor is there a single laser surgical instrument. Efficacy, reliability, flexibility, safety, and sterilizability of lasers continue to offer challenges.

## REFERENCES

Anders A, Aufmuth P (1979) Dye lasers in photodermatology, erythema production, psoriasis treatments and tumor destruction. Laser Elektro-Optik. November 1979, pp. 36–37.

Apfelberg DP, Maser RM, Lash H (1978) Argon laser treatment of cutaneous vascular abnormalities, progress report. Ann Plastic Surg 1:14–18.

Bailin A (1980) Personal communication.

Cong L, Zweibach BW (1979) In vivo and in vitro velocity measurement in microvasculature with a laser. Micro Vasc Res 17(2):131–134.

Ginsbach G, Hohler H, Lemperle G (1977) The treatment of hemangiomas, telangiectasia, radiodermatitis and tattoos with argon laser. In: Waidelich W (ed) Laser 77 Opto-Electronics. IPC Science and Technology Press, Guildford Surrey, p. 1977.

Goldman L (1977) Laser surgery for skin cancer. State J Med 77:1897.

Goldman L (1978) The laser in skin cancer. International Advances in Surgical Oncology 1:217.

Goldman L (1979a) The challenge of biophysics to dynamic dermatology. Cutis 23:224.

Goldman L (1979b) Surgery by laser for malignant melanoma. J Dermatol Surg Oncol 5:2.

Goldman L (1980) The argon laser and the portwine stain. Plastic and Reconstructive Surgery 65:138.

Goldman L, Dreffer R, Rockwell RJ Jr, Perry E (1976) Treatment of portwine marks by an argon laser. J Dermatol Surg 2:5.

Goldman L, Naprestek Z, Johnson J (1977) Laser surgery of a digital angiosarcoma. Report of a case and six-year followup study. Cancer 39:1738.

Goldman J, Goldman L, Jaffe M, Richfield DF (1977) Digital mucinous pseudocysts. Arthritis and Rheumatism 20:997.

Holloway G, Allen J (1980) Cutaneous blood flow response to injection trauma measured by laser Doppler velocimetry. J Moest Dermatol 74:1–4.

Kaufman R, Hillenkamp F, Wechsung R (1979) The laser microprobe mass analyzer (LAMMA): A new instrument for biomedical microprobe analysis. Med Progr Technol 6:109–121.

Mester E, Naglucskay S, Tisza S, Mester A (1980) Neuere Untersuchungen über die Wirkung, der Laserstrahlen auf die Wundheilung: Immunologische Aspekte. In: Waidelich EW (ed) Laser 77 Opto-Electronics. IPC Science and Technology Press, Guildford Surrey, p. 490.

Narong N (1980) Operations perfomed from March 1977 by means of $CO_2$ laser scalpel. Tokai University Hospital. Quoted by Oshiro (1980).

Nath G (1978, 1979) Personal communications.

Oshiro T (1980) Laser Treatment for Nevi. Medical Laser Research Co. Tokyo, Japan.

Ratz JA (1980) Personal communication.

Ueki H, Yoskie H, Kieda A, Nozomi N (1979) A semiquantitative measurement of antinuclear antibody using immunomicrofluorometry. Arch Dermatol Res 265:189–194.

Waidelich W (1980) Personal communication.

Wilson R, Goldman L, Brech F (1967) Calcinosis cutis with laser microprobe analysis. Arch Derm 95:490.

# 19

# The Carbon Dioxide Laser in Head and Neck and Plastic Surgery: Advantages and Disadvantages

*Billie L. Aronoff*

Before one launches into a discussion of the advantages and disadvantages of the carbon dioxide laser, it is quite necessary to know something about the instrumentation. At present, our primary experience has been with the Sharplan 791 laser, which has a flexible arm and a good radius for activity. Various heads have been adapted to the $CO_2$ laser, and some of them have helped considerably; others have been a disappointment. We have had very little experience with the use of the microscope on the $CO_2$ laser but feel that, in certain cases, it would certainly be an advantage. I am sure this will be discussed by others.

## ADAPTING TO A NEW MODALITY

There is a reluctance by surgeons to try new methods, particularly when it is a divorce from the common method of the sharp scalpel. For one thing, the pressure of the knife blade on the skin, which we have all learned these many years, is completely lost when one uses the laser. Rather, it is almost abstract in that the laser barely, if ever, touches the skin, and the amount of pressure that one uses with the laser has no relationship whatever to the depth of the incision. This means that one must learn a completely new modality.

Another problem is one of delicacy of approach with the use of the laser, because most of us trained in general surgery have become accustomed to making sharp incisions and doing delicate dissections, whether they be with the knife or scissors, but always with an excellent view of what is going on and, particularly, a knowledge of how deep a cut will be. With the laser, one can acquire this skill, but it is time-consuming, and there may be injury to certain structures that would not be injured by the more delicate surgery with the knife.

### The Laser Bulk

Many surgeons have complained about the bulkiness of the instrument, and certainly, in some areas, the size of the instrument makes it difficult to see exactly the point of contact. In the oral cavity, if one is to put the head of the laser in, then it frequently will interfere with visualization. Some right-angle lenses and various other headpieces of less than 90% and up to 135% help to some degree. Certainly, if there were a filament that could be seen very easily and the beam were directed off the filament, it would make the use of the instrument much more practical. The use of the laser through the endoscope will be discussed by other contributors.

### Smoke

Also important is the problem of the smoke. One of the main complaints of our resident staff and nurses has been that the smoke is acrid and irritating to a certain extent. Attempts to remove it by various methods are fairly successful, but both the visual and the olfactory senses are impinged upon. There are also complaints by personnel of abdominal cramping after the use of the laser. I, too, noticed this early in the the use of the laser. Either we are getting rid of the smoke more successfully, or I am getting used to it. But certainly, this is a major problem.

## ACQUIRING EXPERIENCE

Our experience has been varied, and, to date, has covered many, many different problems. First of all, the use of the laser for the excision of small skin tumors is very easy and can be accomplished in two different ways. We have done excisions with the laser and primary closure and have also tried vaporization of these tumors. Certainly there is a disadvantage in vaporization in that one does not know about margins, but with some experience one can learn, particularly on basal cells, to get rid of a high percentage of these skin tumors. For the keratotic lesions, the laser is a very satisfactory method of destroying them. Our usual method of treating the people with the so-called "Texas skin" is, first of all, to clean up as much as possible by the application of 5-fluorouracil. We ask the patients to use this twice a day for 3 weeks, then wait a month. Then, either in the office with local anesthesia, we destroy the keratosis with a cautery and excise the carcinomas, or we take the patients to the operating room to excise or to vaporize the lesions with the laser.

A big disadvantage would be the cost. The use of the operating room adds a figure almost the equivalent to the surgical fee, or sometimes greater, for many of these small cases. So, at least from a practical standpoint, this is a lot to do for little skin lesions. For the most part, we have used the laser for skin lesions—first of all, to see how effective it was, and secondly, in those patients on whom other operating procedures are being performed.

To date, I have not noticed an effort to document, with microscopic studies, the ablation of tumor by means of vaporization. We have decided that this would be a good project for us to undertake and are now doing a controlled study. We are vaporizing basal-cell and carcinoma-in-situ lesions in the skin and in-situ lesions and leukoplakia of the oral cavity.

## THE LASER'S INDISPENSABLE QUALITIES

There are certain cases in which the laser is indispensable for any area of the body: (1) in patients who have some sort of blood dyscrasia, or (2) in those people who have bleeding tendencies due to leukemia, who are receiving chemotherapy, or in whom the platelet levels might be low. We have had experience in turning skull flaps (Figs. 19.1–19.3) and other flaps in both of these situations, and find that the control of bleeding is very simple, and that it is maintained. We have not noticed postoperative bleeding, except in very rare instances.

If, indeed, the maintenance of lymphatics is essential for the growth of flaps, then the laser is not the method one should use. It certainly does seem to seal the lymphatics. Our experience to date has shown that there may be slight delay in healing, and this is simply overcome by leaving the sutures in a little longer, or by inserting the sutures in a slightly different fashion. The flaps have healed well; nonhealing has been a rare occurrence.

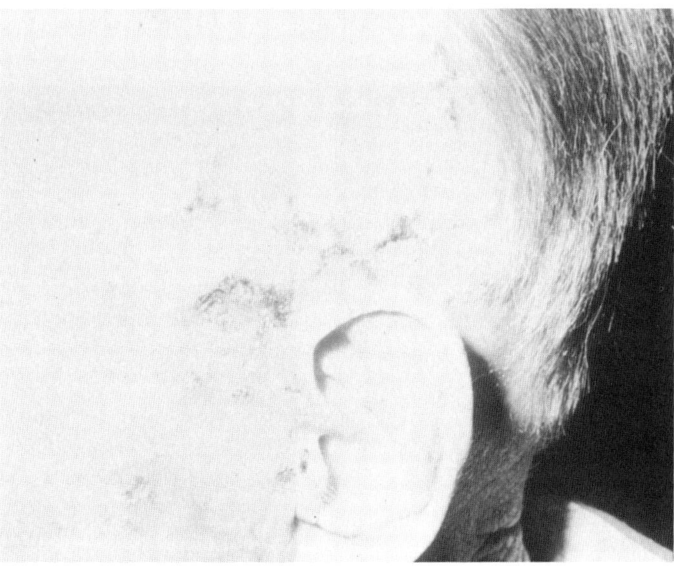

**Fig. 19.1.** Large basal cell of left temple and ear treated previously with irradiation and surgery.

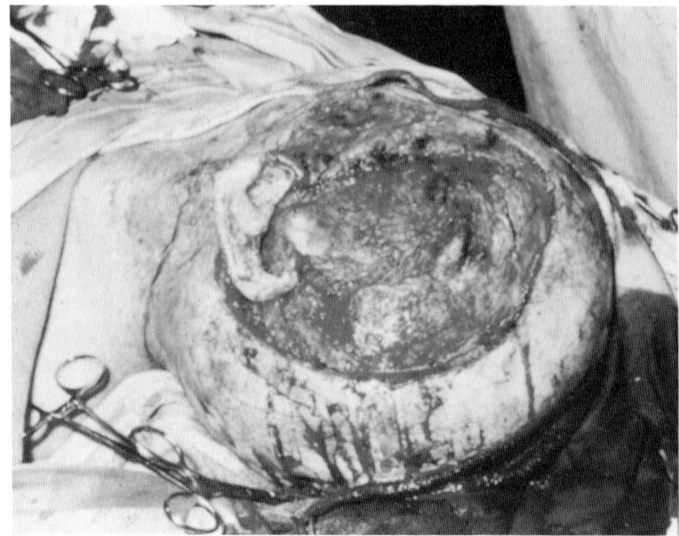

Fig. 19.2. Lesion excised with laser and then large skull flap turned.

## Hemangioma and Lymphangioma

We have been fortunate in having extensive experience with hemangiomas and lymphangiomas in the entire body, but particularly in the head and neck. The laser has been the instrument of choice in treating these lesions. First of all, the laser will seal the smaller vessels, particularly up to 1 mm. Probably it will seal 2-

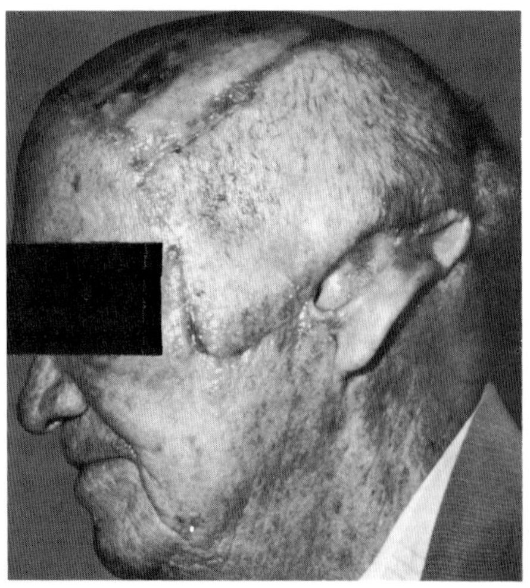

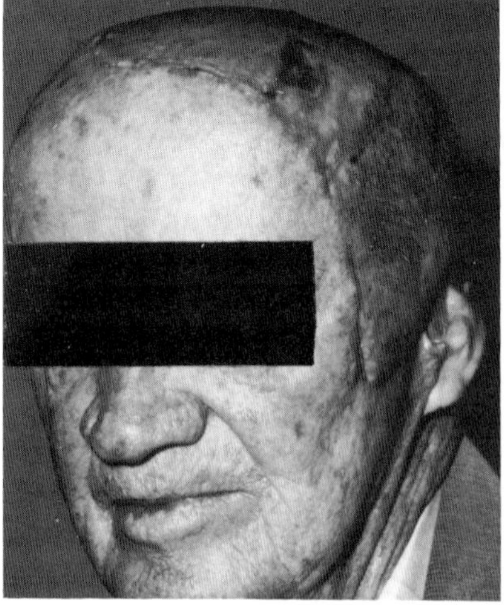

**A** **B**

**Fig. 19.3.** **A.** Postoperative view showing large healed flap. **B.** Ear was advanced recently, with good cosmetic result. Healing was rapid.

mm vessels if they are clamped. Then the larger vessels may be seen more easily, secured, and ligated.

In other lesions around the scalp, where bleeding can be a nuisance, the laser can be used to excise these tumors with primary closure, a split graft, or turned flaps; our experience has been fairly extensive in this type of lesion. When we have used the knife to remove lymphangiomas, the drainage has been fairly considerable. To date, our experience with the use of the laser has resulted in wounds that have very little drainage and have good healing.

## Hemorrhagic Telangiectasia

We have had one case of hereditary hemorrhagic telangiectasia (Rendu-Osler-Weber disease). This was quite interesting in that the patient's primary problem was bleeding from the nose and nasopharynx. With the laser, we were able to destroy the vessels in the nose and, partially, in the nasopharynx. After this bleeding was stopped, of course, other areas started to bleed, in the gastrointestinal and the genitourinary tracts, and the patient eventually developed a cerebrovascular accident and died.

## Birthmarks

The $CO_2$ laser has been used by some for strawberry birthmarks and port-wine stains, but our experience has been minimal and also unsuccessful. We have tried to treat these birthmarks in a kind of tattoo approach, particularly when they were small. Although there was some ablation of the tumor on some patients, the result was usually scarring, and more often, if the treatment was not extensive enough, the hemangioma continued or returned. We have just begun work with the argon laser and believe that it will be a much better instrument for these tumors. Others have had similar results. However, there is certainly a place for the use of both these instruments; first the $CO_2$ laser to get rid of the large part of the tumor and then the argon to take care of the changes in the skin. This would alleviate the problem of having to take wide areas of skin, occasionally necessitating skin grafts. The argon would be the method of treatment if grafts can be prevented. We have several patients receiving treatment at present. It is too early to evaluate results, but I feel confident that if we can reduce the size of the vessels that must be treated and also their depth, the addition of an argon laser to destroy the changes in the dermis will be most beneficial.

## Skin Cancer

One patient with multiple carcinomas of the scalp also had chronic lymphatic leukemia. Although his blood counts, including platelets and clotting times, were reported to be within normal limits, apparently they were not. We excised all three lesions with the laser. Two of them were closed per primum, and the third one we felt would need a skin graft. Since this man wanted as little scarring as possible, we decided to turn a flap. We had already taken the sterile sleeve off the laser and

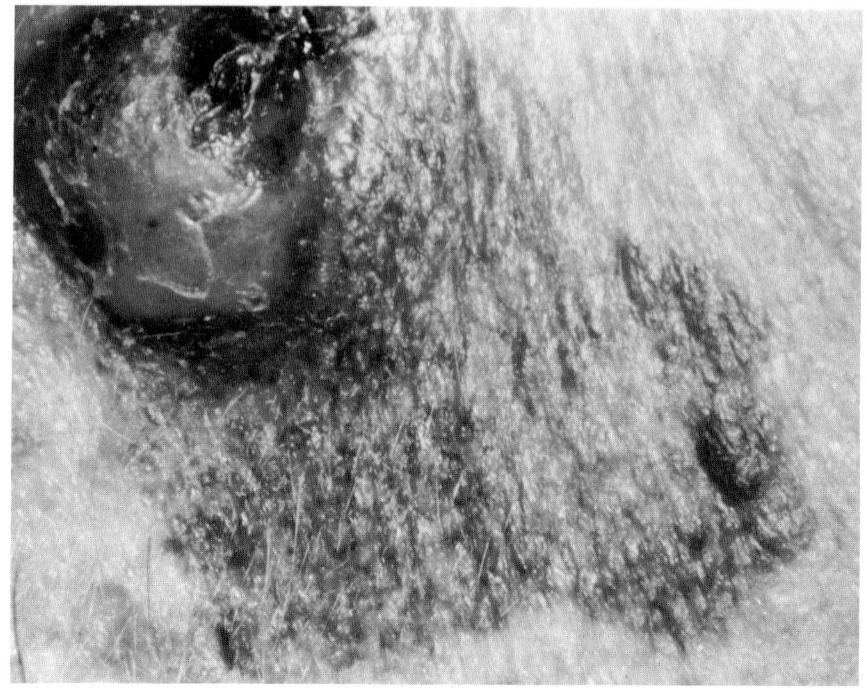

**Fig. 19.4.** Melanoma of right temple.

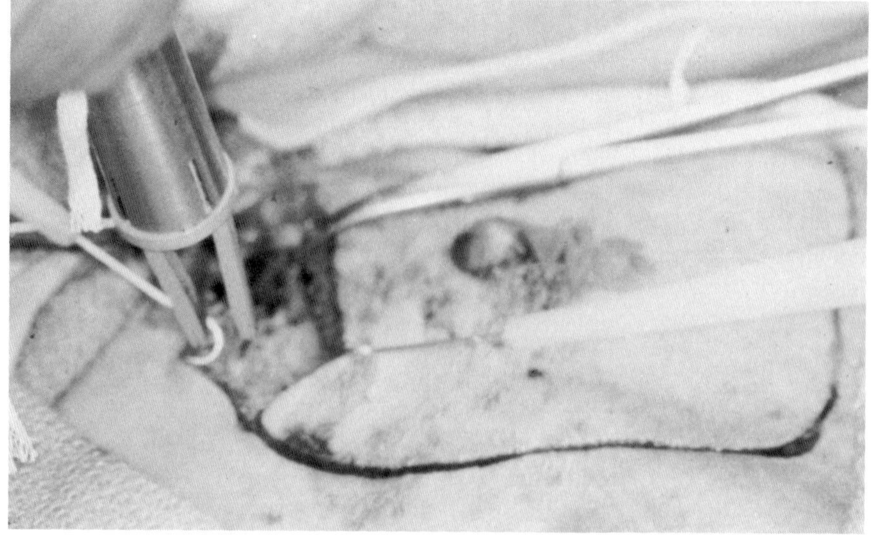

**Fig. 19.5.** Excision of melanoma with laser.

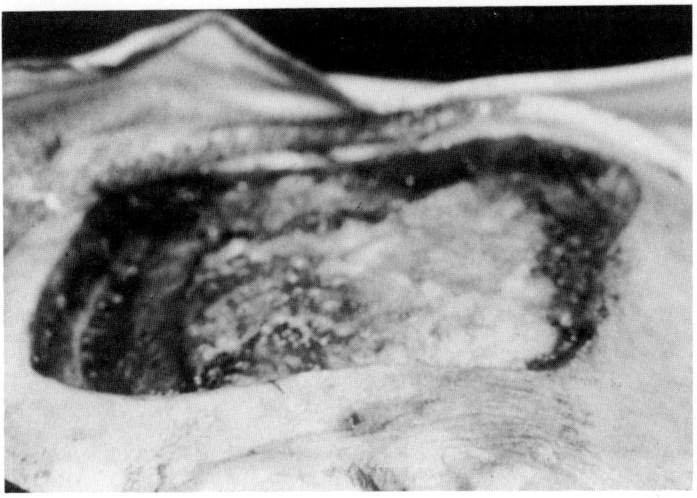

**Fig. 19.6.** Laser excision, including fascia. Parotidectomy and neck dissection were performed in continuity.

decided to use a scalpel. The number of clamps that were necessary to stop the bleeding in this very small flap proved better than anything that I have ever seen the value of using the $CO_2$ laser in this type situation.

We have not attempted to vaporize any melanomas (Figs. 19.4–19.6), for we have felt this is probably not the way to treat them. We have tried to vaporize recurrent tumor in the skin of the head and neck for those people in whom radical surgery has failed, and our results have been very discouraging. Others have reported cases in which vaporization and probably curettage then chemotherapy has worked very well, but in our hands these combined modalities have left a lot to be desired.

## Lesions of the Oropharynx, Nasopharynx, and Hypopharynx

The oral cavity probably gives us the best chance to demonstrate the effectiveness of the laser in head and neck surgery. We have started with the minimal lesions of leukoplakia, erythroplasia, and carcinoma in-situ, and though our experience is probably less than 50 cases, the results have been very gratifying. To date we have had no major recurrences of carcinoma in-situ, and in very few cases has leukoplakia returned.

We feel that if one is going to do this type of work, it should be done with great care to be sure that the tumor is gone, and the patients must be followed up faithfully. To date we know of no controlled series on these cases. Therefore, to be sure that the excision is adequate, we have often taken biopsies of the lasered wound or if we used vaporization, we have obtained frozen sections to be sure that the tumor was completely destroyed.

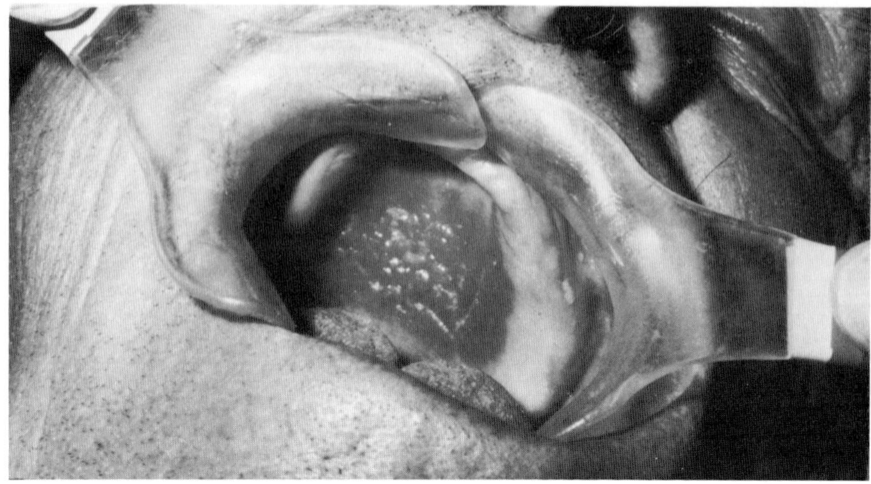

**Fig. 19.7.** Papilloma of palate treated by vaporization with laser.

We are setting up a protocol to compare other modalities, such as the use of cautery versus laser destruction versus surgery, and will, hopefully, have enough information to present in the near future. Certainly on the palate, where skin grafting may be quite difficult and it may at times be necessary to get down to bone with a knife, the use of the laser is par excellence!

**Techniques.** We have tried the laser on various types of benign lesions of the palate (Fig. 19.7) including the papillary tumors that one sees. We have not tried to treat any bony tumors of the palate, but certainly carcinoma in-situ and leukoplakia have been a prominent part of our experience. These are vaporized for the most part. As a rule, we do no biopsies of palate lesions so that it will not be necessary to go too deep. On the buccal mucosa or floor of the mouth, however, we have made it a policy, particularly recently, to vaporize an area with the laser, leaving enough of the leukoplakia or carcinoma in contact on either side. Then, with a knife, we excise this small area to be sure the result is effective (Figs. 19.8–19.10).

During the time of surgery, it is simple to take a dry gauze, or even a wet one if that is preferred, and wipe the tissues clean. After this has been done a few times, one may see that the remaining tissue is normal. This can be proved by microscopy.

Excessive destruction, caused by going down into the fat, is certainly not necessary. That step can result in more scarring than is really desirable, and the deformity that the operator is trying to prevent will occur if the laser has been used for massive destruction. I am referring, of course, to those large patches of leukoplakia in which, in the past, irradiation, cryosurgery, cauterization, and, frequently, excision with skin grafts have been the method of choice. To date, we have been quite successful in avoiding any of these methods, and there has been

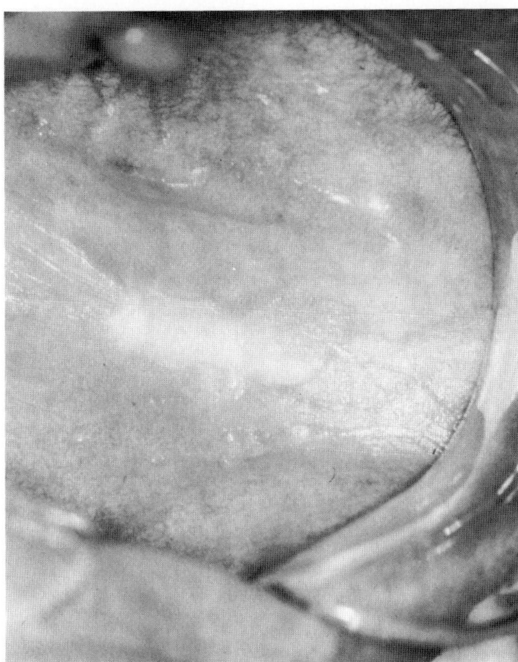

**Fig. 19.8.** Leukoplakia of buccal mucosa.

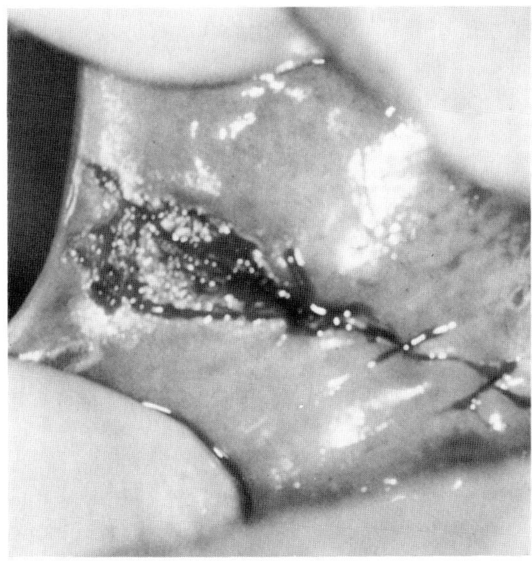

**Fig. 19.9.** Lesion partially vaporized then excised along with nontreated area for microscopic examination.

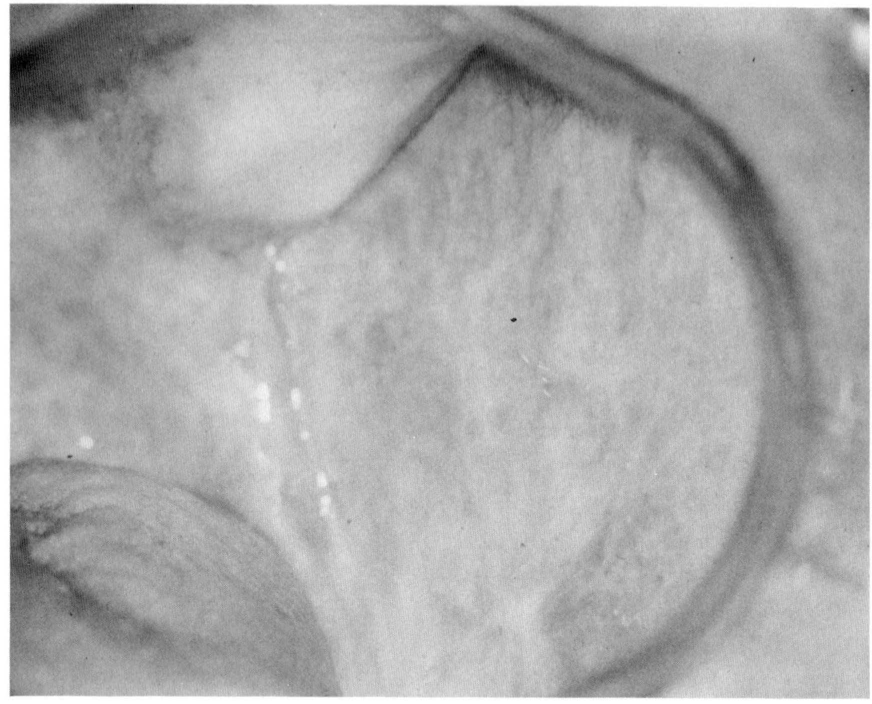

**Fig. 19.10.** At 6 weeks, all lesions have healed.

practically no scarring. The patients have been very happy, with normal contour of both the internal and external surfaces of their faces.

In the South and Southwest United States, where cigarette smoking, snuff dipping, and tobacco chewing are common, extensive leukoplakia occurs very frequently. This large population could certainly be helped by a method that is relatively inexpensive, certainly does not require hospitalization in most cases, and can be carried out under local anesthesia. The morbidity is practically zero, and the mortality should be zero. More importantly, the rehabilitation starts the minute the procedure is finished. These patients can return to work the next day, or even the same day, if they are so inclined. We feel that this is a method of the present, and not of the future, and should be widely used.

We have also used the laser on all other types of intraoral lesions. (Figs. 19.11–19.13). For example, buccal carcinoma has been excised with the laser, and skin grafts have been applied immediately. The bleeding has certainly been much less, the grafts have taken well, and there has been no delay in healing.

## Problem Areas

*The Tongue.* We particularly like to use the laser on carcinoma of the tongue, but in this situation instrumentation can be a problem. We do many intraoral excisions, and in some people whose mouths are not very large, inserting the instrument and

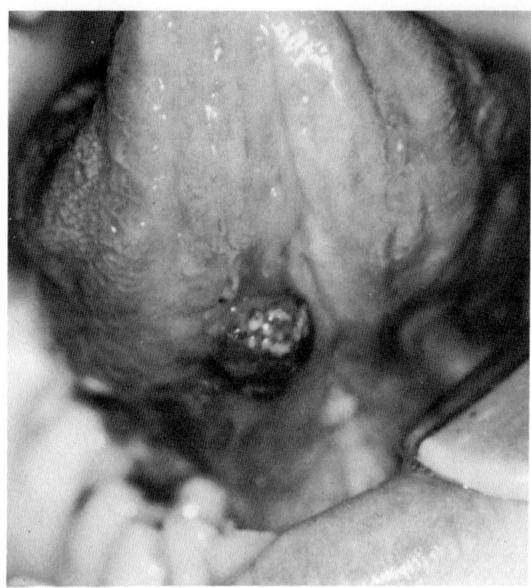

**Fig. 19.11.** Extensive lymphangioma of tongue. Tumor mass of under surface was excised and base was vaporized with laser. No sutures.

obtaining a good view may be quite difficult, particularly in the area of the middle and upper parts, of the posterior third of the tongue. We prop the jaws open as widely as we can (under general anesthesia as a rule), excise the lesions (the pathologist has no difficulty in telling us about the margins), and effect primary closures using some absorbable suture but, for the most part, nonabsorbable, and simply leave them in a few more days. Healing has been good, though a little delayed, and the cosmetic and functional result is good.

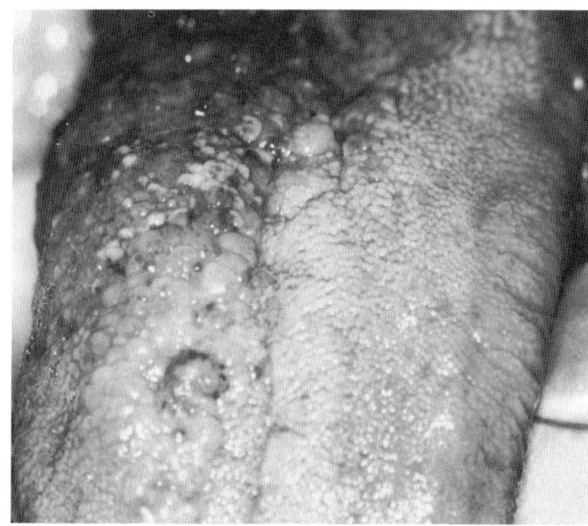

**Fig. 19.12.** Dorsum of tongue treated by vaporization. No bleeding encountered.

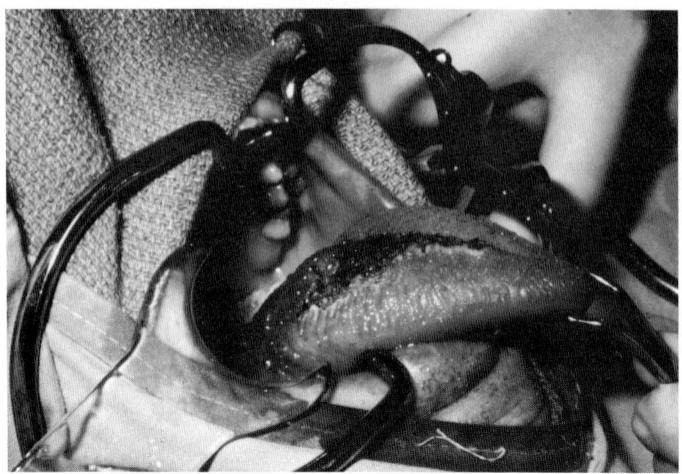

**Fig. 19.13.** Tongue immediately after destruction of lymphangioma.

*The Palate.* Further back on the palate (Fig. 19.14), in the soft palate, or on the pharynx, we often find it quite difficult at times to see what we are doing while the laser is in place, although we certainly use the laser whenever it is possible. Here, certainly, is a place where a fiber-optic instrument or some other instrument may be very beneficial. We have tried using the laser to cut through the bone of the palate while removing malignant lesions and find that it can be done. It is time-consuming, and the big problem, of course, is to get enough retraction so that the bone that has been destroyed is removable. Moreover, the heat is so intense that the adjacent bone is injured, and rongeur forceps must be used to prevent bone from sloughing out later.

*The Mandible.* Early in our experience, we tried to divide the mandible with the laser and found that it was time-consuming, the destruction was great, and healing was definitely prolonged and sometimes did not occur at all. I know of work that has been done in Germany with the use of a different type of gas jet, but to date our experience is limited to the modalities that are common. We have used ice-water slush to try to prevent damage to the surrounding tissues, but our experience is not great enough to evaluate this particular modality. Certainly, some have found it to be of great benefit in preventing thermal damage.

*The Nose.* In treating nasal problems, the laser may be used in many cases. I particularly like it for the vaporization of superficial lesions, but because most nasal lesions must be excised, sometimes the laser is used with fear and trepidation. Many of the patients have already had extensive surgery or irradiation around the nose, and the tissues are thinned. The mucosa may be directly under the skin, with a deficiency of cartilage in that place, or the cartilage may be present and thin, so that if the operator penetrates the skin, the laser has passed through the cartilage and into the mucosa before the operator knows it. This is certainly a drawback in the use of the laser. With the knife, it is often possible to avoid entering the mucosa. Of course, if a through-and-through excision is going to be done, then there is really no problem and the laser is our choice. We do no cosmetic surgery, such as plastic repair of the nose to make it shorter or more cosmetically beautiful, so our evaluation of the laser in this particular situation would be useless.

*The Lips.* The lips offer a challenge to those who use the laser. The laser may be used primarily for vaporization, or it may be used for excision. Excision of the lips with the lasar is quite good (Figs. 19.15–19.17). We find that we had to tie only the marginal artery. Healing has been quite satisfactory, but occasionally it may be delayed.

We have been asked to treat several patients with carcinoma of the lip who have suffered recent heart attacks and are receiving anticoagulant therapy (a mini-heparin dose). We have used the laser to excise these tumors and have been very happy with the minimal amount of bleeding and the highly satisfactory healing of these wounds. For those patients, as well, in whom platelets are decreased as a result of disease or medication, the laser may be used with great confidence that bleeding will be for the most part controlled.

*The Neck.* One cannot talk about surgery of the head and neck without including neck dissections. We have mixed emotions about the use of the laser on the neck. The incision for neck dissection is very simple and may be done with either the laser or the knife. (It has been said many times by many people using the laser

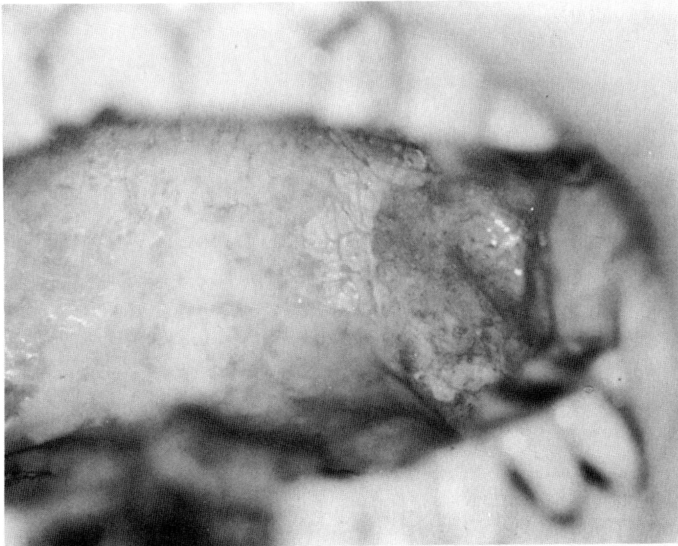

**Fig. 19.14.** Carcinoma of palate and anterior pillar. The tumor was excised with the laser. The jaw was not divided, hence the procedure was more difficult because of the instrument. A split graft was placed with excellent healing.

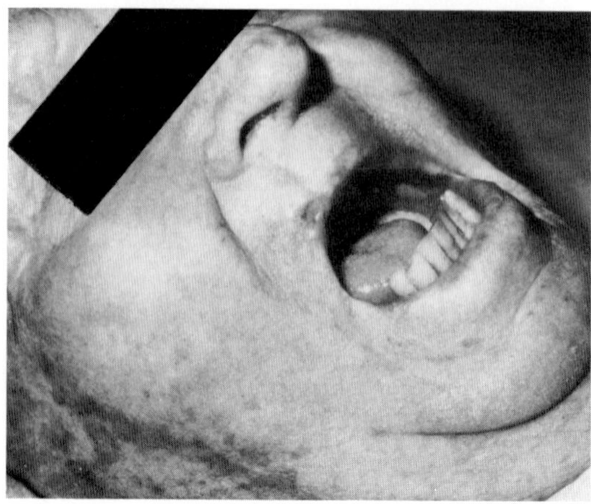

**Fig. 19.15.** Recurrent carcinoma of upper lip in elderly patient.

that it is not the only instrument one has, and the other modalities may be as good as the laser or better.)

Certainly, with adequate assistance, one may make all the incisions necessary for a neck dissection with a minimal amount of bleeding. The flaps may be turned more easily—in my experience, at least—with the knife, and the amount of blood loss with the laser is really comparable to the minimal blood loss that one has with sharp dissection with the scalpel.

One early and discouraging problem we had in using the laser was that fre-

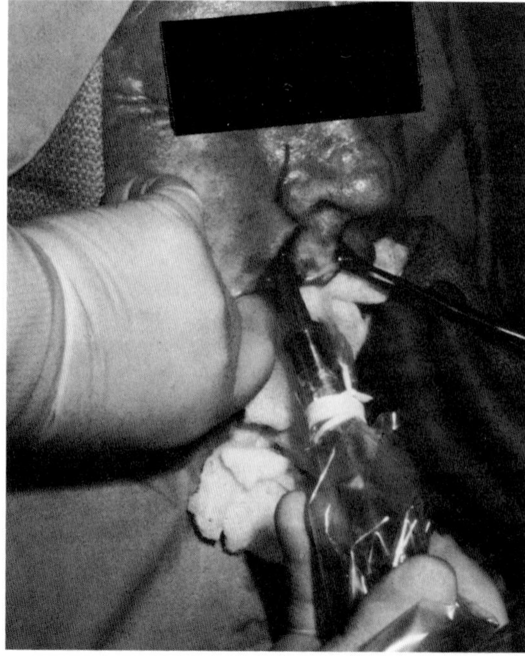

**Fig. 19.16.** Local anesthesia and laser excision. Only marginal vessels were ligated.

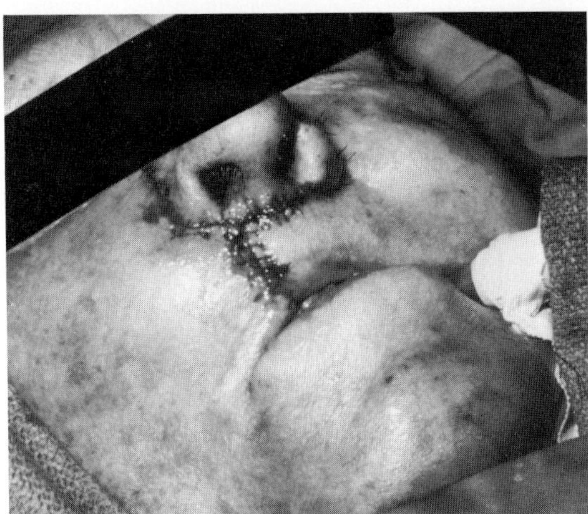

**Fig. 19.17.** Closed wound after creation of ala nasae flaps. Healing was excellent.

quently, in making incisions (particularly transverse incisions), the external jugular vein would be punctured with laser before we were really ready for that experience. Moreover, in turning flaps, it would be very difficult to avoid the external jugular vein, whereas with the knife or the scissors this particular problem could be averted.

When one approaches the vicinity of the brachial plexus or the carotid vessels or even the internal jugular vein, the laser must be used with a great degree of delicacy. Nevertheless, there is a chance that injury may occur much more frequently than when conventional means are used. We have tried putting instruments behind the sternocleidomastoid when it is divided, and in this way we could certainly prevent injury to the structure behind it. However, the procedure is so simple with conventional means that we have just about abandoned the use of the laser for it. Occasionally, if a patient is suffering with any sort of blood dyscrasia, we return to use of the laser, but with the many tools that the surgeon has at his command it is not necessary. I am speaking, of course, of means for lowering the blood pressure or, by gravity, inducing some of the venous drainage away from the neck so that the amount of bleeding during surgery may be minimal.

*Vascular Tumors.* The vascular tumors that one encounters may make it very desirable to have the laser, but on some of these it can almost be disastrous. I am referring to patients who present with tremendous hemangiomas of the head and neck, in which the veins just beneath the skin may be as much as 1 cm or more. When the surgeon has penetrated the skin, the patient's vessels are entered immediately. I know of no one who can really control the laser well enough to prevent this and the loss of a large amount of blood. Still, to some extent, there are exceptions. On one patient, we started with the laser on two different occasions but met with this problem. The third time, when we decided to resect part of the lip where the major vessels had been destroyed, we used the laser and bleeding was minimal. Even though the laser may not be beneficial throughout the case, it may be indispensable in certain areas (Fig. 19.18).

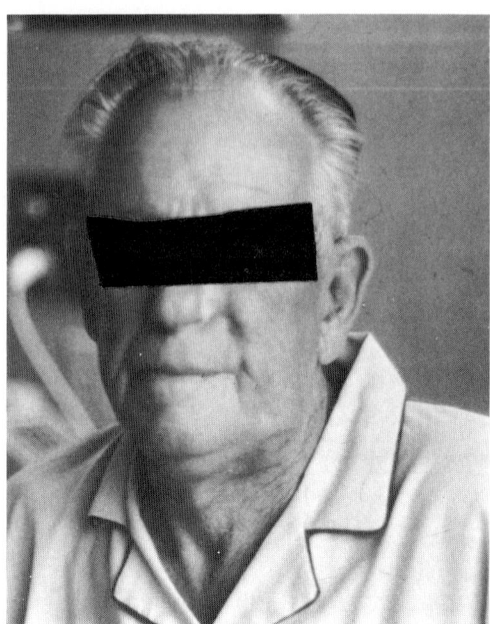

**Fig. 19.18.** Recurrent carcinoma of nose with large submandibular node. Laser resection of area included part of nose and adjacent cheek in continuity with neck dissection. Plastic repair. Ideal case for laser surgery.

## SUMMARY

The $CO_2$ laser is a very diverse and accurate instrument. It may be used in most any type of procedure where a scalpel could be used. Big disadvantages are the departure from conventional means of incision by the surgeon and, more important, unawareness of the possibility of using the laser both to incise and to vaporize tissue. Certainly, in vascular tumors the laser is essential and may, in many cases, convert the patient's problem from an inoperable one to one that may be accomplished with little risk. With the addition of the argon laser, I feel thay many who have suffered for years with horrible deformities can be returned to a normal, active life.

The instrumentation offers problems in certain areas, particularly in the deep part of the oral cavity, but this can partially be alleviated by using a microscope. More importantly, future advances in the instrument will make it more desirable. In the treatment of leukoplakia and carcinoma in-situ of the buccal cavity, the instrument is one that must be used if many of the deformities are to be prevented that could result from extensive resection and grafting. The laser has been shown to seal lymphatics, and this should really reduce the seeding of wounds.

It has been our intention to try to prove that the laser does not interfere with the immune response, but to date our experiments have not been accomplished. Hopefully, this will be something to be done in the immediate future. The $CO_2$ laser is an instrument of today and should be used widely.

# 20

# The Technique of Gastrointestinal Laser Endoscopy

*Richard M. Dwyer*

Application of the laser to the problem of gastrointestinal bleeding was first conceived by three separate groups: (1) the University of Washington group with Drs. Silverstein and Rubin; (2) Dr. Peter Kiefhaber at the University of Munich in Germany; and (3) our group in Los Angeles, California. The first successful application of endoscopic argon laser photocoagulation for bleeding in humans was accomplished by our group in 1974. Subsequently, in 1975, Dr. Peter Frühmorgen et al. in Erlangen, Germany, reported endoscopic coagulation by the argon laser. In 1975, Dr. Peter Kiefhaber first began using the neodymium-YAG laser, and most groups have since followed his lead. The argon laser was first adopted because it was easily focused with the current fiber-optic technology. In addition, the blue-green light of the argon laser is maximally absorbed in things that are colored red, leading to the assumption that since bleeding vessels produce red blood this would be an ideal hemostatic laser, selectively depositing energy in the blood. However, the argon laser's lack of penetration without overlying-tissue vaporization minimizes its ability to stop massive hemorrhages from large-bore vessels such as esophageal varices or large arteries in the gastric and duodenal mucosa. The neodymium-YAG laser, which has greater penetrating power giving uniform heating and coagulation of deep large-diameter vessels, enables the therapeutic endoscopist to control esophageal varices and other massively bleeding vessels.

Therapeutic endoscopy developed because of the lack of any consistently effective alternative modality between the ice-water lavage routinely carried out on bleeding patients and open surgery. Good, flexible fiber-optic endoscopes became available in the late sixties and early seventies, providing adequate visualization of the bleeding sites. Endoscopists endeavored to locate an effective treatment deliverable through the endoscope, including electrocautery, injection of vasoactive substances or sclerosing solutions, tissue adhesives, heater probes, and thrombin spray. With the technical advance represented by coupling lasers to flexible fiberoptic endoscopes, the next priority became the development of a technique for safe coagulation of the largest variety and number of bleeding patients.

## ENDOSCOPY AS A THERAPEUTIC PROCEDURE

Therapeutic endoscopy requires a complete change in the gastroenterologist's approach to gastrointestinal bleeding. New habits must be formed, for one must develop a surgical approach to the problem of gastrointestinal hemorrhage. One must also become familiar with the development of new equipment, such as lasers and other heretofore unorthodox pieces of equipment in the endoscopy suite, to assist in the isolation and treatment of the bleeding points. Physical changes must be made to adapt the standard diagnostic endoscopy suite to the therapeutic endoscopy suite. Finally, proper utilization of the therapeutic facilities must be learned along with the technique of performing therapeutic endoscopic procedures.

To become a therapeutic endoscopist, one has to sail on uncharted waters and cross from simple diagnostic endoscopy into a futuristic area. The development of a surgical approach means the endoscopist must be as available as a surgeon for emergency treatment. This means that if a bleeding patient comes into the hospital and continues bleeding bright-red blood uncontrollably for more than 30 min from the nasogastric tube, the patient should undergo an emergency diagnostic procedure and (if actively bleeding) a therapeutic laser coagulation procedure. The amount of blood transfused and overall morbidity can only be decreased by early endoscopy and coagulation of all bleeding points. The ability to perform emergency endoscopy is also very critical. A person who performs emergency endoscopy does not become proficient enough to attempt laser endoscopy until after completing 100 emergency endoscopic procedures. In general, there is 1 emergency procedure for every 10 elective procedures. The difficulty in performing therapeutic endoscopy lies with the ability of the physician to perform accurate emergency endoscopy and isolate the bleeding point. Approximately 85% of the challenge involved is in being able to perform an accurate and fast emergency endoscopy, while 15% of the work involves using the laser properly. In the past it was adequate to identify the general location of the bleeding point and the probable source of the bleeding. The therapeutic endoscopist must identify the point source of bleeding within the lesion or area of hemorrhage. Then the endoscopist must shoot the point source, which is usually moving with respiration and periodic contractions.

The endoscopist must be able to aggressively and properly manage bleeding and shock with massive replacements of intravenous fluid, colloids, and blood. In general, each patient needs at least two large-bore intravenous lines. It is important, also, to have a team accustomed to therapeutic endoscopy and the proper management of critically ill patients. These patients are either too dangerously ill for surgery or they have a surgically treatable problem making them surgical candidates. Therapeutic endoscopy and emergency surgery have similar requirements for personnel, equipment, space, and even, perhaps, an anesthesiologist for some patients.

It has been speculated that transmural necrosis is a negative result of laser endoscopy. The work of John Dixon et al. (1979) at the University of Utah in dogs showed the absence of any morbidity or mortality from transmural necrosis. Clinically, it is known that thousands of patients who have had gastric surgery and suture lines have a much larger area of transmural necrosis than the laser-treated group.

## EQUIPMENT FOR LASER ENDOSCOPY

The new equipment in the endoscopy room that is of great value in therapeutic endoscopy is large-bone gastric-lavage tubes, such as the Dwyer tube (Fig. 20.1) which has a 58 Fr outer diameter. This tube enables the endoscopist to clear out massive quantities or clots in the stomach by pouring ice saline into a 1-liter funnel, lifting the funnel up to deliver the saline into the stomach, and then lowering the funnel into a 5-gallon reservoir or container which by siphon action, suction, or gravity drains the stomach contents. If this tube becomes obstructed, an atmospheric vacuum suction pump can be applied to the tube removing large clots and debris. The atmospheric vacuum suction is another piece of equipment that is critical for the performance of these techniques. It can be attached to the endoscopic suction to assist evacuation of remaining stomach contents during endoscopy. Isolation of the bleeding point within the area of hemorrhage can be facilitated by either gas or water jets, coaxial or noncoaxial with the laser fiber. The neodymium-YAG laser has the additional advantage of being able to coagulate tissue and effect hemostasis even through a covering of blood. Large-bore channel endoscopies,

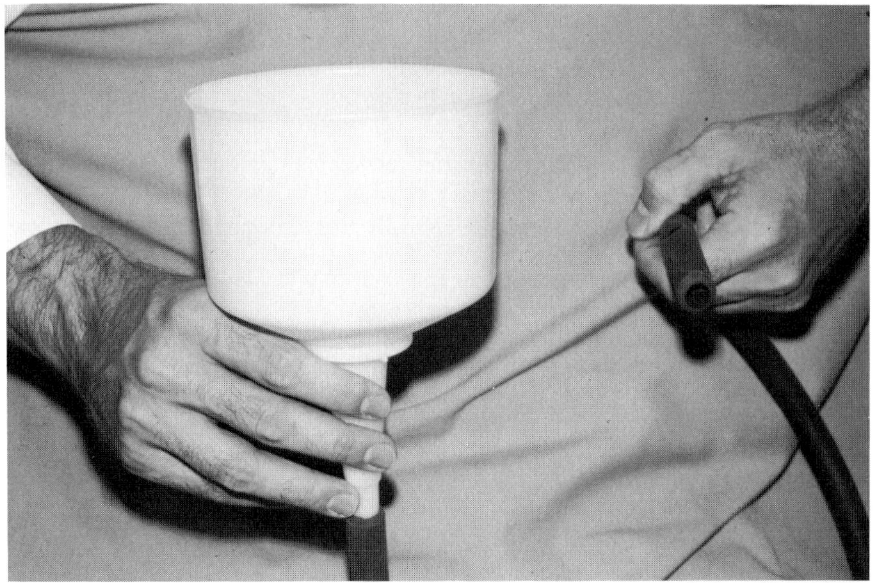

**Fig. 20.1.** Dwyer lavage tube for massive gastrointestinal hemorrhage.

such as the Olympus TGF 1 D, can more rapidly clear accumulated material in the upper intestinal tract and thereby hasten the application of the laser energy. This endoscope is capable of evacuating 80%–90% of large organized clots through its 5-mm suction channel.

There are three endoscopic lasers currently available: one argon laser and two neodymium-YAG lasers. The argon laser requires a greater amount of exposure on target than the neodymium-YAG laser. The argon laser is unable to consistently coagulate massive large-vessel hemorrhage on unselected bleeding patients, however, a high rate of success is observed while using the neodymium-YAG laser on unselected bleeding patients.

The argon laser is produced by Spectra Physics; the neodymium-YAG laser is produced by both Molectron and Messerschmidt. A variety of technical developments are available with these systems. The argon laser system has a coaxial carbon dioxide gas jet around its quartz fiber in order to protect the tip from debris and subsequent burning. This fiber may be inserted into the biopsy channel of most upper endoscopes. The protective carbon dioxide gas flow requirements of this system are approximately 20–60 cc/s with massively bleeding patients. The neodymium-YAG laser produced by Molectron also has a coaxial carbon dioxide gas jet with similar requirements of 20–60 cc/s flow to protect the tip of the fiber. These gas jets, in addition to protecting the tip of the fiber, also may be used to clear blood and debris from the surface area of the target lesion. Two types of gas-protected fibers are offered by Molectron. One fiber has an 8° beam divergency (approximately) and may be inserted into the biopsy channel of most standard endoscopes. The other fiber may only be used in an endoscope with a channel size greater than 3.3 mm and has a lens on the distal end which reduces the beam divergence to approximately 4°. A reduction of beam divergence enables the endoscopist to maintain a coagulation power-density at a greater distance from the target area.

Messerschmidt has developed a carbon-dioxide–protected quartz fiber system that has a nozzle (Fig. 20.2) which reduces the amount of protective gas required to less than 5 cc/s. This fiber has an 8° divergence and may be inserted into any endoscope with a channel of 2.5 mm. They also developed a dedicated laser endoscope from several standard double-channel endoscopes produced by ACMI, Pentax, and Olympus. This endoscope has a 4° beam-divergent fiber mounted in an air- and water-tight channel behind an optically coated disposable quartz window.

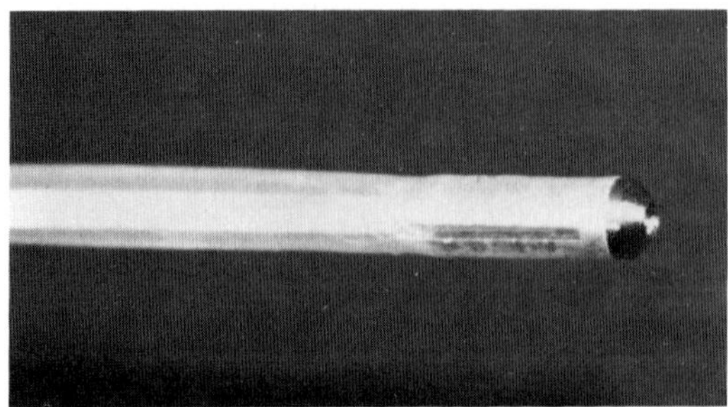

**Fig. 20.2.** Low-flow nozzle tip for $CO_2$-protected laser fiber optic (Messerschmidt).

This packaged laser endoscope frees the endoscopist from any fiber manipulation during laser phototherapy, and with a 4° beam divergence the endoscopist is able to operate at a distance away from the bleeding lesion and still maintain adequate coagulation power-density. They have also developed a third channel in this endoscope which may be used to clear the laser target with a noncoaxial carbon dioxide gas or a water jet.

There are some disadvantages to the higher-flow carbon dioxide gas jet offered by Spectra Physics and Molectron. This flow rate can lead to overdistension of the stomach, resulting in respiratory distress and thinning of the stomach wall and predisposing the tissue to laser perforation. Severe abdominal cramps have been reported with large volumes of carbon dioxide gas in the upper intestinal tract, and respiratory acidosis from absorption of this gas has been observed. The carbon dioxide gas should not be turned on nor the gas-assisted fibers mounted in the endoscope during esophageal intubation because of possible pulmonary complications such as hypoxia or pneumothorax.

Aiming beams are used by all laser endoscopic systems to pinpoint the impact area prior to irradiation. The argon laser system leaves the blue-green light on a lower-power output setting which is easily visualized. The Molectron aiming system uses the white light spot of a xenon lamp directed through the fiber system. The Messerschmidt aiming system uses a helium-neon low-power laser directed through their fiber delivery system, which produces a bright-red spot in the laser impact area.

Laser eye protection is provided by optical filters for the appropriate laser wavelength, which shield the eye while allowing observation of the endoscopic view. The argon laser shield is provided by a mounted, electronically timed and controlled shutter over the eyepiece of the endoscope. When the dense orange filter covers the eyepiece, vision is reduced by almost half. The neodymium-YAG protection filters are 95% transparent and snap on and off the eyepiece easily.

## OPERATING ROOM

Physical room changes are important before attempting therapeutic endoscopies. Requirements for laser endoscopy include: a large room of at least 250–300 $ft^2$; anesthesia capability with an anesthesiology machine in the room; and preparation of the room in the manner of a surgical suite with cardiac monitoring, defibrillator, and crash cart. It is also preferable to have two or three atmospheric vacuum suctions with 3000-cc reservoir bottles in the room and a xenon light source for proper endoscopic illumination in massively bleeding patients.

## TECHNIQUE

The technique initially requires cardiovascular stabilization of the patient with proper fluids and appropriate laboratory studies. The patient's respiratory status must be secure, especially if obtundation is present or when massive gastric lavage will have to be administered in weakened patients. Iced saline should be stored in the endoscopy-room refrigerator at 4°C. This refrigerator should have a capacity of 50 liters or more at any one time. Usually a quick diagnostic endoscopy is performed in bleeding patients to determine the area, and perhaps even the exact point source, of the bleeding site. Proper positioning of the patient may be helpful in localizing the bleeding point. The standard endoscopic position starts with the patient lying in the left lateral decubitus position. However, when heavy bleeding is on the greater curvature of the stomach, the right lateral decubitus position allows better visualization. For lesions at the cardioesophageal junction and in the esophagus, the sitting position is sometimes preferable to allow easy visualization in these areas. At the time of observation of the bleeding point, a laser fiber optic can be introduced into the biopsy channel of the endoscope for treatment or, if using a dedicated endoscope, the diagnostic endoscope could be removed and the therapeutic endoscope immediately inserted. The sequence of lavage and endoscopy may need to be repeated as many as six times in difficult bleeding patients. The duration of the procedures of lavage, blood replacement, stabilization, endoscopy, and laser treatment can exceed 4 h.

The impact of laser energy on tissue produces a characteristic blanching or charring easily recognized by visual observation. This change determines when proper coagulation has occurred. If this change is not observed after laser exposure, then the power output of the laser should be checked along with the integrity of the fiber-optic system and the tip of the fiber. Continued operation of the laser in this situation can lead to the destruction of your equipment. Minor emergency repairs during the procedure, such as changing the protective windows or the fibers, may be necessary along with minor adjustments to the laser itself.

At endoscopy, most patients are bleeding from more than one isolated source. All bleeding areas should be treated by the laser. There may be as many as 12–15 total sites with 1 or 2 major bleeding points. The laser treatment technique is unique for each area and lesion.

## Esophageal Varices

In the esophagus, massive hemorrhage can be so great that the laser energy directed at the point source is unable to cause a coagulation because of the heat sink created by the flowing blood. Several techniques to staunch the blood flow have been effective, such as shooting on each side of the esophageal varix adjacent to the bleeding point with an overlap of perhaps 10%–20% of the laser spot on the varix (Fig. 20.3). This causes a tissue edema cuff and compression of the tissue adjacent to the bleeding varix. Then, coagulation of the open site can be accomplished easily (Fig. 20.4). This technique can be used either at the level of the bleeding point or slightly distal in an attempt to slow the blood flow from the inferior portion of the esophagus.

Another technique in the bleeding esophagus is to deliver a crescent burn across one-third of the circumference in a nonbleeding region distally to reduce heavy blood flow from the esophageal varix above. Other nonlaser techniques that temporarily reduce the bleeding points to allow coagulation are the intravenous bolus or submucosal injection of 5–20 units of vasopressin and the placement of a Linton

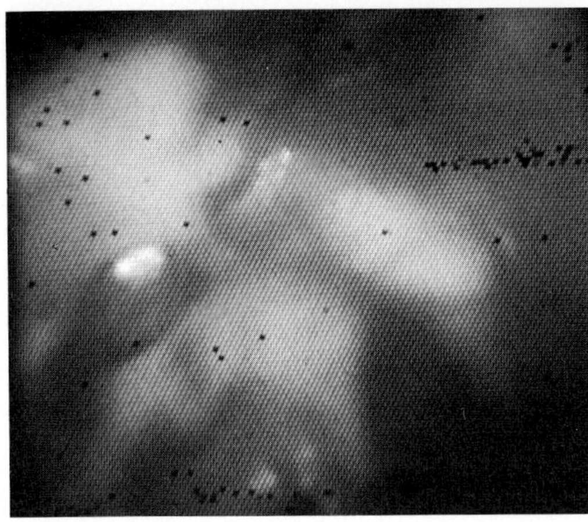

**Fig. 20.3.** Esophageal varix with bilateral adjacent coagulation technique.

tube. The endoscope can be passed beside the Linton tube and coagulation performed. Care must be taken to avoid hitting the Linton balloon or tube with the laser beam, since this might cause a sudden collapse of the balloon with rapid extubation of the Linton tube, resulting in respiratory difficulty and increased hemorrhage.

## Gastric Ulcers

The best technique for coagulating gastric hemorrhage is to shoot the laser beam at the area adjacent to the bleeding point. If this is unsuccessful, shooting at the periphery of the lesion circumferentially may coagulate the feeding vessel or cause a substantial edema cuff to close off or reduce the bleeding point enough for easy coagulation (Fig. 20.5). The edema cuff also protectively increases the thickness of the wall and hopefully reduces the perforation risk. In the case of deep ulcers, both in the duodenum and the stomach, it is wise to shoot the periphery of the ulcer rather than the base. However, if the peripheral coagulation technique is not effective, a pool of blood may be allowed to accumulate in the base of the ulcer and laser impacts may be directed into the ulcer base, coagulating through this film of blood, which then forms a gelatinous coagulum sealing the ulcer.

A B

**Fig. 20.4.** Esophageal varix **(A)** pre- and **(B)** postcoagulation by neodymium-YAG laser.

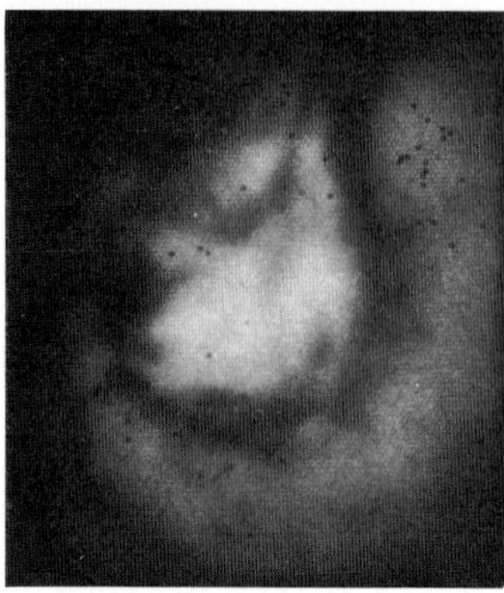

**Fig. 20.5.** Circumferential coagulation of a gastric ulcer.

Sometimes retroflexion of the endoscope is required to coagulate bleeding lesions in the fundus of the stomach. However, this may result in damage to the endoscope if impacted by laser energy. At other times, the angle of the laser beam directed to the target is more tangential than perpendicular. Most of the energy is reflected in this situation, and coagulation can only be accomplished by dragging the endoscope back along the lesion while shooting. Side-viewing endoscopes can be useful if this technique is not successful.

## Other Gastric Lesions

When large areas of diffuse hemorrhage are noted, a Z coagulation technique is recommended. This is accomplished by withdrawing the endoscope while lasering in a back-and-forth motion. This creates a zig-zag pattern across the area of hemorrhage and serves to coagulate vessels feeding into the area of hemorrhage. After slowing of the hemorrhage has been accomplished in this area, individual points within each triangular region of the zig-zag pattern may be coagulated. There are usually two to three points within each triangular area requiring coagulation.

In elective therapeutic endoscopy of lesions, such as hereditary hemorrhagic telangiectasias (Osler-Weber-Rendu) and vascular malformations, it is not advisable to shoot directly at the center of the lesion on the first impact. Initially, the laser energy should be directed circumferentially around the lesion, and the surface of the telangiectasia can be coagulated after the edema cuff has occurred. On occasion, by not following these techniques, one may increase the hemorrhage by vaporizing the clot directly on top of the lesion prior to proper coagulation. After coagulation is completed, water irrigation of the treatment site assists in the cooling, and removal of the insufflated air reduces the distension and tension in the laser-impact area. The collapse of the stomach produces a Z tract of the muscle layers by the horizontal sliding of these layers away from the mucosal area of laser impact. This may also reduce the risk of laser perforation. The important sequence in laser coagulation of all these areas and lesions includes tissue swelling, vessel shrinkage, coagulation, air evacuation, and subsequent surface cooling.

The argon laser can coagulate approximately a 1.5-mm artery, and the neodymium-YAG laser can coagulate approximately a 4-mm artery. The factors in laser tissue coagulation and injury include the wavelength, the optical absorption of that wavelength in a particular tissue, the energy concentration incident on the treatment site (power-density), and the duration of energy concentration on the treatment site (time exposure). The human factor which determines much of the overall success is the ability of the endoscopist to hit a bleeding point amid cardiac, respiratory, and intestinal motions.

## Colonic Hemorrhage

Colonic lesions must be treated differently due to the thinness of the distended colonic wall (Fig. 20.6). Lesions, such as bleeding diverticula and arteriovenous

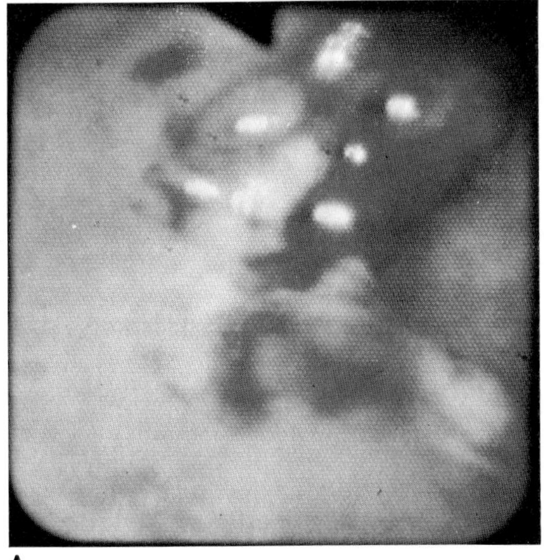

**A**

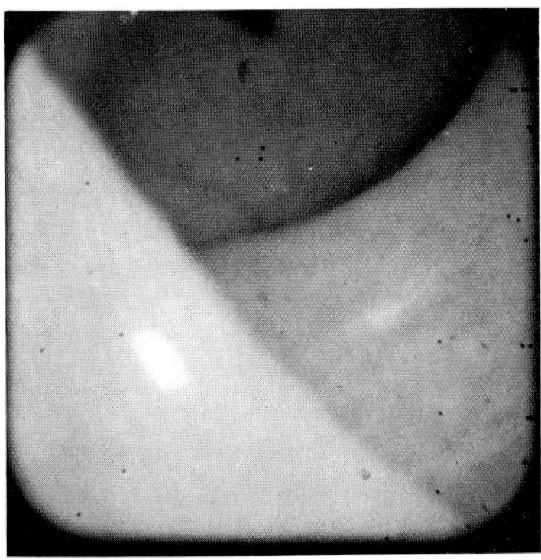

**B**

**Fig. 20.6. A.** Bleeding from nonoperative adenocarcinoma of the colon. **B.** One month postcoagulation with neodymium-YAG laser (biopsies negative for residual cancer). (Courtesy of Dr. Peter Kiefhaber.)

malformations in nonsurgical cases which are unresponsive to conventional therapy, may be coagulated circumferentially by laser energy with an exposure time of 0.1–0.2 s at approximately 60 W throughout of neodymium-YAG energy. The argon laser should have an exposure time of approximately 0.2–0.5 s with a throughout power of approximately 6 W. Colitis is treated with a Z technique and coagulation of all sites visible, as described above. Carcinomas are treated in two ways: by coagulation for hemorrhage and by debulking tumor mass for palliation.

In nonbleeding lesions, such as sessile polyps, coagulation alone without vaporization is adequate for ablation using the neodymium-YAG laser. With the argon laser it is necessary to remove the majority of the lesion by cutting or vaporization to ensure ablation of the lesion.

## PATIENT SELECTION

Patients selected for laser endoscopy treatment are divided into elective and emergency categories. The laser need not be used where other less-expensive, safer, noninvasive, and more effective techniques already exist. Patients selected for elective laser photocoagulation include nonbleeding but recently bleeding patients with a visible vessel, vascular malformations, angiodysplasias, or any chronically bleeding lesion. Patients who have a standard surgical lesion but are not surgical candidates or refuse surgery should be considered for laser treatment. Patients with coagulopathies from any origin and Jehovah's Witnesses (who because of religious reasons refuse all blood and blood-product replacements) who are bleeding should have early and aggressive management with the laser. Patients who do not stop actively bleeding after 30–45 min of gastric lavage and medical management are laser candidates. Patients who present to the emergency room in shock, hemorrhage more than 2 units of blood in the hospital, or rebleed while still in the hospital are emergency laser candidates.

## POSTOPERATIVE CARE

After laser treatment, the patient is given nothing by mouth for 24 h, then placed on a clear-liquid diet and antacids, if tolerated, at 24–48 h posttreatment. Nasogastric tubes are not used to monitor hemorrhage because the mechanical trauma of the tube on the treated site may induce hemorrhage. The nasogastric tube also allows reflux into the esophagus, which may cause subsequent erosions. Routinely, cimetidine is administered intravenously, and then orally when tolerated by the patient, during the entire hospital stay.

## CONTRAINDICATIONS AND COMPLICATIONS

Contraindications to laser endoscopic phototherapy are an uncooperative patient and a poorly trained laser endoscopist. Relative contraindications are an unstable

**Table 20.1.** Complications of Laser Endoscopy

| | |
|---|---|
| Perforation, free and delayed | 1%–2% |
| Increased hemorrhage | |
| Vaporization—higher laser power density | |
| Vasodilatation—low laser power density | |
| Rebleeding | |
| Same location | $<2\%$ |
| New location | $<10\%$ |
| Delay of healing (theoretical) | |
| Overdistension by high-flow $CO_2$ gas | |

patient; a moribund patient; and lesions unusual in size, location, or number. Complications of endoscopic laser phototherapy, other than the standard mechanical and cardiopulmonary complications of emergency endoscopy, are listed in Table 20.1.

## SUMMARY

Lesions suitable for elective laser phototherapy are listed in Table 20.2, and lesions suitable for emergency laser endoscopy are listed in Table 20.3. The worldwide experience with laser endoscopy for gastrointestinal hemorrhage was summarized

**Table 20.2.** Indications for Elective Laser Phototherapy

| |
|---|
| Chronic bleeding lesions |
| Nonbleeding but recently bleeding lesions |
| Vascular malformations |
| Visible vessel |
| Angiodysplasias and telangiectasias |
| Sessile polyps |
| Obstructing carcinomas |
| Infundibulotomy |

**Table 20.3.** Indications for Emergency Laser Phototherapy

| Esophagus | Stomach | Duodenum | Colon |
|---|---|---|---|
| Varices | Varices | Ulcers | Colitis, ulcerative or radiation |
| Esophagitis | Gastritis | Erosions | Diverticula |
| Carcinoma | Ulcers | Postsphincterotomy | Vascular malformations |
| Mallory-Weiss tears | Erosions | Carcinomas | Polyps |
| Vascular malformations | Vascular malformations | Vascular malformations | Carcinomas |
| | Carcinomas | | Postpolypectomy |
| | Postpolypectomy or biopsy | | |

**Table 20.4.** Worldwide Experience with Laser Endoscopy for Gastrointestinal Hemorrhage[a]

| Argon Laser | | | | |
|---|---|---|---|---|
| Unselected patients | | Bleeding episodes | No. patients | Success rate (%) |
| Kiefhaber | Munchen | 587 | 459 | 94 |
| Schonekas | Nurnberg | 334 | 298 | 93 |
| Dwyer | Los Angeles | 106 | 71 | 87 |
| Posl/Sander | Munchen | 83 | 61 | 97 |
| Rhode | Marburg | 83 | 61 | 92 |
| Ramirez | Mexico | | 80 | |
| Weinzierl | Munchen | 77 | 70 | 74 |
| Ghezzi | Mailand | 75 | 65 | 87 |
| Vantrappen | Lowen | 53 | 50 | 96 |
| Wotzka/Kaes | Munchen | 48 | 35 | 81 |
| Ultsch/Bader | Munchen | 37 | 27 | 88 |
| Stauber | Steyr | 30 | 28 | 80 |
| Fiedler/Waldm | Freiburg | 30 | 25 | 80 |
| Kreutzer | Wien | 29 | 25 | 90 |
| Richter | Mannheim | 25 | 20 | 92 |
| Escourrou | Toulouse | 22 | 20 | 75 |
| Immig | Koln | 22 | 14 | 82 |
| Know/Hausaman | Dortmund | 22 | 20 | 82 |
| Marcon | Toronto | 20 | 18 | 75 |
| Ihre | Stockholm | 15 | 15 | 93 |
| Dixon | Utah | 15 | 12 | 100 |
| Troidl | Kiel | 12 | 10 | 85 |
| Viets | Bremen | 11 | 11 | 100 |
| Beckly | Plymouth | 11 | 9 | 82 |
| Classen/Wurbs | Frankfurt | 10 | 10 | 100 |
| Zimmermann | Munchen | 5 | 5 | 100 |
| Sochendra | Hamburg | 3 | 3 | 100 |
| Stadelmann | Furth | 3 | 3 | 100 |
| Tijtgat | Amsterdam | 3 | 3 | 75 |
| Devhle | Zurich | 3 | 3 | 100 |
| Mockel | Koln | 2 | 2 | 100 |
| | | 1776 | 1533 | 90 |

| Nd-YAG Laser | | | | |
|---|---|---|---|---|
| Selected patients | | Bleeding episodes | No. patients | Success rate (%) |
| Brunetaud | Lille | 87 | 80 | 87 |
| Waitman | New York | 50 | 20 | 94 |
| Fruhmorgen | Erlangen | 43 | 41 | 83 |
| Dwyer | Los Angeles | 34 | 21 | 70 |
| LcBodic | Nantes | 18 | 14 | 82 |
| Laurence | London | 12 | 10 | 70 |
| Manegold | Mannheim | 10 | 10 | 100 |
| | | 254 | 196 | 84 |

[a] Data Courtesy of Dr. Peter Kiefhaber.

by Dr. Peter Kiefhaber, and his data are reproduced in Table 20.4. The success rate for the argon laser on selected bleeding patients is 84%, while the success rate of the neodymium-YAG laser on unselected bleeding patients is 90%.

The advantage of laser endoscopy is that it incorporates a therapeutic technique into a commonly used diagnostic procedure. It offers a reliable alternative to emergency surgery for bleeding. Laser endoscopy is safer and can reduce the morbidity and mortality. Reductions in hospital stay, blood transfusions, and days out of work will greatly diminish the skepticism with which this procedure was initially met, and at the same time reduce the cost of management for patients with gastrointestinal hemorrhage.

In the future, we can look forward to such laser applications as cutting through the duodenum into an obstructed common bile duct (infundibulotomy) and vaporizing a channel through an obstructing carcinoma of the esophagus.

## REFERENCES

Allan R, Dykes P (1976) A study of the factor influencing mortality rates from gastrointestinal hemorrhage. Quart J Med 45:533–550.

Baum S, Nusbaum M (1971) The control of gastrointestinal hemorrhage by selective mesenteric arterial infusion of vasopressin. Radiology 98:497–505.

Bown SG, Salmon PR (1979) The factors determining the safety and efficiency of Argon and Nd:YAG laser photocoagulation. Presented at the International Medical Laser Symposium, Detroit, Michigan, March 1979.

Boyce HW (1980) Upper gastrointestinal bleeding evaluation and treatment. Practical Gastroenterology 4:38–44.

Brunetaud JM (1979) Argon laser coagulation of acute gastrointestinal bleeding. Therapeutic Gastrointestinal Laser Endoscopy Course, San Francisco, California, April 1979.

Brunetaud JM (1979) Argon laser sphincterotomy or infundibulotomy for ampullary obstruction. Therapeutic Gastrointestinal Laser Endoscopy Course, San Francisco, California, April 1979.

Dixon JA, Berenson MM, McCloskey DW (1979) Neodymium: YAG laser treatment of experimental canine gastric bleeding. Acute and chronic studies of photocoagulation, and perforation. Gastroenterology 77:647–651.

Dotter CT, Goldman ML, Rosch J (1975) Instant selective arterial occlusion with isobutyl 2-cyanoacrylate. Radiology 114:227–230.

Douglass, H Jr (1974) Levarterenol irrigation. JAMA 230:1653–1647.

Dunn DH, et al. (1977) The treatment of hemorrhagic gastritis with H-2 blocking antihistamine, cimetidine. Gastroenterology 72:1053.

Dwyer RM (1976) Treatment of upper gastrointestinal bleeding by endoscopic submucosal injection of vasopressin. Gastrointest Endosc 22:223.

Dwyer RM, Bass M (1977) Lasers in Medicine. Academic Press, New York.

Dwyer RM, Bass M (1978) Laser phototherapy in man using argon and Nd:YAG lasers. Gastrointest Endosc 24:195–196.

Dwyer RM, Bass M, Van Stryland E (1979) Safe and effective laser phototherapy in man using the Nd:YAG laser. Presented at the International Medical Laser Symposium, Detroit, Michigan, March 1979.

Dwyer RM, Haverback BJ, Bass M, Cherlow J (1975) Laser induced hemostasis in canine stomach. JAMA 231:486–489.

Dwyer RM, Yellin AE, Cherlow J, Bass M, Haverback BJ (1975) Laser induced hemostasis in the upper gastrointestinal tract using a flexible fiberoptic. Gastroenterology 68:888.

Dwyer RM, Yellin AE, Crag J. Cherlow J, Bass M (1976) Gastric hemostasis by laser phototherapy in man. JAMA 236:1383.

Eastwood GL (1977) Does early endoscopy benefit the patient with active upper gastrointestinal bleeding? Gastroenterology 72:737.

Frühmorgen P, Boden F, Reidenbach HD, et al. (1975) The first endoscopic laser coagulation in the human GI tract. Endoscopy 7:156–157.

Frühmorgen P, Bodem F, Reidenbach HD, et al. (1976) Endoscopic laser coagulation of bleeding gastrointestinal lesions with report of the first therapeutic application in man. Gastrointest Endosc 23:75–78.

Gaisford WD (1976) A new prototype 2-channel upper gastrointestinal operating fiberscope. Gastrointest Endosc 22:148–150.

Goodale RL, Okada A, Gonzales R, et al. (1970) Rapid endoscopic control of bleeding gastric erosions by laser radiation. Arch Surg 101:211–214.

Griffiths W, Neumann D, Welsh J (1979) The visible vessel as an indicator of uncontrolled or recurrent gastrointestinal hemorrhage. N Eng J Med 300:1411–1413.

Hastings P, Skillman J, Bushnell L, et al. (1978) Antiacid titration in the prevention of acute gastrointestinal bleeding. N Eng J Med 298:1041–1045.

Hellers G, Ihre T (1975) Impact of change to early diagnosis and surgery in major upper gastrointestinal bleeding. Lancet 20:1250–1251.

Jensen DM, Machecado G, Tapia J, et al. (1980) Endoscopic coagulation of telangiectasia with Argon laser photocoagulation and bipolar electrocoagulation in patients with chronic gastrointestinal bleeding. Clin Res 28:29A.

Johnston GW, Rodgers HW (1974) A review of 15 years experience in the use of sclerotherapy in the control of acute haemorrhage from oesophageal varices. Br J Surg 60:797–800.

Johnston J, Jensen D, Mautner W, et al. (1980) YAG laser treatment of experimental canine gastric ulcers. Gastroenterology 79:1252–1261.

Katon RM (1976) Experimental control of gastrointestinal hemorrhage via the endoscope: A new era dawns. Gastroenterology 70:272.

Katon RM, Smith FW (1973) Panendoscopy in the early diagnosis of acute upper gastrointestinal bleeding. Gastroenterology 65:728–734.

Kiefhaber P (1976) Endoskopische Blutstillung mit Laserstrahlen. Fortschr Med 94:656.

Kiefhaber P, Nath G, Moritz K (1977) Endoscopic control of massive gastrointestinal hemorrhage by irradiation with a high power neodymium-YAG laser. Prog Surg 15:140–155.

Kiefhaber P, Nath G, Moritz K, et al. (1975) Program Congress Gastroenterology and Endoscopy 7th, Vienna.

Kiselow MC, Wagner M (1973) Intragastric instillation of Levarterenol. Arch Surg 107:387–389.

Knoblauch M, Stevka E, Lammli J, et al. (1976) The Mallow-Weiss syndrome: A clinical study of 20 cases. Endoscopy 8:5–9.

Lucas CE, Sugawa C, Riddle J, et al. (1971) Natural history and surgical dilemma of "stress" gastric bleeding. Arch Surg 102:266–273.

Macoomb RK (1960) Polyurethane foam (Ostamer): Its use in experimental animals and in the investigation of tissue reactions. Surg Forum 11:454.

Matsumoto T, Hardaway PM, Heisterkamp A, et al. (1967) Higher homologous cyanoacrylate tissue adhesives in surgery of internal organs. Arch Surg 94:861.

Meyer HJ, Haverkamp F, Drake KH (1979) Optical and thermophysical tissue characteristics. Presented at the international Medical Laser Symposium, Detroit, Michigan, March 1979.

Midgley R, Cantor D (1977) Upper gastrointestinal hemorrhage—diagnosis and management. West J Med 127:371–377.

Nath G, Gorisch W, Kiefhaber P (1973) First laser endoscopy via a fiberoptic transmission system. Endoscopy 5:208–213.

Palmer ED (1969) The vigorous diagnostic approach to upper gastrointestinal tract hemorrhage. JAMA 207:1477–1480.

Papp J (1976) Endoscopic electrocoagulation of upper gastrointestinal hemorrhage. JAMA 236:2076–2079.

Piercey JRA, Auth DC, Silverstein FE, et al. (1978) Electosurgical treatment of experimental bleeding gastric ulcers: Development and testing of a computer control and a better electrode. Gastroenterology 74:527–534.

Rosch J, Dotter CT, Brown MJ (1972) Selective arterial embolization: New method for control of acute gastrointestinal bleeding. Radiology 102:303–306.

Rossi N, Green E, Pike J (1968) Massive bleeding of the upper gastrointestinal tract due to Dieulafoy's erosion. Arch Surg 97:797–800.

Sandlow LJ, et al. (1974) A prospective randomized study of the management of upper gastrointestinal hemorrhage. Am J Gastroenterol 61:282.

Silverstein FE, Protell RL, Gilbert DA, et al. (1978) Argon vs laser treatment. III. Development and testing of a gas-jet assisted argon laser wave-guide in control of bleeding experimental ulcers. Gastroenterology 74:232–239.

Sugawa C, Shier M, Lucas CE, et al. (1975) Electrocoagulation of bleeding in the upper part of the gastrointestinal tract. Arch Surg 110:974–979.

Welch AJ (1979) Interaction of light with biologic tissue, part 2. Presented at the International Medical Laser Symposium, Detroit, Michigan, March 1979.

# 21

# A Review of Soviet Techniques in Laser Instrumentation for Medicine and Biology

*Nikolai F. Gamaleya*

The first lasers appeared in the Soviet Union in 1960. Their production was based on the fundamental research in the field of quantum radiophysics by Basov and Prokhorov (Lenin and Nobel Prize winners) (Basov and Prokhorov, 1954; Basov et al., 1959, 1961) and other Soviet physicists. In 1963–1965 research into the biomedical applications of laser radiation was started, and the first attempts in development of laser systems especially for medical purposes were made.

This review is confined to laser systems that are already produced industrially, and no equipment is presented that is undergoing development.

## THE PRINCIPAL PURPOSES OF BIOMEDICAL APPLICATIONS OF LASERS

All applications of the laser in medicine and biology may be divided quite conventionally into two main groups: (1) the laser as a tool for research (i.e., laser spectroscopic investigation, microbeam systems, holography, etc.) and (2) the laser as an instrument for influencing an organism and its components. There is actually no specially manufactured equipment in the first category. The second category comprises three types (Fig. 21.1):

The first type consists of equipment for coagulating pathologic foci, such as a detached retina, skin tumor, or similar defect. This equipment is based on the pulsed or continuous-wave (CW) lasers. The power-density obtained is not sufficient to induce deep dehydration of tissues, and their evaporation is not substantial.

The second type comprises the surgical instruments for various branches of medicine. The CW or pulsed generators with a sufficient frequency of high-pulse repetition used in

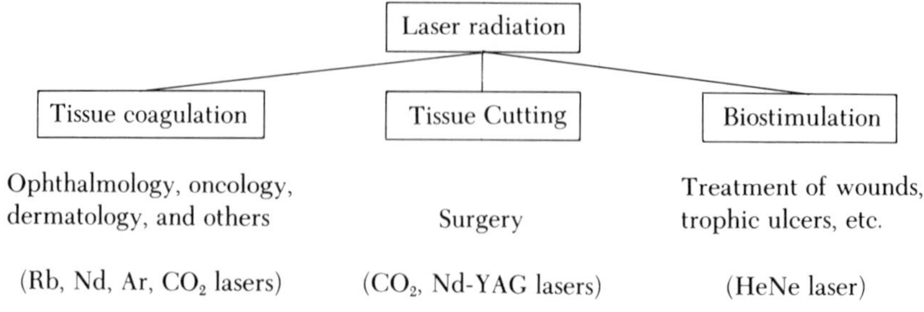


**Fig. 21.1.** Diagram of principal directions of laser medical application.

these instruments (up to now, CW $CO_2$ lasers have been used mostly) permit the achievement of greater power-densities than are possible with the coagulating devices and provide the cutting effect. More flexible devices for laser-beam manipulation are also characteristic.

The third type is equipment for biostimulation with the laser. Following the discovery of a phenomenon of favorable influence that a red laser beam can exert upon an organism, special equipment was developed employing low-intensity HeNe lasers.

## OPHTHALMOLOGIC LASER SYSTEMS

The road to the application of laser coagulation in ophthalmology was paved by Xe-arc coagulators, beginning in 1964 with the use of the OK-1 ruby-laser photocoagulator (Linnik, 1966; Puchkovskaya et al., 1966), which was succeeded by an improved model—the OK-2.

### The OK-2 Ruby-Laser Ophthalmocoagulator

The OK-2 photocoagulator[1] (Linnik, 1972) is intended for the treatment of retinal detachments and tears and for coagulation of intraocular tumors. The construction of the apparatus provides means for ophthalmoscopic investigation and coagulation of the lesions situated in the region of the macula or in the peripheral zone of the retina. The position of the optical head in vertical and horizontal planes is regulated automatically by buttons placed on the frame of the head. The radiation energy is set smoothly or in steps. The patients are treated in the recumbent position.

The technical characteristics of the OK-2 ruby-laser ophthalmocoagulator are as follows:

Wavelength of radiation, 694.3 nm
Pulse duration, 1 ms

[1]Advertisement for the laser ophthalmocoagulator OK-2 (1978) Quantum Electronics 5:239–240.

Pulse energy, 0.3–1.5 J
Pulse-repetition frequency, 50/s
Cooling system, water
Transmission coefficients of light filters, 0.2, 0.4, 0.6, 0.8

The magnifications of visual systems of the equipment are the following:

Monocular, 10×, 20×, 27×
Binocular, 3.5×, 5×
Supply voltage, 220 V (50 Hz)
Supply power, 2.5 kW
Overall dimensions, 550 × 650 × 1500 mm
Mass, 250 kg

The OK-2 ophthalmocoagulator and its predecessor (the OK-1) were used extensively for the treatment of retinal detachments (Linnik, 1969), for melanoblastomas of the choroid (Terent'eva, 1971, 1973), and for prophylactic irradiation of patients with cystic degeneration of the retina (Lebekhov and Kerova, 1973). An experimental and clinical comparison of laser and Xe-arc coagulation was presented by Libman (1973); see also a survey by Gamaleya (1977).

As a result of preliminary clinical applications of other generators besides the ruby laser (especially argon lasers) (Filimonova, 1973; Krasnov et al., 1973b; Belyaeva et al., 1974; Saprykin et al., 1974) a photocoagulator of a new type was tested recently in which three different lasers (ruby, neodymium, and argon) are used.

## The Yataghan-1 Laser Ophthalmologic Apparatus

The apparatus (Fig. 21.2) is used for the microsurgical interventions on the anterior region of the eye without disturbance of its integrity. The creation of the Yataghan-1 apparatus is related to research by Krasnov and his collaborators (Krasnov, 1973a,b,c; Krasnov et al., 1973a; Krasnov et al., 1974a,b). They showed that irradiation, by means of a Q-switched ruby laser, of the superior angle of the anterior chamber in patients with glaucoma produced a temporary hypotensive effect. The operation, called laser goniopuncture, induced widening of the tissue spaces in the filtering zone, apparently as a result of the mechanical effect of laser radiation. As the thermal factor can lead, in an opposite way, to a coagulating effect and obliteration of filtering space, the use of a laser operating in Q-switched mode is essential.

The technical characteristics of the Yataghan-1 laser ophthalmologic equipment are as follows:

Radiation wavelength, 694.3 nm
Pulse duration, 50–70 ns
Pulse power, 0.5–0.8 mW

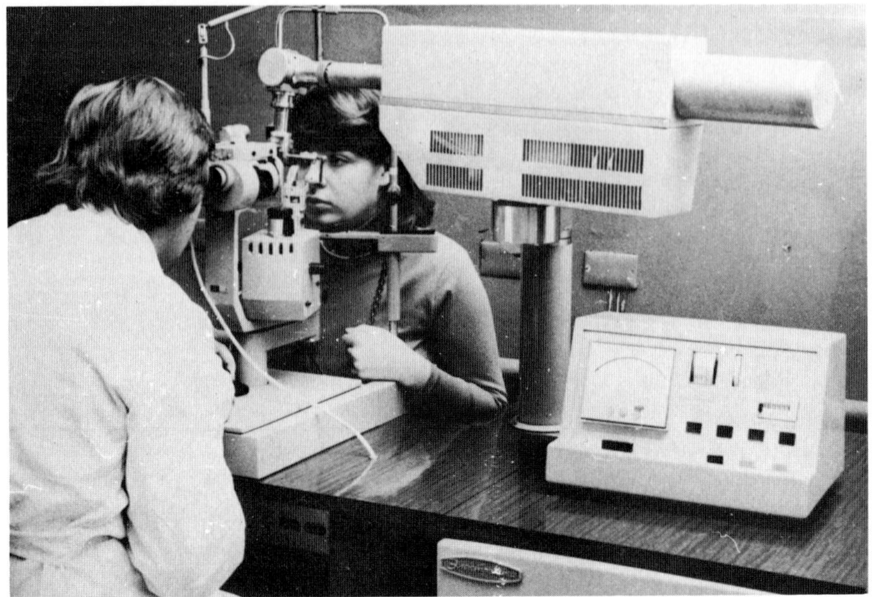

**Fig. 21.2.** Yataghan-1 laser ophthalmologic apparatus.

Energy of radiation (a train of not less than 3 pulses), 0.1–0.2 J
Pulse-repetition frequency, 1/5 Hz
Spot diameter, 0.3–0.5 mm
Beam divergence, not more than 9 mrad

The Yataghan-1 apparatus consists of the emitter, including ruby and HeNe lasers, a supply unit, a control panel, an ophthalmologic slit lamp, and a binocular microscope (Malishev et al., 1976). The HeNe laser (The LG-56 model) serves as a part of the aiming system. The physician's eyes are protected from reflected light with a shutter that shields the microscopic objective automatically in the moment of irradiation.

The Yataghan-1 system is recommended for the treatment of open-angle and closed-angle primary glaucoma in an initial phase, the various kinds of secondary cataracts, some types of "mild" childhood and juvenile cataracts, and cysts of the iris. The operations for open-angle glaucoma are performed after local anesthesia, which is necessary for the introduction of a special spherocylindrical lens (goniolens) suggested by Krasnov (irradiation itself is painless). From 15 to 20 pulses in the form of a continuous chain are applied during the session. The mean duration of the hypotensive effect from one session was 2–3 months (Krasnov, 1973b,c).

The treatment of closed-angle glaucoma is carried out by irradiation of the areas of the iris that have been pretreated with an argon laser. The procedure does not require anesthesia (Krasnov et al., 1974a). The irradiation of patients suffering secondary cataracts and cysts of the iris also is given without anesthesia.

The Yataghan-1 is the original apparatus, with worldwide priority, and has been patented in several countries.

## THE EQUIPMENT FOR DERMATOLOGY, ONCOLOGY, AND SURGERY

On the basis of the diverse laser experiments with animals (Kavetskii et al., 1969; Gamaleya, 1972; Kromov, 1973; Pletnev et al., 1978), several laser systems for dermatology, oncology, and surgery were constructed and are undergoing clinical tests. In these systems, pulsed Nd or CW $CO_2$ lasers are utilized, providing tissue coagulation or cutting. Some of these are briefly described: the Impulse-1, the Pulsar-1000, the Scalpel-1, the LGM, and the Effect.

### The Impulse-1 Laser Apparatus

The Impulse-1 apparatus (Rosenfeld et al., 1973) is based on a pulsed Nd laser (wavelength, 1060 nm; maximum energy, 1000 J; pulse duration, 2 ms). The optical head is adapted so that it can be moved back and forth and around its axis. This freedom of movement, added to the swinging movements of the apparatus stem, facilitates direction of the radiation at any point of the operating field. The installation is equipped with a water-cooling system, energy-measuring devices, and television and radio communication between technical and control sections.

The Impulse-1 apparatus is used for the irradiation of skin tumors. Attempts were made also to evaluate the possibility of treating Meniere's syndrome (Nikolaev et al., 1976).

### The Pulsar-1000 Laser Medical System

The Pulsar-1000 system (Vaniukov et al., 1975), like the Impulse-1, is designed for coagulation of biologic tissues. It includes a pulsed Nd laser (wavelength, 1060 nm; exit energy, 1000 J; pulse duration, 1 ms). The system features a water-cooling device with a pump and a thermostat; a light guide by which the beam may be moved over an operating area of $400 \times 700 \times 500$ mm and directed at an angle of $\pm 90°$; a built-in energy meter; an aiming light beam supplied by an incandescent lamp with a special optical system; and the main and distant control panels.

The Pulsar-1000 system was used most extensively in Petrov's Oncological Institute of Leningrad, where hundreds of patients with malignant and benign skin tumors were treated (Wagner et al., 1974, 1975, 1977). In dermatology, the system was applied for irradiation of hyperkeratosis, tattoo marks, etc. (Rakcheev et al., 1976).

### The Scalpel-1 Laser Apparatus

The Scalpel-1 (Fig. 21.3) was one of the first laser surgical apparatuses produced commercially. It is based on the CW $CO_2$ laser with output power not less than 25

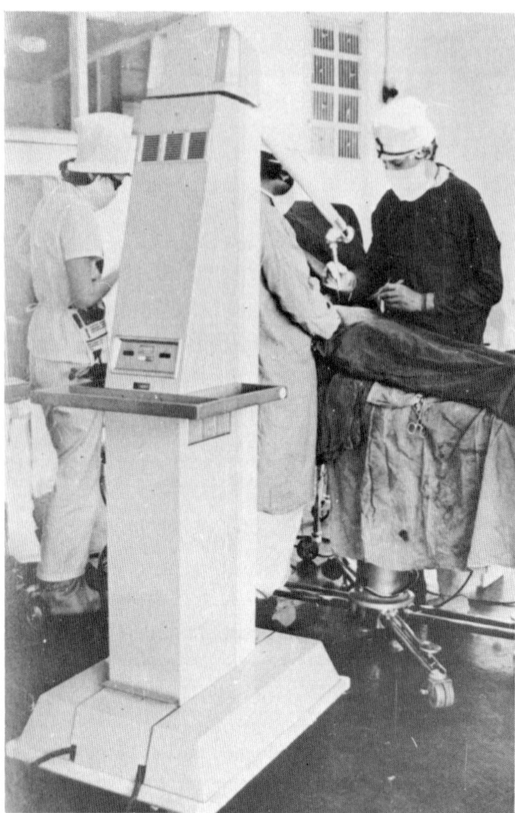

**Fig. 21.3.** Operation with Scalpel-1 laser apparatus.

W. The apparatus is fitted with a light guide that provides free manipulation of the beam, focused to a spot of 0.5 mm, over an area 200 × 500 mm. The maximum power at the light guide exit is not less than 20 W and may be regulated to levels of 20%, 40%, 60%, and 80% of maximum power.

In spite of comparatively low power of radiation, the apparatus was used quite successfully for performing various surgical interventions, especially in operations on alimentary canal (Skobelkin et al., 1976). For this purpose, the laser apparatus was used in combination with appliances that were specially designed for use with the laser instruments: clamps for stomach and intestine, a mending device for hollow organs, etc. The instruments were intended to provide local compression of organs, precise mechanical movement of the beam, and complete isolation of it from bordering tissues, and also to facilitate rapid cutting and closure of tissues.

Patients with stomach ulcers and cancers of the esophagus, stomach, and rectum underwent operation. The irradiation proved effective in providing hemostasis, in preventing abdominal-cavity infection, and in creating optimal conditions for the application of anastomosis of any kind.

## The LGM Laser Surgical Apparatuses

The apparatuses of this family, incorporating the CW $CO_2$ lasers, were created as a result of joint work of engineers and scientists at Herzen's Oncological Institute of Moscow (Belyaev et al., 1976; Abdurazakov et al., 1976). The first model of the LGM apparatus had the following main characteristics:

Radiation power at manipulator exit, not less than 20 W
Focused-beam diameter, not more than 0.3 mm
Operating-area dimensions, 400 × 400 × 200 mm

The apparatus was used for the treatment of skin tumors by coagulation with unfocused radiation or (more seldom) by tumor tissue excision with focused beam (Pletnev et al., 1978). In our department at the Kavetskii Institute for Oncology Problems, the apparatus was applied with good results in the irradiation of females with epithelial dysplasias of the cervix uteri (Milianovskii et al., 1976; Polishchuk et al., 1977).

Recently, clinical tests of the second model of the LGM apparatus were started. This model has a maximum radiation power 100 W, regulated smoothly or in steps. There is a system of automatic exposures to irradiation from 40 to 80 s. The dimensions of the operating field are extended to 500 × 500 × 250 mm.

## The "Effect" Medical Installation

The most important distinctive features of the Effect medical installation are (1) the joining up of two different types of lasers (pulsed and CW) and (2) the availability of an automatic mode of operation (Isakov et al., 1976). The lasers are usually installed in a separate room. There are a pulsed Nd laser (with an output energy of 1000 J, pulse duration of 2 ms) and a CW $CO_2$ laser (with an output power of 50W). The laser radiation is transmitted by two light guides (separate for Nd and $CO_2$ lasers) to a scanning device (Fig. 21.4). The light guide from the $CO_2$ laser has an additional flexible two-jointed arm. By its optics, the laser beam can be focused to a spot diameter of 0.2–0.5 mm and directed to any point within an area 500 × 500 × 200 mm. Actually the scanning device may be used with any other laser besides the Nd and $CO_2$ lasers. The scanning device is operated manually, semiautomatically (with aid of a remote control panel), or automatically by a computer, in accordance with a coded program of irradiation. The lasers are supplied with a water-cooling system. The equipment includes a vacuum trap for smoke, energy meters, an aiming device with a HeNe laser as a light source, and a radio and television communication system between the control section and the operating theater.

My coworkers and I have used the Effect medical installation for the treatment of patients with different forms of malignant and benign skin tumors (Gamaleya and Polishchuk, 1977, 1978). The Effect equipment has been patented not only in the Soviet Union, but also in the United States and the Federal Republic of Germany.

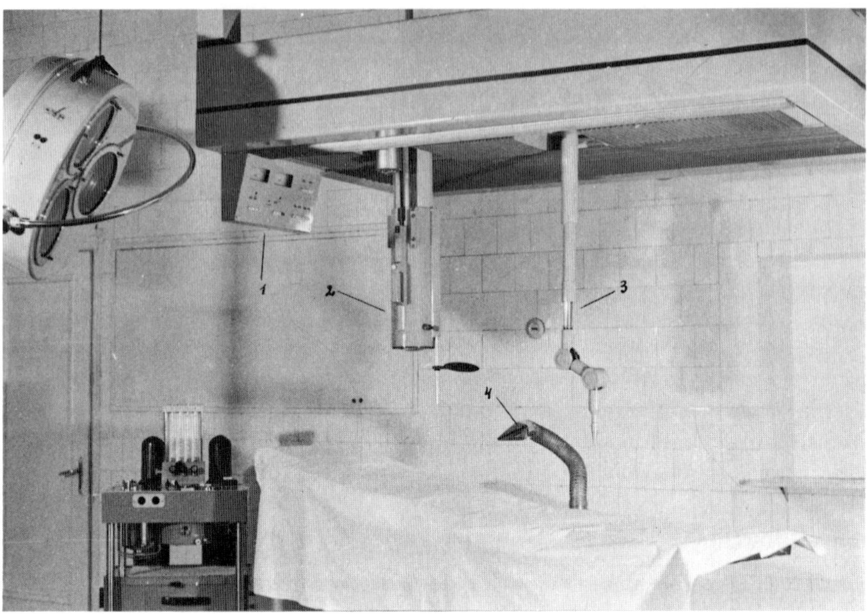


**Fig. 21.4.** The Effect medical installation: *1*, control panel; *2*, light guide of Nd laser; *3*, manipulator of $CO_2$ laser; *4*, vacuum trap for smoke.

## THE APPARATUSES FOR LASER BIOSTIMULATION (LASER PHYSIOTHERAPEUTICS)

The original direction of laser medical instrument-making was brought about by the discovery of the stimulating effect of HeNe laser radiation (wavelength, 632.8 nm) on different biologic processes, which was nevertheless not explained satisfactorily (Gamaleya, 1977). In dermatology, stomatology, orthopedics, and other branches of Soviet medicine, a vast amount of material was accumulated on the favorable action of low-power red laser light in patients suffering from various local injuries and even systemic diseases (Babayants et al., 1974, 1976; Koshelev et al., 1974; Inyushin and Chekurov, 1975; Bogdanovich and Karimov, 1978; Korytnyi, 1979). The most convincing results were presented on the treatment of indolent wounds and trophic ulcers.

In the majority of cases the investigators utilized usual HeNe lasers, as such, or with the addition of simple optical systems. The method of treatment was very simple: The pathologic foci were irradiated once or repeatedly by a laser beam with a power of a few milliwatts and exposures ranging from several seconds to several minutes. In other cases, especially in patients with systemic diseases, the irradiation of biologically active (acupuncture) points was performed.

Lately, special physical-therapy apparatuses have been designed in which CW

HeNe lasers are fitted with focusing lenses, fiber light guides, and devices for automatic exposures (Boyarskih et al., 1976). Some of the models are intended for irradiation of biologically active points and are supplied with a device for spotting such areas on the basis of their different electric potential.

## SUMMARY

Two tendencies may be noted in working out the laser ophthalmologic systems: (1) further perfection of apparatuses with a coagulating action, and (2) the designing of systems with a mechanically altering effect. Perhaps both effects could be achieved by one apparatus—for example, one based on the Nd-YAG laser (Saprykin and Tarkhov, 1976). The compactness of this laser, its ability to generate in CW and pulse modes, and the availability of the harmonic radiations possibly make it the most universal laser for ophthalmologic applications.

Also two types of equipment (with coagulating and cutting actions) are used in dermatology, oncology, and surgery, but the first combined systems have already been constructed. New lasers (Ar, Nd-YAG) are being tested parallel to the traditional ones—Nd and $CO_2$ lasers.

A new, very specific direction in laser medical industry has been born, making use of biostimulating effects of low-power HeNe laser radiation. Its development, however, is hampered by vagueness concerning the mechanism of the phenomena.

## REFERENCES

Abdurazakov MS, Belyaev VP, Martinov VF, Pletnev SD, Felianin YA (1976) Laser apparatus LGM-1 for medical practice. Electronics Industry 52(4):61–62.

Babayants RS, Rakcheev AP, Konstantinov AV, Ivanov OL, Makeeva NS, Shchur VV (1974) On the use of lasers with low radiation output in some dermatoses. Vestn Dermatol 48(4):7–13.

Babayants RS, Vorontsova GM, Makeeva NS, Shchur VV (1976) The application of the laser physiotherapeutic system in dermatology. Electronics Industry 52(4):62–63.

Basov NG, Krokhin ON, Popov YM (1961) The production of states with negative temperature in p-n-transitions of degenerate semiconductors. Zh Eksp Teor Fiz 40:1879–1880.

Basov NG, Prokhorov AM (1954) The use of molecular bundles for radiospectroscopic study of the band spectra of molecules. Zh Eksp Teor Fiz 27:431–438.

Basov NG, Vul BM, Popov YM (1959) Quantum-mechanical semiconductor generators and amplifiers of electromagnetic waves. Zh Eksp Teor Fiz 37:587–588.

Belyaev VP, Martinov VF, Pletnev SD, Felianin YA (1976) In: Means and Methods of Quantum Electronics in Medicine. Saratov University Publishing House, Saratov, pp. 12–13.

Belyaeva MI, Saprykin PI, Simonova KK (1974) In: Proceedings of the 3rd Scientific Conference of Ophthalmologists of Georgia, Tbilisi, pp. 58–63.

Bogdanovich UY, Karimov MG (1978) Lasers in Orthopedy and Traumatology. Kasan University Publishing House, Kasan.

Boyarskih GV, Zausaev VI, Makeeva NS, Sidorova TA, Ushakov AI (1976) Small therapeutic laser apparatus. Electronics Industry 52(4)59–60.

Filimonova NM (1973) Laser coagulation in the optic fundus by reverse microscopy with a positive lens. Vestn Oftal'mol 5:75–77.

Gamaleya NF (1972) Lasers in Experimental Researches and Clinical Practice. Meditsina, Moscow.

Gamaleya NF (1977) Laser biomedical research in the USSR. In: Wolbarsht ML (ed) Laser Applications in Medicine and Biology, vol. III. Plenum Press, New York and London, pp. 1–173.

Gamaleya NF, Polishchuk EI (1977) Treatment of skin tumors by pulsed neodymium and continuous wave carbon dioxide lasers. Dermatol Dig Nov, 43–50.

Gamaleya NF, Polishchuk EI (1978) The skin tumor's treatment by a pulsed laser. Vopr Oncol 24:76–81.

Inyushin VM, Chekurov PR (1975) Biostimulation by Laser Radiation and the Bioplasma. Kazakhstan, Alma-Ata.

Isakov VL, Kavetskii RE, Kaznacheev VP, Kochnev VA, Koba AI, Lazarev IR, Pavlov KA, Pozmogov AI, Hliviniuk BG (1976) In: Means and Methods of Quantum Electronics in Medicine. Saratov University Publishing House, Saratov, pp. 8–9.

Kavetskii RE, Chudakov VG, Sidorik EP, Gamaleya NF, Kogut TS (1969) Lasers in Biology and Medicine. Zdorov'e, Kiev.

Korytnyi DL (1979) Laser Therapy and Its Application in Stomatology. Kazakhstan, Alma-Ata.

Koshelev VN, Papaev BA, Stepanenko SG, Basharova TV, Tsapko AI (1974) In: Transactions of the Conference on Problems of Suppurative Surgery. Saratov University Publishing House, Saratov, pp. 23–25.

Krasnov MM (1973a) In: Current Problems in Ophthalmic Surgery. Kuibyshev Medical Institute, Kuibyshev, pp. 7–11.

Krasnov MM (1973b) Laser microsurgery of the eye. Vestn Oftal'mol 1(1):3–11.

Krasnov MM (1973c) Laser puncture of anterior chamber angle in glaucoma. Am J Ophthalmol 75(4):674–678.

Krasnov MM, Klatt A, Saprykin PI (1973) Ocular hydrodynamics in laser goniopuncture. Vestn Oftal'mol 86(3):13–15.

Krasnov MM, Klatt A, Mamedov NG, Saprykin PI, Yarygin VN (1974) Modulated laser goniopuncture of the simian eye. Preliminary report. Vestn Oftal'mol 87(1):13–16.

Krasnov MM, Saprykin PI, Klatt A (1974) Laserogonioplasty in glaucoma. Vestn Oftal'mol 87(2):30–34.

Krasnov MM, Saprykin PI, Nikol'skaya GM (1973) Coreoplasty with the argon laser. Vestn Oftal'mol 86(4):43–45.

Kromov BM (1973) Lasers in Experimental Surgery. Meditsina, Leningrad.

Lebekhov PI, Kerova IK (1973) Late results of prophylactic laser photocoagulation. In: The Use of Optical Quantum Generators in Modern Science and Technology. Znanie, Leningrad, p. 94.

Libman ES (1973) Comparative study of laser (ruby) and xenon coagulation in ophthalmology. Experimental and clinical investigation. (Abstr) Doctoral dissertation, Moscow.

Linnik LA (1966) Indications and method of photocoagulation using radiation of optical quantum generators for detachment of the retina. Proceedings of the 3rd Congress of Ophthalmologists of the USSR, Volgograd, vol. 2, pp. 324–326.

Linnik LA (1969) Five years of experience of the use of laser coagulation in the clinical treatment of detachment of the retina. Oftal'mol Zh 3:171–176.

Linnik LA (1972) Laser coagulators and their applications in ophthalmology. Oftal'mol Zh 27(3):208–213.

Malishev BN, Saliuk VA, Prosorov VN, Fundator JV (1976) In: Means and Methods of Quantum Electronics in Medicine. Saratov University Publishing House, Saratov, pp. 17–18.

Milianovskii AI, Stepankovskaya GK, Polishchuk EI, Gamaleya NF (1976) (Abstr) Proceedings of 13th All-Union Congress of Obstetricians, Gynaecologists, Moscow, pp. 443–444.

Nikolaev MP, Tverskoi JL, Rodionova LP, Demin VK (1976) In: Means and Methods of Quantum Electronics in Medicine. Saratov University Publishing House, Saratov, pp. 58–61.

Pletnev SD, Devyatkov ND, Belyaev VP, Abdurazakov M (1978) Gas Lasers in Experimental and Clinical Oncology. Meditsina, Moscow.

Polishchuk EI, Stepankovskaya GK, Milianovskii AI, Dudnichenko VN (1977) In: Oncology. Interdepartmental Republican Collection, vol 8. Naukova Dumka, Kiev, pp. 88–90.

Puchkovskaya NA, Pakhomova AI, Terent'eva LS, Linnik LA, Tverskoi YL (1966) Proceedings, 3rd Congress of Ophthalmologists of the USSR, Volgograd, vol 2, pp. 208–210.

Rakcheev AP, Fedorovskaya RF, Cherniaev YS (1976) In: Means and Methods of Quantum Electronics in Medicine. Saratov University Publishing House, Saratov, pp. 63–64.

Rosenfeld EB, Malishev BN, Razigrin BA, Prosorov VN (1973) The laser medical systems. In: The News of Medical Instrument-making, vol. 3. All-union Research Institute for Medical Instrument-making, Moscow, pp. 6–11.

Saprykin PI, Tarkhov GN (1976) In: Means and Methods of Quantum Electronics in Medicine. Saratov University Publishing House, Saratov, pp. 13–16.

Saprykin PI, Simonova KK, Belyaeva MI (1974) Argon laser in the treatment of diabetic retinopathy (preliminary communication). Vestn Oftal'mol 2:78–81.

Skobelkin OK, Brekhov EI, Parhomenko YG, Ovsiankin VM, Danilin NA, Fomin SA, Malishev BN, Saliuk VA, Shapovalov AM (1976) In: Means and Methods of Quantum Electronics in Medicine. Saratov University Publishing House, Saratov, pp. 39–41.

Terent'eva LS (1971) Destruction of melanoblastomas of choroid by laser irradiation. In: Abstracts of Proceedings of an All-Union Symposium on the Biological and Antitumor Action of Laser Radiation. Moscow, pp. 50–51.

Terent'eva LS (1973) The therapeutic use of light energy of various sources in melanoblastomas of the choroid. In: The Use of Optical Quantum Generators in Modern Science and Technology. Znanie, Leningrad, p. 96.

Terent'eva LS (1976) In: Means and Methods of Quantum Electronics in Medicine. Saratov University Publishing House, Saratov, pp. 100–102.

Vaniukov MP, Gavrilov NI, Serebriakov VA, Ilchenko AM, Liubavskii YV, Kozlov AP, Moskalik KG, Pertsov OL (1975) Optical quantum generator for oncology: "Pulsar 1000." Opt Mech Industry 12:31–33.

Wagner RI, Kozlov AP, Moskalik KG, Khachaturian LM (1974) On treatment of pretumor and tumor diseases of skin by laser "Pulsar-1000" radiation. Vopr Onkol 4:11–16.

Wagner RI, Kozlov AP, Moskalik KG, Khachaturian LM (1975) Laser therapy of human benign and malignant neoplasms of the skin. Acta Radiol 14(5): 417–423.

Wagner RI, Kozlov AP, Moskalik KG, Khachaturian LM, Motus IY, Lipova VA (1977) On the treatment of the skin melanoblastoma by means of pulse laser radiation. Vestn Khir 119(12):56–61.

# 22

# Tissue Diagnosis by Laser Transillumination and Diaphanographic Methods

*David B. Greenberg*
*Michael D. Tribbe*

Advancements in surgical techniques for the treatment of breast cancer have not resulted in a significant improvement in the survival rate over the last 20 years. A female who developed a stage II breast cancer in the early 1970s had the same 5-year relative survival rate by stage as a female afflicted in the early 1950s.

Since advancements in treatment appear to be at a statistical standstill, the American Cancer Society (ACS) and the National Cancer Institute (NCI) have taken another route to curb mortality—earlier detection. The two organizations hope that with earlier detection the cancers will be smaller and more confined, thus making treatment more successful.

Therefore, in 1973, the ACS and NCI at a cost of $45 million, implemented breast cancer detection programs throughout the country. The programs' principal tool—mammography—allows one to detect potential precursors as small as 0.1 mm in size. The participants in the experiment are screened once a year, and changes from checkup to checkup are carefully analyzed.

The impact of earlier detection is obvious. Before mammography, most females became aware of breast cancer from self-examination for subtle changes in the breast: lumps, indentations, etc. To be found by this palpation, the cancer had to be relatively large, at least 5 mm in size. With a tumor this size, from a purely statistical standpoint, a female has roughly a 63% chance of survival for 10 years. Now, however, mammography can spot 0.1-mm in-situ or preinvasive cancers, and survival rates have jumped appreciably. Letton et al. (1977) report an 87.1% cure rate and Shapiro (1975) a 97% cure rate for tumors of this size.

A problem arises since x rays from the mammography may themselves induce incipient cancers. More explicitly, one might ask if the tradeoff between potential cancer inducement and cancer detection by mammography is reasonable.

The exact extent of genetic damage is unknown. Some scientists, such as Dr. G.

Timothy Johnson (1979), indicate that it would take 500 x rays (at 0.2 mR each) to equal the dose of radiation that we receive from natural sources each year, and therefore, the damage is insignificant. It has also been reported that a single transcontinental flight exposes a person to as much radiation as that of 12 chest roentgenograms (Johnson, 1979).

On the other hand, in an article by Starr (1978), Dr. William Bross of the Roswell Park Memorial Institute for Cancer Research in Buffalo, New York, warns that as many as 1:20 persons undergoing x-ray examinations experience the genetic damage that may lead to leukemia. The same article reports that a well-accepted British study cited in a recent survey showed that children of women x-rayed during pregnancy had a 40% higher leukemia risk than others.

Most physicians acknowledge that there is at least some risk in x rays and would welcome an alternative but equally sensitive means of early detection if it included only minimal side effects. For the past 50 years, transillumination has been regarded as such a method but one offering only limited success. With the recent discovery of a coherent and intense light source in the laser, transillumination procedures are being investigated anew, and detection techniques using both visible and infrared light are being explored. The early work accomplished at the University of Cincinnati provides a significant improvement in resolution of tumors to be used in conjunction with such transillumination techniques.

## HISTORY OF TRANSILLUMINATION

Transillumination, the passage of light through a part of the body to discover or examine a pathologic condition, has been used for breast cancer detection since 1929, when Cutler (1929) first published the results of clinical examinations that he and his associates Ewing and Adair performed, using this technique. Their illuminating source was a Cameron transilluminating electric lamp, used at that time to study inflammatory diseases of the sinuses. By placing the lamp against the undersurface of the breast and moving it over the surface to place the particular portion in question directly between the light and the examiner's eye, they found marked variation in the degree of translucence among different sections of normal and pathologic tissue. In the 174 cases studied from 1926 through 1929, these investigators found transillumination particularly valuable for the detection of cystic and solid tumors, hematomas, and bleeding nipples.

The following conclusions drawn by Cutler and his associates from the results of this study show the capabilities of the method.

1. Solid tumors show an intermediate degree of opacity. Cysts are translucent and blood intensely opaque. These can be differentiated.
2. The visible character of the opacity does not itself permit differentiation between benign and malignant solid tumors.
3. Traumatic hematoma has a characteristic appearance of intense opacity with irregular outlines.

4. Intracystic or duct papillomas associated with bleeding nipples also have a characteristic appearance. Furthermore, they can be more precisely located, and papilloma number and extent of spread can be estimated for proper surgical removal.

Despite these assets, transillumination was progressively abandoned for many reasons: the need to carry out the observations in total darkness, which requires long adaptation times; the poor contrasts in images; the subjective nature of prognosis; and the high heat output of the lamp, which caused considerable discomfort to patients.

## DIAPHANOGRAPHY

Major improvements by Gros et al. (1972) in France were made on the illuminating equipment as well as on the protocol. They found that the light frequencies at the two ends of the visible spectrum were undesirable for transillumination, and by using an arc lamp they were able to eliminate them. Blue and violet radiation appeared to be more scattered in the tissue, thereby causing deterioration of the contrast. Infrared, on the other hand, although less scattered through tissue, was still undesirable since it produced large quantities of heat, resulting in difficulty for the patient.

Other modifications by these French investigators included water cooling of the illuminating source; a variable voltage to prolong the life of the instrument, as well as to permit regulation of light intensity as a function of the tissue transparency; a more mobile unit; and recording of the transillumination examination on ordinary color film, which eliminated the need for total darkness. This procedure of recording the transillumination field on film is now known as diaphanography. The improvements by Gros et al. (1972) did not substantially increase disease detection and differentiation. A recent breakthrough in 1978, however, appeared to do so.

After a 2-year double-blind, controlled study in Sweden, Gunderson et al. (1979) have introduced a new diaphanographic method that they found to be more sensitive than mammography when a tumor could not be palpated. The novelty in this approach is that a diffuse, low-intensity light transmitter with built-in flash is the source, and sensitive infrared film is used for photographic registration. With this technique, malignant and benign tissue can surprisingly be differentiated. The former appears in a brown-black color scale, whereas the latter appears red in the infrared photograph. This further suggests the possibility that different absorption may occur in preneoplastic and neoplastic tissue within the breast.

These investigators have made diaphanographic examinations and diagnoses on 107 patients prior to operation and then compared the diagnoses with the histologic findings in the excised tissue. Evaluation of the actual results (Tables 22.1 and 22.2) best demonstrates the capability of the method. In two cases out of three, diaphanography appears to be more accurate than mammography.

Goldman (1967, 1978) made the first studies of lasers for transillumination. Using a 75-mW CW HeNe laser and later a 0.5-W CW krypton system, he

**Table 22.1.** Results of Diaphanographic Investigation and Histologic Examination in 112 Biopsies (107 Patients)*

| Diaphanographic investigation | Histologic findings (no. of patients) | | | |
|---|---|---|---|---|
| | Benign change | Precancerous change | Malignancy | Total |
| Malignancy | 4 | 2 | 15 | 21 |
| Suspicious malignancy | 20 | 4 | 5 | 29 |
| Benign change | 60 | 1 | 1 | 62 |
| Totals | 84 | 7 | 21 | 112 |

*Based on data of Gunderson J, Nilsson DM, Ohlsson B (1979) Lakartidninger 76:1425–1427.

obtained soft-tissue penetration through 7 cm of tissue but found that the resolution of masses within was relatively poor. He noted, however, that the longer wavelength HeNe irradiation source resulted in better resolution than the krypton laser. An extension to clinical diagnosis was not made at that time.

The scanning technique that we now have under development at the University of Cincinnati shows promise toward increased resolution of breast tumors when used with the detection methods of Cutler et al. (1929), Gros et al. (1972), Gunderson et al. (1979), and Goldman (1967, 1978).

## SCANNING WITH LASER LIGHT

The idea to scan developed from the observations of transillumination users who found it necessary to have the particular portion of the breast in question directly between the light source and the examiner's eye. This suggested that the underside

**Table 22.2.** Diagnosis by Three Types of Examination: Analysis of Seven Mammary Tumors in Six Patients*

| Patient | Diagnosis† | | |
|---|---|---|---|
| | Cytology | X ray | DPG‡ |
| 1 | Neg | Pos | Pos |
| 2 | Pos | Pos | Pos |
| 3 | Neg | Neg | Pos |
| 4 | Pos | — | Pos |
| 5 | Neg | Pos | Pos |
| 6 (both breasts) | Neg | Neg | Pos |
| | Pos | Neg | Neg |
| Totals | 3/7 | 3/6 | 6/7 |

*Based on data of Gunderson J, Nilsson DM, Ohlsson B (1979) Lakartidninger 76:1425–1427.
†Pathology reports showed positive results in all seven cases.
‡DPG, diaphanography.

of the breast could be scanned in a grid pattern by means of laser light, while on the upper side of the breast, by appropriate masking, only the light directly across from and with the same area as the impinging laser light be allowed to reach a recording photographic film.

In the laboratory at the University of Cincinnati, human tissue phantoms were scanned in 3 × 3 mm blocks with a pulsed organic-dye laser capable of 60 mJ output with rhodamine 6G dye. Actual intensities needed for scanning through the 3-cm thicknesses studied were considerably lower at 10–15 mJ. Even lower intensities were possible because the recording was on film that allowed successive shots at the same scanning position to be superimposed. For example, good results were obtained at 3–4 mJ per pulse through addition of four shots. Literature searches have revealed no findings of detrimental effects on tissue exposed to visible light even at intensities higher than the 60 mJ.

In this study, the investigators assumed that cancerous areas in the breast would be distinguishable from normal tissue by means of the different absorptions of visible light. The procedure was simulated by embedding opaque and partially transmitting artifacts in one of two phantoms: (1) pathologic specimens of human breast tissue from mastectomies preserved in formaldehyde; and (2) a homogeneous mixture of wax, animal fats, and dye formulated to yield a substance analogous to female breast tissue, through which light would be transmissible. The transmittance curve for each is given in Figure 22.1.

The transillumination technique of Cutler et al. (1929), which can be compared to shining a flashlight through one's hand, was used, but 3 × 3 mm square metal displays under ordinary light illumination could not be distinguished with the eye through either phantom for thicknesses greater than 1 cm (the displays were positioned midway through the sample).

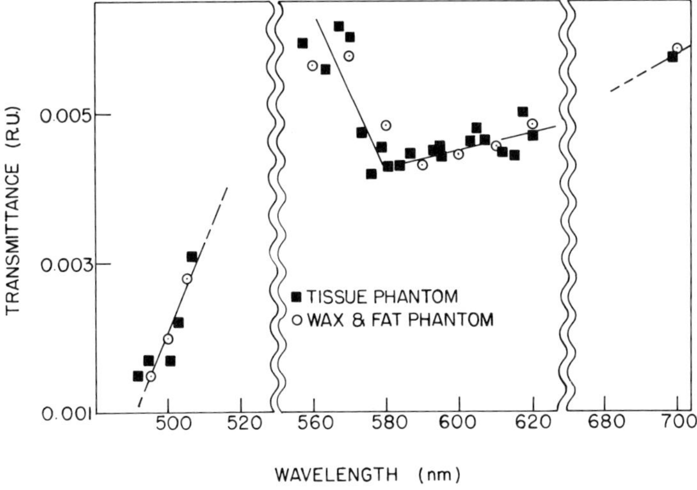


**Fig. 22.1.** Transmittance as a function of wavelength for the tissue in formaldehyde and animal fat/wax phantoms used in the dye laser study (Greenberg and Tribbe, 1979).

With the scanning method, the same 3 × 3 mm nontransmitting displays were readily detectable, located at the center of 2.7 cm of the formaldehyde-tissue phantom and 2.8 cm of the homogeneous phantom using rhodamine dye (570–618 nm). Moreover, a 3-mm square, 36% light-transmitting display was easily discerned, but not one of 50% through 1 cm of the first phantom.

Detection was achieved by finding numerical values of transmittance (the ratio of output to input) for each 3 × 3 mm square of the scanned grid and analytically comparing the squares for significant density differences (Fig. 22.2). This provided a statistically determined image, which was then compared to the known display location, shape, and size. This statistical protocol eliminated the normal bias of subjective diagnosis.

To maintain resolution through increased thicknesses, an attempt was made to optimize the wavelength and the intensity of the transilluminating light. On the basis of previous studies by Buckley and Grum (1964) and the transmittance curves generated in the current work at the University of Cincinnati, wavelengths were chosen that demonstrated the least scattering in fat tissue and showed the best penetration. In scans performed at these wavelengths, however, reasonable detection was not obtained past 2.8 cm. Input intensities were varied between 10 and 50 mJ (per 3 × 3 mm square), and filters were placed after the tissue but before the film to ensure uniform exposure between intensities. Resolution or detection does not seem to rely on input power within this range. The 2.8-cm thickness is the maximum through which a 3 × 3 mm display can be detected at this time.

Since the average breast can be compressed to a thickness of about 6 cm or less,

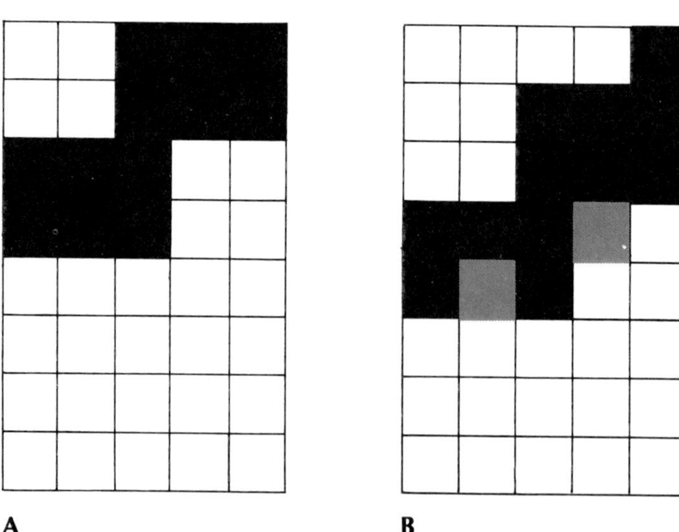


**Fig. 22.2.** Detection of display through 2.5 cm of breast tissue phantom. Each small square is 3 × 3 mm. **A.** Position of actual display is black. **B.** Detected display, based upon statistical evaluation of transmittance data. Gray areas, at 95% confidence levels, could be either display or nondisplay.

the method at this state of development is not capable of providing the detail and resolution achieved by mammography. However, the limited successes thus far achieved in terms of improved resolution, coupled with other inherent advantages of the technique, point to a need for further work, followed by clinical testing. These advantages include the following:

1. The examiner's subjective diagnosis is partially eliminated.
2. The light and intensities used are considered safe and do not induce genetic damage.
3. Discomfort to the patient from the heat of the earlier transillumination lamps is minimized since the pulses are short and low in energy (30–40 mJ/cm$^2$ is sufficient to penetrate the normal 6-cm breast).
4. Lower input energies are needed since output from two or more subsequent low-energy pulses are additive to produce a viable image on photographic film.

The details of this work have been reported elsewhere (Greenberg and Tribbe, 1979).

## OTHER CURRENT WORK

Other researchers are currently exploring the use of monochromatic light sources for cancer detection.

Thomas J. Dougherty and coworkers (1978) at Roswell Memorial Park Institute in Buffalo, have shown that cancerous cells are stained selectively with the dye hematoporphyrin. In their study, Dougherty et al. used this to irradiate the malignant cells. By illuminating with laser light at 620 nm and 640 nm at intensities of about 10 mW/cm$^2$, they found that hematoporphyrin was ionized, producing singlet oxygen which selectively denatured the malignant cells. Normal cells did not appear to be so affected.

In an earlier study, it was reported that detection of cancerous cells using this same dye had been achieved by D. R. Sanderson et al. (1972) of the Mayo Clinic. Under ultraviolet light, the porphyrin dye within the cell fluoresces, and this emitted light is used to map the shape and location of tumors. A diagram of the technique (Fig. 22.3) shows monochromatic laser transillumination with fluorescence of light at different frequencies from cancerous tissue. A filter before the recording medium would prevent the incident laser light frequencies from being recorded.

It may be that the introduction of dye into the breast is not necessary to obtain fluorescence. Cancerous cells may naturally fluoresce. Gibson (1963) showed that biologic samples, such as animal tumors, aorta, and even dead teeth, fluoresced in the infrared range.

More recently, researchers at Lawrence Livermore Laboratory in California (Energy Insider, 1978) have shown that a carcinogen-producing enzyme (AHH) absorbs blue light and fluoresces in the ultraviolet. This suggests, therefore, that tumor discrimination may be achieved and could be used as a means of cancer detection.

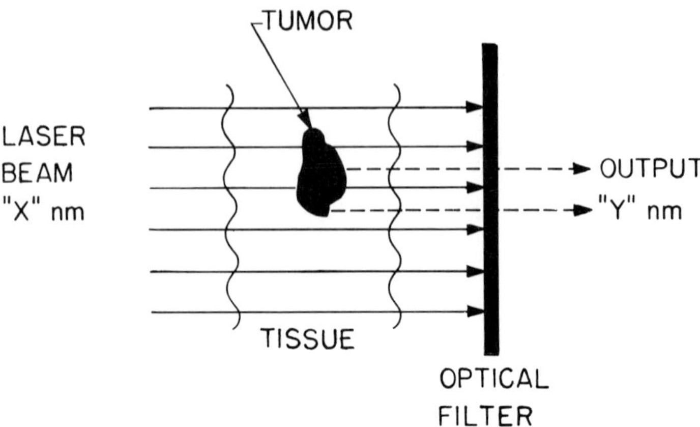


**Fig. 22.3.** Detection of tumor by fluorescence techniques. Laser light at "X" nm is absorbed by tumor and induces fluorescence at wavelength "Y" nm. Only "Y" wavelength reaches film, as other exiting frequencies are absorbed by a discriminating filter.

## CONCLUSIONS

The advent of the laser and the recent successes in transillumination and cancer detection using laser light will no doubt lead to further activity in this area. The largest driving force will be the new detection methods utilizing laser irradiation, which, at low levels, is considered harmless.

We do not mean to imply that laser techniques will replace x rays for resolving cancers in the 0.1-mm range. There appears to be no window through which visible light is not scattered in tissue like radiation in the x-ray range.

Hope for lasers as a safe and widespread detection technique lies with the absorption and fluorescence techniques previously discussed. In this application x rays are not capable of utilizing these properties. Although they can be used to detect 1-mm size tumors and calcifications and map their location and borders, wavelength ranges in the visible spectrum can be absorbed and reemitted. Such changes, when detected, provide basic clues as to the malignancy of the tumor. This information is of signal importance, more so than tumor size or location, for, although location is required before surgery, knowledge of the malignancy is needed to determine whether surgery is needed.

Resolution improvements in the visible range, such as those developed in the University of Cincinnati work are, of course, still welcome. However, the potential of this methodology will be realized only when coupled with further absorption and fluorescence studies.

## SUMMARY

There has been a renewal in the development of early breast cancer detection by transillumination methods to supplement surgical techniques and mammography, both of which have obvious drawbacks. Initial transillumination studies with infrared sources demonstrated some success; however, in practice, the method was difficult for both the clinician and the patient.

Major equipment modifications and improvements in the 1970s and better clinical protocol have led to modest recent breakthroughs by several teams of researchers. These include photographic-image registration (known as diaphanography) and the use of monochromatic coherent (laser) light sources.

Although improved resolution has been achieved by these methods, light scattering becomes a limiting factor as transillumination is attempted through longer tissue-path lengths. Therefore, the ultimate success of transillumination as a viable technique for breast cancer detection will depend upon the development of the method in conjunction with absorption and fluorescence. Current researchers are already exploring these coupled phenomena.

## REFERENCES

Buckley WR, Grum F (1964) Reflection spectroscopy. III. Absorption characteristics and color of human skin. Arch Dermatol 89:110–116.

Cutler M (1929) Transillumination as an aid in the diagnosis of breast lesions, with special reference to its value in cases of bleeding nipple. Surg Gynecol Obstet 48:721–729.

Dougherty TJ, Kaufman JE, Goldfarb A, Weishaupt KR, Boyle D (1978) Photoradiation therapy for the treatment of malignant tumors. Cancer Research 38:2628–2635.

Energy Insider (1979) July 24, p. 3.

Gibson H (1963) The photography of infra-red luminescence part II. Investigation of infra-red phosphorescence. Med Biol Ill 13:18–26.

Goldman L (1967) Biomedical Aspects of Laser. Springer-Verlag, New York.

Goldman L (1978) Personal communication.

Greenberg DB, Tribbe M (1979) Scanning technique for breast cancer detection. 32nd Annual Conference on Engineering and Medicine in Biology Transactions 16(4):49.

Gros C, Quenneville Y, Hummel Y (1972) Diaphanologie Mammaire. J Radiol Elect Med Nucl 53:297–306.

Gunderson J, Nilsson DM, Ohlsson B (1979) Diafanografi for bedömning av bröstförändringar. Lakartidningen 76:1425–1427.

Johnson GT (1979) Cincinnati Enquirer, Jan. 16.

Letton AH, Wilson JP, Mason EM (1977) The value of breast screening in women less than fifty years of age. Cancer 20:1–3.

Sanderson DR, Fontana RS, Lipson RL, Baldes EJ (1972) Hematoporphyrin as a diagnostic tool; a preliminary report of new techniques. Cancer 30:1365–1372.

Shapiro S (1975) Screening for early detection of cancer and heart disease. Bull NY Acad Med 51:80–95.

Starr D (1978) Cincinnati Post, July 8.

# 23

# Investigative Studies of Laser Technology in Rheumatology and Immunology

*John A. Goldman*

The use of the laser in investigative studies in rheumatic and immunologic diseases is very new. Various laboratory methods have been developed using lasers to help identify and quantitate many components of immunologic reactions. Very few clinical studies are available outlining the immunologic effect of laser radiation on human tissue or on patients with specific immunologic or rheumatic problems.

## LASER MEASUREMENT OF IMMUNE RESPONSE

### Quantitative Determination of Immune Associated Proteins with a Laser Nephelometer System

A solution that is cloudy or turbid as a result of the presence of particles will scatter light when it is placed in the path of a light source. Nephelometry measures light that is diffusely scattered by particles in solution (Laser Bulletin No. 1[1]). Initially, the light-scattering measurements were made at a 90° angle but were constantly unreliable in antigen excess and difficult to keep clean. Recently, instruments that utilize laser light sources and measure light scattering at much lower angles have been developed.

I would like to thank Ms. Jennie Crook and Miss Esther Lawson for their help in the development and typing of this manuscript, and also Sandra Stahl, Ph.D., of Nashville, Tennessee, for translating the Russian literature. I would like to thank E. E. Uzgiris, Z. Darzynkiewicz, J. C. Ruckdeschel, and E. D. Kloszewski for their aid in the research of this chapter. I would also like to acknowledge the continued support of the A. Ward Ford Memorial Institute, Wausau, Wisconsin, and the Irvine Young Foundation, Palmyra, Wisconsin.

[1]Quantitative Determination of Proteins with Calbiochem-Behring Corp. Laser Nephelometer System. Laser Bulletin No. 1, Calbiochem-Behring Corp. Immunological Technical Services, LaJolla, California.

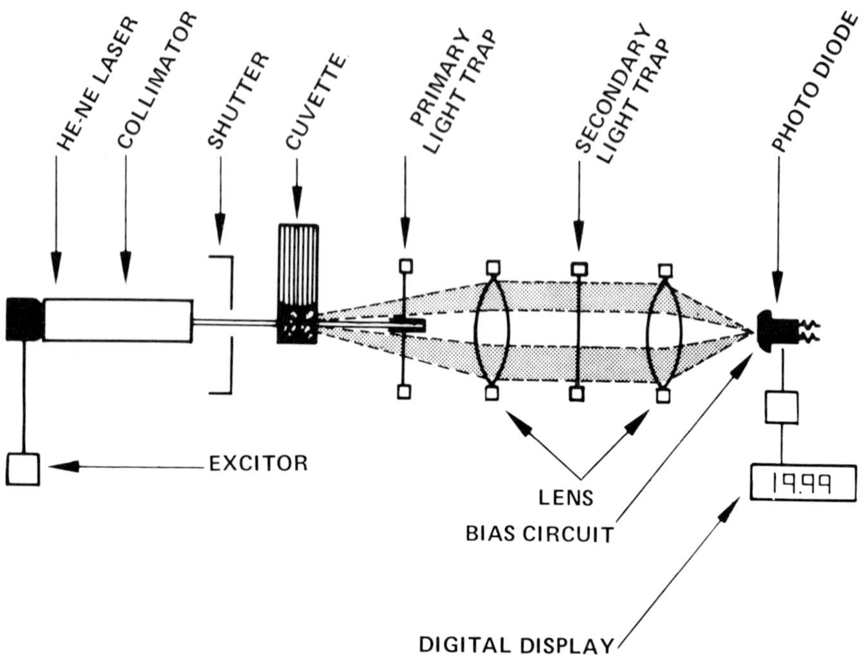


**Fig. 23.1.** Schema of laser nephelometer. (Laser Bulletin #1, Calbiochem-Behring Corp., Immunology Technical Services.)

The nephelometric assay requires a diluted antigen solution, which may be a standard or test serum, mixed with small amounts of diluted antiserum. The mixture of antigen and antibody produces immune complexes in the solution that can then be measured by light scattering and compared to known standards.

The laser nephelometer uses a helium-neon (HeNe) laser that emits light of 632.8-nm wavelength, which is intensive, monochromatic, and yields a very low beam divergence. The light from the laser passes through the sample, which is in a cuvette, and is scattered into a detector placed at an angle of 0° with respect to the transmitted beam (Fig. 23.1).

According to the particle size, characteristic patterns of distribution of scattered light emerge from the lamp source. The extremely narrow beam helps to reduce light scattering due to dust particles and air bubbles in the samples. Although the nephelometer measures the direct forward light scatter (0° angle), the primary light is prevented from reaching the detector device by a light trap. The actual forward light scatter is measured at approximately 5°–12° angles, providing for a high input signal. Light scattered beyond these angles is also trapped. The background noise is extremely low. Because of the forward-light–scattering system of the laser nephelometer, a photodiode may be used to record the scattered light. The incoming light is several magnitudes higher than that of light scattering at angles such as 31° or 90°, which occurs in other laser and nonlaser nephelometers. Those nephelometers that use light-scattering measurements at 31° and 90° use only a small part of the scattered light signal, and some means of amplification such as a photomultiplier must be employed. The use of the photomultiplier, however, also amplifies the background signal, and readings are more difficult, with the result that laser nephelometers that scatter and read light at low angles are now becoming standard.

Because light scattering is the basis of laser nephelometry, anything that erroneously increases light scattering will interfere with the accuracy of the technique. Certain M proteins will be cloudy because there is a high amount of antigen excess, and the readings are therefore inaccurate. If one wishes to use a laser nephelometry technique to measure M proteins, an extra dilution of the patient's serum must be made. Other substances that may increase light scattering include scratches on the cuvette surface, lipoproteins that give a lipemic turbid specimen, bacterial contamination, and desiccation of the solution if the serum is incubated too long.

Proteins associated with immune reactivity that can be measured by laser nephelometry include the following (Buffone et al., 1974; Deaton et al., 1976; Walsh et al., 1979):

IgG
IgA
IgM
IgD
C3
C4
C3 proactivator (properdin factor B)
C1 esterase inhibitor
C-reactive protein
$Alpha_1$-antitrypsin
$Alpha_1$ acid glycoprotein (Orosomucoid)
$Alpha_2$-macroglobulin
Albumin
Transferrin
Haptoglobin

## Differentiation and Quantitation of Lymphocytes

**Laser Doppler Spectroscopy.** Laser Doppler spectroscopy is a technique that permits rapid and precise measurement of the distribution of electrophoretic mobilities in a population of suspended particles (Uzgiris and Cluxton, in press). By characterizing the spectrum of light scattered from particles on an electric field, the technique permits a very rapid measurement of the distribution of the particles' electrophoretic mobilities. The electrokinetic motion induced by the electric field will cause a Doppler frequency shift of scattered light. The spectrum of the photocurrent will have a peak that will be shifted from the origin (on the frequency axis) when an electric field is applied. Laser light from a HeNe laser is scattered by an angle $\theta s$, which can be detected by a photomultiplier (Fig. 23.2). Part of the scattering of light at this angle is due to the particles moving in the applied electric field. As a consequence, this light will be Doppler-shifted in fre-

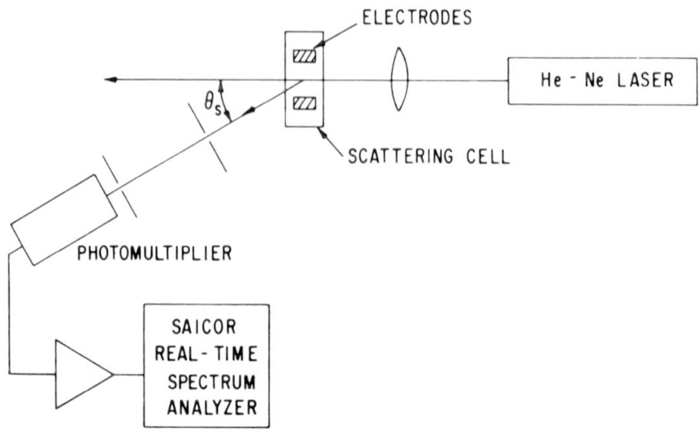


**Fig. 23.2.** Schema of laser Doppler spectrometer. Laser light (Spectra Physics 124A) is scattered by an angle $\theta s$, defined by a pair of 0.5-mm slits, and is detected by a photomultiplier (RVA7265). Part of the light scattered at this angle is due to particles moving in the applied electric field. Consequently, this light will be Doppler-shifted in frequency. The other component of detected light arises from stationary scattering centers on glass windows of the cuvette (Luminon Inc., 2 mm $\times$ 10 mm $\times$ 45 mm, optical cell, type 26) and this light is not shifted in frequency. These two scattered light components beat with each other in the process of photodetection, giving rise to a photocurrent that is modulated at the Doppler frequency. The spectrum of the photocurrent will thus have a peak shifted from the origin by an amount equal to the Doppler shift. We normally use a 10-cm-focal-length lens to focus the incident beam. The $\sim$ 2-mm and 10-mm-long electrodes of a 1-mm gap spacing were immersed into the cuvette so that the electric field (Wavetek 112 square wave generator source) was perpendicular to the short 2-mm axis of the cuvette, as shown. The photomultiplier was approximately 40 cm from the scattering region. [Kaplan JH, Uzgiris EE (1975) The detection of photomitogen-induced changes in human lymphocyte surfaces by laser Doppler spectroscopy. J Immunol Methods 7:337–346.]

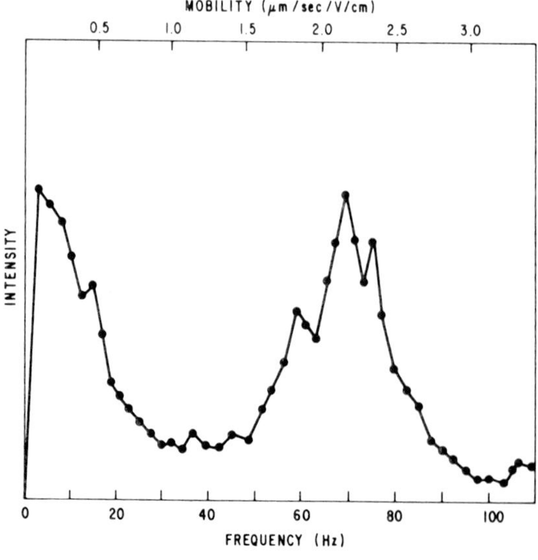


**Fig. 23.3.** Doppler spectrum for a Ficoll-Hypaque cell preparation containing $1 \times 10^6$ cells per milliliter. In addition to the usual mobility components (235 and 2.15 $\mu$m/sec/V/cm), there is resolved in this sample a cell population of 1.85 $\mu$m/sec/V/cm mobility. This spectrum was determined with an incident wavelength of 632.8 nm. The scattering angle $\theta$ was 12.9° and the electric field was 72.4 V/cm. (Kaplan and Uzgiris, 1976.)

quency. If the sample under study contains a heterogeneous population, there will be a series of peaks in the spectrum of scattered light, each of which will be proportional to the number density of the particular type of particles and the position of the peak on the frequency axis.

By means of this technique, lymphocytes can be identified separately from other cells in the bloodstream, such as erythrocytes (Uzgiris and Kaplan, 1974). Major lymphocyte subpopulations can also be characterized and identified (Kaplan and Uzgiris, 1976; Kaplan et al., 1979; Uzgiris et al., 1978, in press). Not only can B cell and T cells be identified, but two types of T-cell subpopulations have also been revealed. Laser Doppler techniques to identify T-cell subpopulations can be used because there is a difference in electrophoretic mobility between these populations. This parameter reflects the surface-charge density in proportion to the cell surface lying close to the hydrodynamic shear boundary, and its value depends upon differences in types and distribution of cell-surface components.

Electrophoretically different lymphocyte subpopulations have been identified in human peripheral blood. Electrokinetic measurements by a laser Doppler technique have identified these subpopulations by enriching them and then depleting them through various surface-marker–dependent reactions. Two of the cell populations have high mobility and appear to be T cells, whereas those of the low-mobility subpopulation are B cells (Kaplan and Uzgiris, 1976) (Fig. 23.3).

The fastest cell subpopulation (M 25° sucrose = 2.35 $\mu$/s/V/cm) is separated from the other cell populations that have mean mobilities of 2.15 and 1.85 $\mu$m/s/V/cm. The two slower mobility subpopulations can be removed by passage through a nylon-fiber column (Fig. 23.4). Those cells with the slowest mobility have both surface-immunoglobulin markers and complement receptors on their surface and, hence, are B cells.

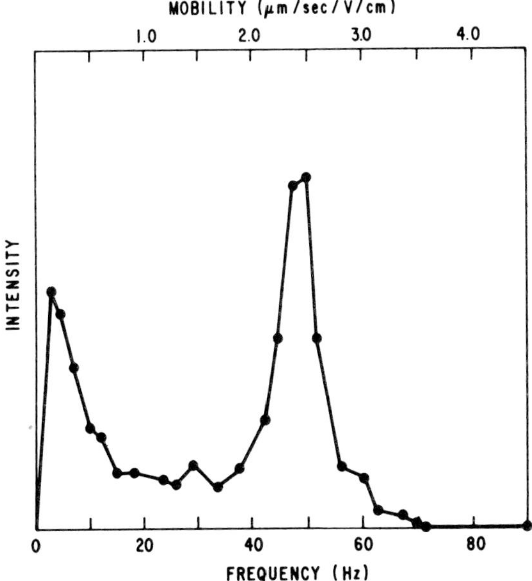


**Fig. 23.4.** Doppler spectrum of lymphocytes (5 × $10^5$/ml) that were isolated on a Ficoll-Hypaque gradient followed by passage through a nylon-fiber column. Only one major mobility component (2.35 $\mu$m/sec/V/cm) passed through. The scattering angle and electric field were 13.1° and 44 V/cm, respectively. [Kaplan JH, Uzgiris EE (1976) Identification of T and B cell subpopulations in human peripheral blood: Electrophoretic mobility distributions associated with surface marker characteristics. J Immunol 117:1731–1740.]

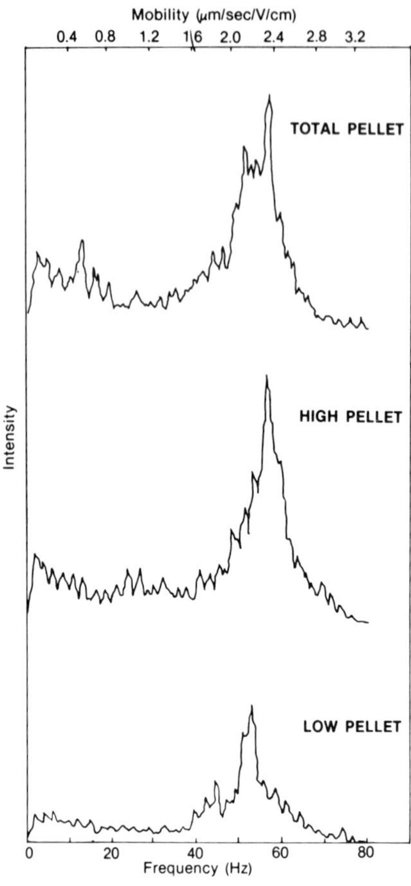


**Fig. 23.5.** Comparison of laser Doppler spectra of isolated high-affinity, low-affinity, and total ERFC pellets. The ERFC fractions are referred to as pellets because they represent cells that originally were recovered in the rosette pellet following Ficoll-Hypaque gradient separation of ERFC from non-ERFC. [Kaplan JH, Uzgiris EE, Lockwood SH (1979) Analysis of T cell subpopulations by Doppler spectroscopy and the association of electrophoretic mobility differences with differences in rosette-forming affinity. J Immunol Methods 17:241–255.]

The T lymphocytes have also been divided into subpopulations of active T cells and total T cells. Active T cells have a capacity to bind to sheep red blood cells (SRBC) to form rosettes after a short period of incubation (e.g., 5 min) whereas 60-min incubation is required for all T cells to rosette. Other studies, in which the temperature and ratio of SRBC to lymphocytes were varied, have demonstrated different binding capacities of T cells for SRBC. Erythrocyte rosette-forming cells (ERFC) of high affinity form rosettes at 29° with a limited number of SRBC, whereas low-affinity ERFC require incubation at lower temperatures (e.g., 4°), with larger SRBC: lymphocyte ratios.

High-affinity ERFC correlate with those T cells that have higher electrophoretic mobility. Low-affinity ERFC bear receptors for the Fc portion of IgG and belong to the T-cell subpopulation of lower mobility (Kaplan et al., 1979) (Fig. 23.5). There seems to be correlation between the cell charge and cell-surface markers on T cells. The low-affinity ERFC that are Fc-receptor–bearing can mediate antibody-dependent cellular cytotoxicity (ADCC). Thus, laser Doppler spectroscopy and cell electrophoretic mobility measurements can give immunologically relevant delineations of lymphocyte subpopulations. The procedure is also being developed to evaluate leukemic cells (Kaplan and Uzgiris, 1979). This development will enable the investigator to observe electrophoretic mobility distribution of different T cells in a heterogeneous population of blood cells and laser Doppler spectroscopy can be used to complement the more time-consuming surface-marker techniques (e.g., erythrocyte rosetting tests). This technique will help to complement the more traditional tests in evaluating patient populations.

**Determination of T-Cell Subpopulations by Laser Cytofluorometry.** The T lymphocytes are responsible for cell-mediated immunity. Those having receptors for IgG, T$\gamma$ cells, are suppressor lymphocytes, and those having receptors for IgM, T$\mu$ cells, are helper lymphocytes. Acridine orange, a metachromatic dye, differentially stains DNA and RNA. The dye intercalates into the double helix of DNA as a monomer that fluoresces green (530 nm), whereas electrostatic dye binds to the phosphates of single-stranded nucleic acids such as RNA and involves dye aggregation ("stacking") and dye-dye interactions that result in red fluorescence (640 nm). Simultaneous measurements of DNA and RNA can be made by laser flow cytofluorometry measuring green ($F = 530$) and red ($F > 600$) fluorescence and low-angle (1°–19°) forward light scatter from cells (Andreef et al., 1978). The fluorescence generated by each cell as it travels in single-file fashion through the focused beam of an argon-ion laser (488 nm) is separated optically into two wavelength bands, $F = 530$ (515–570 nm) and $F > 600$ (600–650 nm), quantified by separated photomultipliers, digitized and recorded for further analysis. Background fluorescence is automatically subtracted.

The pulse width of green fluorescence, i.e., the time taken by the cell nucleus to pass through the illuminating beam, is also recorded and is used to distinguish single cells from cell doublets, as well as to estimate nuclear size. Nonstimulated lymphocytes from peripheral blood, when compared with other cell types (i.e., blastoid cells, tissue culture cell lines), have very low quantities of RNA per cell and thus exhibit low intensity of red fluorescence ($F > 600$) after acridine-orange staining.

When T cells are separated from other lymphocytes by rosetting with sheep erythrocytes and stained with acridine orange, RNA histograms show a bimodal shape indicating at least two T-cell subpopulations (Andreef et al., 1978) (Fig. 23.6). When T$\gamma$ or T$\mu$ cells are separated by incubating T-lymphocyte suspensions with ox erythrocytes prepared with IgM or IgG and stained with acridine orange, each subpopulation displays a unimodal RNA distribution. The T$\gamma$ cells have a peak value at low fluorescence intensity skewed to the right; the T$\mu$ cells have high fluorescence, and the distribution is skewed to the left (Fig. 23.7).

Measurements of nuclear diameters by use of the green pulse width show the mean value of T cells to be 37.8 and the mean value of non-T cells to be 39.1. No difference was found between T$\gamma$ and T$\mu$ cells. The mean RNA content of T$\gamma$ lymphocytes is slightly lower than that of non-T cells, whereas T$\mu$ lymphocytes have twice the RNA content of T$\gamma$ cells. The distribution of RNA content in both T$\mu$ and T$\gamma$ cells is nongaussian and may be the consequence of either incomplete separation of the two populations by the rosette technique employed or the exis-

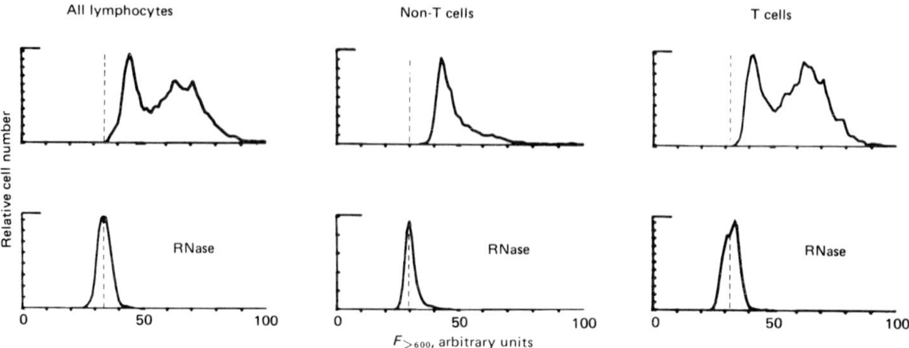


**Fig. 23.6.** Computer-drawn histograms displaying red fluorescence (F > 600) measurements of human peripheral blood lymphocytes stained with acridine orange. Lymphocytes of one subject were measured under identical conditions: *All lymphocytes*, mononuclear cells after depletion of monocytes; *non-T cells*, nonrosetting lymphocytes; and *T cells*, rosetting lymphocytes. *Dashed lines*, mean values of F > 600 after RNase treatment (F > 600 unspecific for RNA). These values can be used as a zero point to rescale the ordinate. After RNA treatment, peak value of non-T cells is slightly higher than that of the first peak of T cells. [Andreeff M, Beck JD, Darzynkiewicz Z, Traganos F, Gupta S, Melamed MR, Good RA (1978) RNA content in human lymphocyte subpopulations. Proc Natl Acad Sci 75:1938–1942.]

tence of different functional states within each population. It may also reflect the existence of additional T-cell subpopulations not yet identified.

The RNA content can separate T-cell subpopulations but is not adequate to distinguish between Tγ and non-T cells. Distinctions between T- and non-T-cell subpopulations can be made by their esterase activity, which can also be quantified by flow cytometry. Thus the combination of laser flow cytofluorometry and flow cytometry may provide a method for separating and analyzing these three lymphocyte subpopulations: non-T cells, Tγ cells, and Tμ cells.

## Measurement of Lymphocyte Stimulation

Lymphocytes can be stimulated in vitro by agents to transform into blastoid cells and undergo mitosis. During stimulation, RNA synthesis is initiated at an early stage and is followed by protein and DNA synthesis. The most common methods of assaying stimulation are based either on measurements of the synthetic activities of cell DNA by radioactive tracers or on changes in cell morphology as visualized by light microscopy.

**Measurement by Laser Doppler Spectroscopy.** The interaction of a specific stimulant with the cell surface can proceed through a succession of stages before the transformation. These stages include binding to receptor sites, changes of configuration on surface macromolecules, surface migration and capping, endocytosis, and microvilli production. Using Doppler spectroscopy following incubation with stimulating agents resulted in stable and reproducible decreases in electrophoretic mobility and increases in the isoelectric point. Incubation with the mitogens phytohemagglutinin (PHA) and concanavallin A (CON A) show these characteristic changes (Kaplan and Uzgiris, 1975).

When laser Doppler spectroscopy was used to measure the electrophoretic mobility of sensitized lymphocytes incubated with the tuberculin antigen, purified protein derivative (PPD), in 75% of the cases a new high-mobility cell subpopulation was shown (Fig. 23.8). This did not occur in a control population. The finding indicates that the high-mobility subpopulation arose from specific interactions between the antigen and sensitized cells. The sensitivity of this assay may need to be improved, but it does indicate specificity (Uzgiris and Kaplan, 1976).

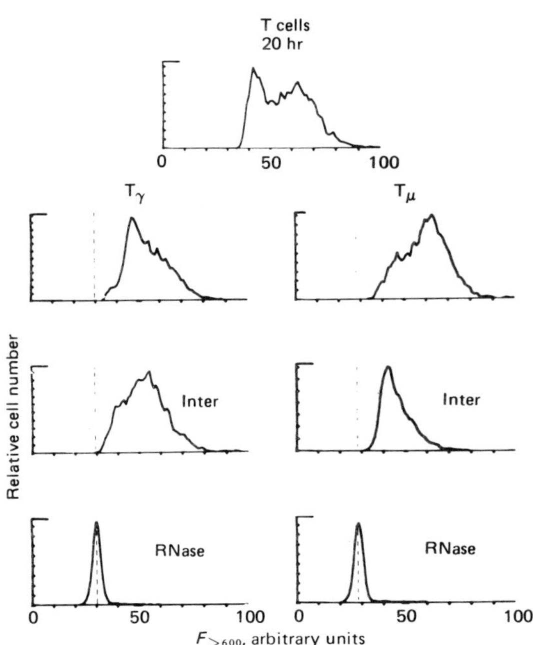


**Fig. 23.7.** Computer-drawn histograms displaying red fluorescence (F > 600) of acridine-orange–stained T lymphocytes from human peripheral blood. Separated T cells (Fig. 23.6) were incubated in RPMI-1640 medium, supplemented with 20% fetal calf serum at 37° for 20 h. Bimodal distribution of these cells is still apparent following incubation. Incubation of these cells with ox erythrocytes coated with either IgM or IgG results in rosette formation. Rosetting cells were separated from nonrosetting cells by Ficoll-Hypaque gradient centrifugation. Rosetting cells, found in the pellet, were either Tμ or Tγ. Their F > 600 histograms are unimodal and skewed either to the right (Tγ) or to the left (Tμ). Cells found in interfaces of gradients display reversed F > 600 distributions. Incubation of Tμ and Tγ cells with RNase results in narrowly distributed histograms with lower peak values *(bottom row)*. *Broken lines* can be used to rescale the ordinate. [Andreef M, Beck JD, Darzynkiewicz Z, Traganos F, Gupta S, Melamed MR, Good RA (1978) RNA content in human lymphocyte subpopulations. Proc Natl Acad Sci 75:1938–1942.]

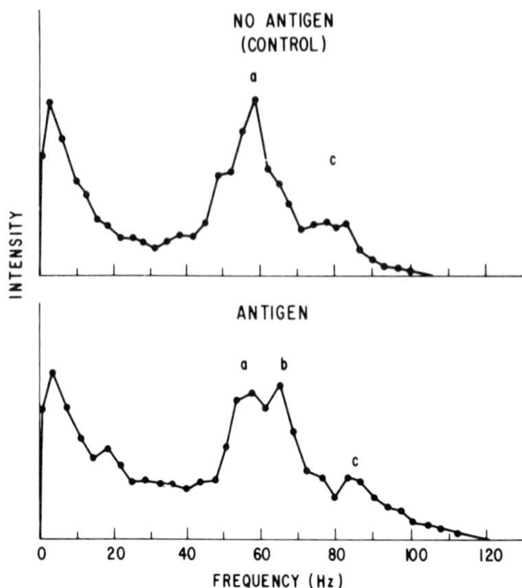


**Fig. 23.8.** Doppler spectra of lymphocytes incubated with PPD (experiment) and without PPD (control). Donor was former tuberculosis patient. In controls, peak *a* is due to lymphocytes, and peak *c* is due to residual erythrocytes. In experimental samples, there appears a new high-frequency, high-mobility subpopulation of lymphocytes (*b*). The scale calibration factor is 65 $Hz^{+}$ 2.35 μm/sec/V/cm (25°C, sucrose buffer). Measurements were made in 0.005 ionic strength isoosmotic sucrose buffer at pH 7.3. (Uzgiris and Kaplan, 1976.)

**Measurement by Laser Flow Cytofluorometry.** During lymphocyte stimulation, RNA synthesis is initiated in an early stage and is followed by protein and DNA synthesis. The metachromatic dye, acridine orange, which stains DNA and RNA preferentially to other cellular polyanions, can be used in laser cytofluorometry to assay lymphocyte stimulation (Darzynkiewicz et al., 1976, 1977). Studies with RNase and DNase treatments of lymphocytes indicate that 87% of the red fluorescence of stimulated cells is due to RNA, and 88% of the green fluorescence induced by acridine-orange interactions is due to cellular DNA.

By choosing the appropriate thresholds for DNA ($F = 530$) and RNA ($F > 600$), it is possible to obtain in a single measurement the following results for analyzing the progress of lymphocyte stimulation (Traganos et al., 1977):

1. Total number of measured cells
2. Total number of stimulated cells, i.e., cells that initiate RNA synthesis, as determined by $F > 600$ values over control
3. Number of nonstimulated cells—gauss zero (G0)
4. Number of the G1-stimulated cells
5. Number of cells in S phase
6. Number of cells that are in G2 + M phase
7. Extent of RNA accumulation per cell in a particular class of stimulated cells (mean or histogram distribution of $F > 600$ for G1, S, and G2 + M)
8. Number of dead cells

This method has many advantages including the following:

1. The simultaneous analysis of parameters of lymphocyte stimulation related to both DNA transcription and replication
2. Recognition of lymphocyte differentiation into blastoid cells, compared to plasmacytoid cells

3. Evaluation of number of cells triggered into stimulation cultures
4. Greater safety and economy in comparison to radioisotopes
5. No need for scintillation counts, which do not provide information regarding individual cells and necessitate autoradiography, which is tedious and time-consuming
6. No need for cell rinsing, fixation, or centrifugation

**Analysis of Lymphocyte Blastogenesis by Laser Cytometry.** The major component of the cytometer is a flow system wherein the cell suspension is introduced into a flowing sheath of filtered water, such that the column of cells is progressively constricted to a 30- to 50-$\mu$m core at the point of interception of the laser beam (Ruckdeschel et al., 1979; Shu et al., 1978). Large numbers of cells ($10^4$, $10^5$) can be counted in less than a minute. The cells intersect a HeNe laser-beam wavelength at 632.8 nm. This wavelength avoids the absorption spectrum of hemoglobin, and consequently, contaminating erythrocytes do not cause undue absorption. The forward angle scatter (transmittance) is monitored, and a pulse is generated inversely proportional to the transmittance. The height of the pulse is directly proportional to cell size and can readily distinguish lymphoblasts and lymphocytes (Figs. 23.9 and 23.10) (Ruckdeschel et al., 1979). Direct quantitation of lymphocyte responsiveness had disclosed that a substantial number of small lymphocytes

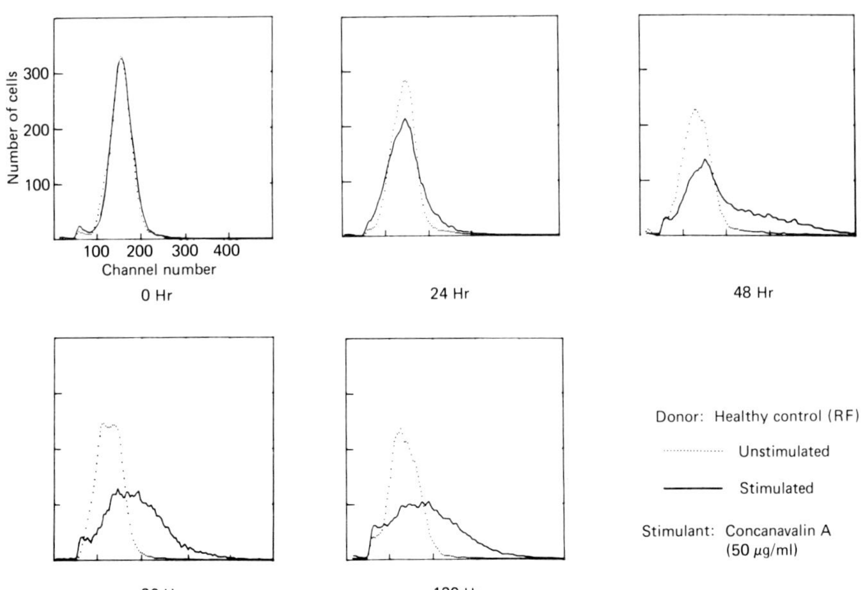


**Fig. 23.9.** Lymphocyte transformation following in-vitro mitogenic stimulation. Ficoll-Hypaque–separated lymphocytes peak in channels 100–190 at time 0. Platelets and debris appear below channel 100 and are windowed out electronically. It is clear that following con A stimulation, a population of large cells (channel number $> 190$) appears in the stimulated cultures. [Ruckdeschel JC, Lininger L, Bryzyski H, Miani M, Becker J (1979) Re-analysis of in vitro lymphocyte blastogenesis using the laser cytometry assay. In: Baum SJ, Ledney DG (eds) Experimental Hematology Today 1979. Springer-Verlag, New York.]

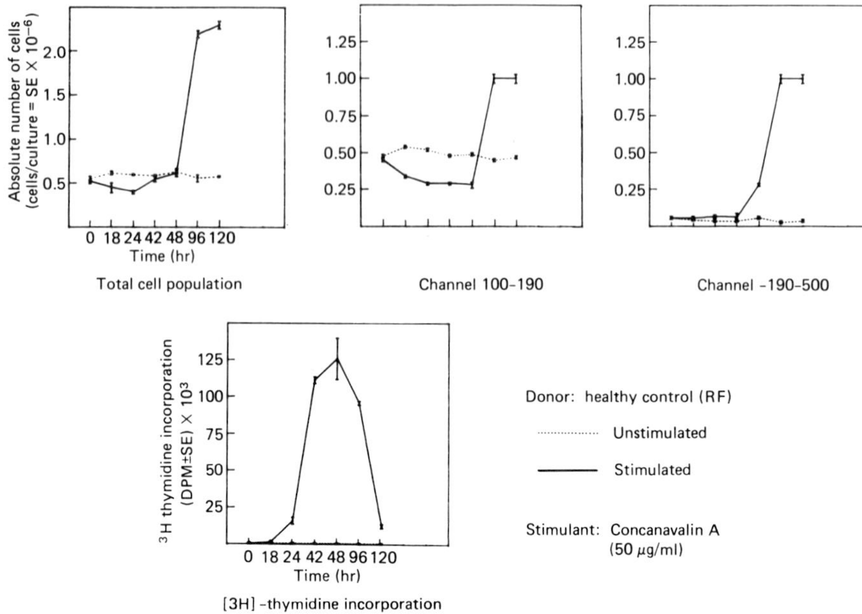


**Fig. 23.10.** Time-course of lymphocyte stimulation as measured by laser cytometry. Absolute numbers of lymphoblasts (channels 190–500) and small lymphocytes (channels 100–190) are determined from percentages on the distribution and the volume-specific cell counts. All cell populations plateau as the peak response is reached. [$^3$H]-thymidine incorporation precedes cell proliferation by 12 to 24 hr and drops off sharply following peak responsiveness. [Ruckdeschel JC, Lininger L, Bryzyski H, Miani M, Becker J (1979) Re-analysis of in vitro lymphocyte blastogenesis using the laser cytometry assay. In: Baum SJ, Ledney DG (eds) Experimental Hematology Today 1979. Springer-Verlag, New York.]

are produced during in-vitro stimulation with mitogen or antigen in addition to the expected increase in lymphoblasts. This suggests a total cellular response (lymphocytes plus lymphoblasts) by both antigen and mitogen stimulation. This technique can also measure the number of cells per unit of time. In facilitating comparison of laser cytometry versus radionucleotide incorporation, in terms of reducibility, the laser cytometry assay is significantly superior to the latter. Assays for both total cell number and total lymphoblast number are superior, with total cell numbers being slightly more stable over time (Doukas et al., 1977; Ruckdeschel et al., 1977, 1979; Shu et al., 1978).

## Rheumatoid Factor: Quantitation and Characterization

Laser detection of rheumatoid factor can be done with laser nephelometry, but it can be both measured and characterized by a recent innovation of multiparameter cell sorting technology (Horan et al., 1979). Immunoglobulin G or one of its various subclasses, IgG1, IgG2, IgG3, is bound to polystyrene microspheres of uniform size.

Microspheres are then placed in serum from patients suffering rheumatoid arthritis, who have rheumatoid factor, so that the factor will react with the immunoglobulins. After free unbound proteins have been washed off, fluorescein-conjugated antirheumatoid factor (IgM) is reacted. These microspheres are then washed and examined by laser-activated flow cytometry (Coulter TPS-1) (Fig. 23.11). Individual microspheres float through a flow chamber in a saline solution. An argon-ion-laser light beam simultaneously measures intensity of emitted fluorescent light and particle size (by low-angle light scatter). This can be done at rates of 50,000–100,000 cells (or subcellular particles) per minute. Any particles that are of interest are electrostatically charged negatively or positively as they pass through a charging collar. As the droplets continue to fall, they pass through a pair of charged flexion plates. Negatively or positively charged droplets (and particles that are of interest) are deflected, retained, and collected separately. Droplets that are not charged are not deflected and thus not kept. In this way, not only the amount of rheumatoid factor can be measured, but specific aliquots can be further evaluated (Fig. 23.12). The method compares with measurements in laboratories using titer dilutions. The specificity for rheumatoid factor (RF) can also be mea-

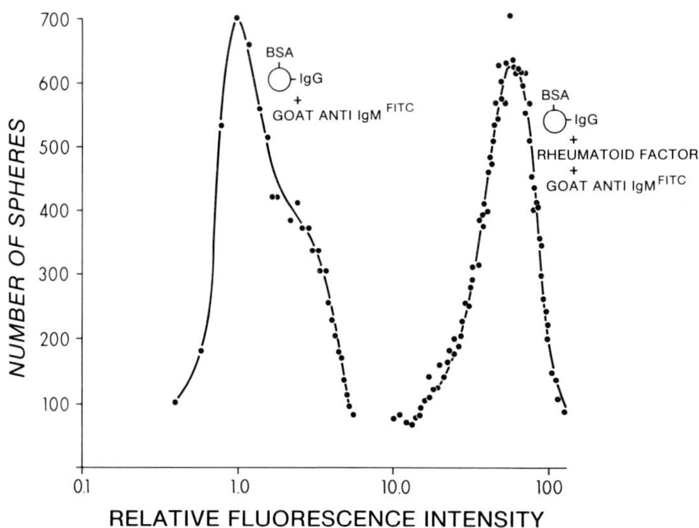


**Fig. 23.11.** Detection of rheumatoid factor. One aliquot of IgG-BSA microspheres was placed into serum containing rheumatoid factor (RF). After being washed to remove unreacted RF, the microspheres were placed into fluorescein-conjugated goat anti-IgM. A second aliquot was placed in fluorescein conjugate only. Fluorescence of each microsphere was analyzed by means of a flow cytometer. Microspheres exposed to RF fluoresce 60 times more brightly than the control *(at left)*. [Horan PK, Schenk EA, Abraham GN, Kloszewski ED (1979) Fluid phase particle fluorescence analysis: Rheumatoid factor specificity evaluated by laser flow cytophotometry. In: Nakamura RM, Dito WR, Tucker ES II (eds) Immunoassays in the Clinical Laboratory. Laboratory and Research Methods in Biology and Medicine, vol. III. Alan R. Liss, New York.]

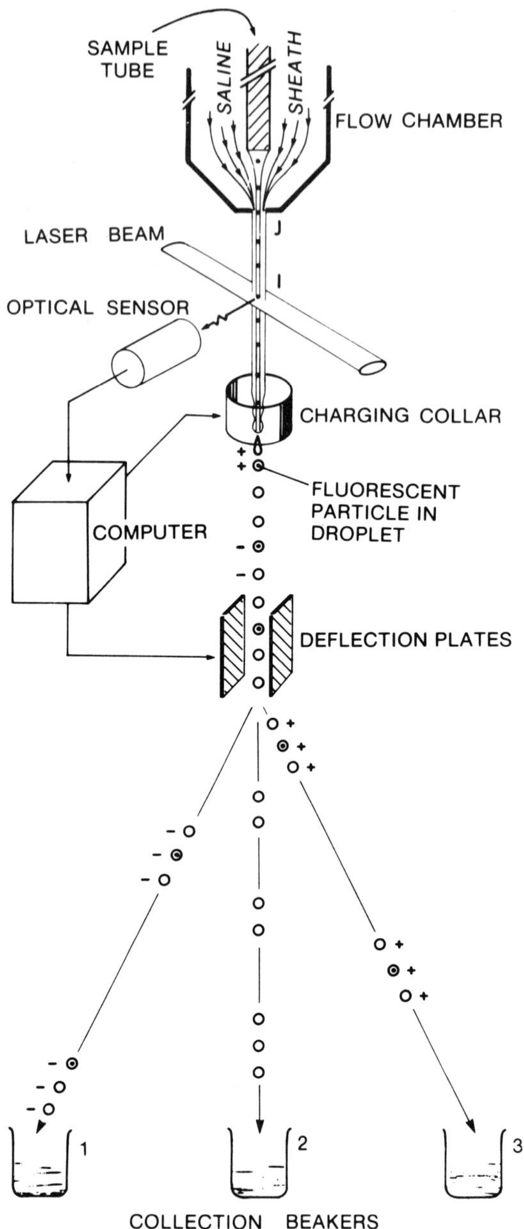


**Fig. 23.12.** Schema of a flow cytometer and sorter. Microspheres enter flow chamber through hypodermic needle and are centered by sheath of saline and resemble beads on a necklace. The exiting stream carries fluorescent particles from flow chamber through argon-ion laser beam. Two-color fluorescence emission and low-angle light scatter (1°–20°) are recorded for each cell. Uniform droplets that contain particles of interest can be charged electrostatically and sorted from the main stream. [Horan PK, Schenk EA, Abraham GN, Kloszewski ED (1979) In: Nakamura RM, Dito WR, Tucker ES II (eds) Immunoassays in the Clinical Laboratory, Laboratory and Research Methods in Biology and Medicine, vol. III. Alan R. Liss, New York.]

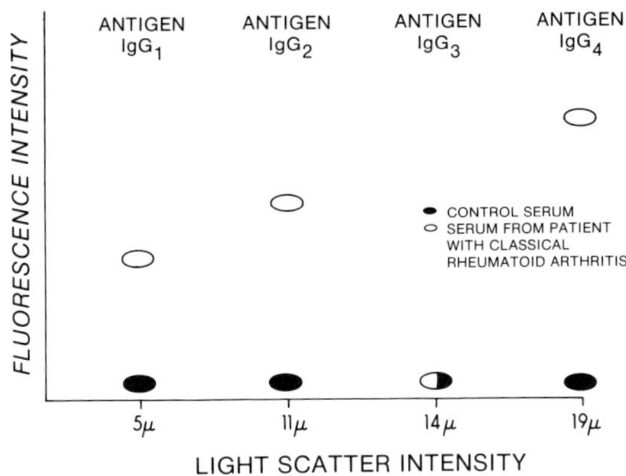


**Fig. 23.13.** Idealized simultaneous detection of IgM anti-$IgG_1$, $IgG_2$, and $IgG_3$. The $IgG_1$ would be adsorbed to 5-μm polystyrene spheres; $IgG_2$ would be adsorbed to 11-μm spheres; and $IgG_3$ would be adsorbed to 14-μm spheres. Equal numbers of each size microspheres would be placed in patient's serum, washed, and then reacted with fluorescein-conjugated anti-IgM. By means of a flow cytometer, size (and therefore the adsorbed antigen) could be identified by light-scatter intensity, and fluorescence intensity (and therefore RF binding) could be measured using the photomultiplier tube. *Solid ovals*, control serum; *open ovals*, serum from patient with autoimmune dysfunction. [Horan PK, Schenk EA, Abraham GN, Kloszewski ED (1979) Fluid phase particle fluorescence analysis: Rheumatoid factor specificity evaluated by laser flow cytophotometry. In: Nakamura RM, Dito WR, Tucker ES II (eds) Immunoassays in the Clinical Laboratory; Laboratory and Research Methods in Biology and Medicine, vol. III. Alan R. Liss, New York.]

sured and indications noted of which subclasses of IgG may be preferentially bound (Fig. 23.13).

The ability to define and collect specific antigen subpopulations is important, for it allows for the detection of antigen-specific antibodies, which are of pathologic importance. The ability to measure and quantitate this information rapidly is important. The method could also be used to measure IgG, IgA, and IgE rheumatoid factors. By characterizing the nature of specificity of the rheumatoid factor in the serum of patients, much may be learned about the pathologic process of arthritis and other conditions that are associated with the presence of rheumatoid factor.

Any protein antigen could be absorbed to the microspheres. With the availability of various size microspheres, absorption of different antigens could be bound to different size spheres. Moreover, the antibodies against the antigens could be conjugated with fluorescein, which fluoresces green, or rhodamine, which fluoresces red. The flow cytometer can determine both green and red fluorescence intensity and size simultaneously on each microsphere at rates up to 50,000/s. This simultaneous measurement of size and fluorescent intensity can provide good information as to which antigen binds antibody and at what titer it is present.

Thus, the ability of the laser to make rapid immunologic measurements of pathologic importance is highlighted by this technique.

## LASER EFFECT ON HUMAN TISSUE

### T and B Lymphocytes

There appear to be many immunologic consequences of various types of laser irradiation. The simultaneous application of HeNe and pulsed lasers can achieve an immunosuppressive effect with minimal cell loss. The immunosuppressive effect involves both T as well as B lymphocytes (Mester et al., 1977). Ruby-laser radiation of the spleen of white rats given injections of *Brucella abortus* 19 demonstrates that nonfocal splenic laser radiation suppresses the immunocellular reaction and function of immune cells. This affects the synthesis of the antibodies after the first antigen challenge and also after the second immunization. Thus, primary and anamnestic responses are involved. There is a decrease in both the number of antibody cells and the titer of *Brucella* antibodies noted (Zlatev et al., 1976). The number of antibody-forming cells in the spleen increased 7–14 days after radiation of experimental tumors on mouse hindlegs with a neodymium (Nd) glass laser (Moskalik et al., 1977). The number of rosette-forming cells, as well as the capacity for T lymphocytes to undergo blast transformation, was also decreased. With time, all these signs returned to pretreatment values. The HeNe laser treatment in combination with immunosuppression by antithymocyte serum of Swiss male albino mice showed a marked graft-protecting effect of transplanted tail skin from CBA male mice. This combination was greater than either immunosuppression or laser treatment separately (Namenyi et al., 1975).

### Laser Treatment of Rheumatoid Arthritis

The effect of laser exposure on the arthritic joints of people with rheumatoid arthritis has been the subject of two studies (Goldman et al., 1977, 1980). In both studies, the patients improved. The earlier study documented improvement of the joints, and the second study sought to compare the improvement of joints exposed to laser with joints that had not been lased and served as controls. An American Optical 641SB high-radiance Nd glass laser that operated in the Q-switch mode at 1.06 $\mu$m was used to evaluate 30 people with rheumatoid arthritis. These patients had the metacarpal, phalangeal (MCP), and proximal interphalangeal (PIP) joints of one hand lased, while the other hand served as a control. Left and right hands were alternated in this group of 30 right-handed patients. The lasing was performed once a week for 10 weeks, and the patients were seen by both a physician and an occupational therapist at each visit to evaluate the effect of the lasing. The patients were not told which hand was lased, and laboratory personnel evaluating the patients did not know which hand was being lased. Only the laser instrument supervisor knew the code. The patients were evaluated by the occupational therapist with range of motion of the MCP and PIP joints, circumferential measurements, tip pinch in pounds, lateral pinch in pounds, grip strength in pounds, and measurement of the distance of flexion from the tip of the fingers to the distal palmar crease. The physician measured heat, erythema, tenderness, pain on motion, and swelling in each of the joints.

Laboratory studies indicating activity of disease and measurement of rheumatoid factor, cryoglobulins, and circulating immune complexes were also performed. The data were collected, keypunched on computer cards, and statistically analyzed.

The results of this investigation indicated that patients underwent improvement in both the lased and nonlased hands. These changes were highly significant over time, and the degree of improvement of erythema and pain was significantly different between the lased and nonlased hands. Grasp and tip pinch also improved more on the lased than the nonlased hand, whereas circumferential measurement and flexion improved on both sides. Laboratory data showed no significant changes except that immune complexes, as measured by platelet aggregation, decreased during the period of lasing. No evidence of adverse effects was observed in laboratory or x-ray studies. However, all patients experienced stinging during the laser treatment; two noted erythema, and two noted hyperpigmentation at the laser impact site.

Exactly how the laser may have helped improve people with rheumatoid arthritis is still unclear. The rationale for a laser for rheumatic disease includes its heat effect; laser shock wave; selective pigment absorption; immunosuppression and immunostimulation of laser upon tissue; stimulation of wound healing that occurs with laser irradiation; and the facts that sites beyond those directly lased have been noted to improve in people with laser therapy and pain relief occurs, somewhat akin to laser acupuncture.

Thus people with rheumatoid arthritis receiving laser therapy noted improvement of their arthritis by both activity and hand-function evaluations. Even though these changes were usually bilateral, there was more improvement in grip strength and tip pinch, and less erythema and pain on the lased side. There was also a decrease in titer of circulating immune complexes measured by platelet aggregation, a finding that may indicate a general improvement in the overall activity of the rheumatoid disease or reflect immune modulation by laser exposure. Thus these preliminary results indicate some effect upon patients with rheumatoid arthritis by laser therapy.

## SUMMARY

The data discussed in this chapter suggest tremendous potential for the use of lasers for investigation and treatment of immunologic disease. Major advances in the use of lasers for this area of medicine and biology are expected.

## REFERENCES

Andreef M, Beck JD, Darzynkiewicz Z, Traganos F, Gupta S, Melamed MR, Good RA (1978) RNA content in human lymphocyte subpopulations. Proc Nat Acad Sci 75:1938–2941.

Buffone GJ, Savory J, Cross RE (1974) Use of a laser-equipped centrifugal analyzer for kinetic measurement of serum IgG. Clin Chem 20:1320–1323.

Darzynkiewicz A, Traganos F, Sharpless TK, Melamed MR (1976) Lymphocyte stimulation. A rapid multiparameter analysis. Proc Nat Acad Sci 73:2881–2884.

Darzynkiewicz Z, Traganos F, Sharpless TK, Melamed MR (1977) Cell cycle-related changes in nuclear chromatin of stimulated lymphocytes as measured by flow cytometry. Cancer Res 37:4635–4640.

Deaton DC, Maxwell KW, Smith RS, Creveling RL (1976) Use of laser nephelometry in the measurement of serum proteins. Clin Chem 22:1465–1471.

Doukas JG, Ruckdeschel JC, Mardiney MR Jr (1977) Quantitative and qualitative analysis of human lymphocyte proliferation to specific antigen in vitro by use of the helium-neon laser. J Immunol Methods 15:229–238.

Goldman JA, Muehlenbeck EC, Muckerhiede MD ((1977) Laser treatment of rheumatoid arthritis. Electro/Optics Laser 77:496–498.

Goldman JA, Chiapella J, Casey HL, et al. (1980) Laser therapy of rheumatoid arthritis. Lasers in Medicine and Surgery 1:93–101.

Horan PK, Schenk EA, Abraham GN, Kloszewski ED (1979) Fluid phase particle fluorescence analysis. Rheumatoid factor specificity evaluated by laser flow cytophotometry. In: Nakamura RM, Dito WR, Tucker ES II (ed) Immunoassays in the Clinical Laboratory. Laboratory and Research Methods in Biology and Medicine III. Alan R. Liss, New York.

Kaplan JH, Uzgiris EE (1975) The detection of phytomitogen-induced changes in human lymphocyte surfaces by laser Doppler spectroscopy. J Immunol Methods 7:337–346.

Kaplan JH, Uzgiris EE (1976) Identification of T and B cell subpopulations in human peripheral blood: Electrophoretic mobility distributions associated with surface marker characteristics. J Immunol 117:1731–1740.

Kaplan JH, Uzgiris EE (1979) Electrophoretic mobility comparison of normal blood lymphocytes and lymphocytes from patients with chronic lymphocytic leukemia. In: Nieburgs HE (ed) Prevention and Detection of Cancer, Part II. vol. II. Marcel Dekker, New York.

Kaplan JH, Uzgiris EE, Lockwood SH (1979) Analysis of T cell subpopulations by laser Doppler spectroscopy and the association of electrophoretic mobility differences with differences in rosette-forming affinity. J Immunol Methods 17:241–255.

Mester E, Nagylucskay S, Tisza S, Mester A, Toth J, Laczy I (1977) Current studies on the effect of laser beams and wound healing immunological effects. Z Exp Chir 10:301–306.

Moskalik KG, Kislow AP, Statschkow AP, Laso WW (1977) Immunological process noted after laser radiation of experimental tumors. Laser Electro Optics 4:34–35.

Namenyi J, Mester E, Földes I, Tisza A (1975) Effect of laser irradiation and immunosuppressive treatment on survival of mouse skin allotransplants. Acta Chir Acad Sci Hungaricae 16:326–335.

Ruckdeschel JC, Doukas JG, Drake WP, Mardiney MR (1977) Application of laser cytometry to the analysis of immunologically induced in vitro lymphocyte responsiveness. Transplantation 23:396–403.

Ruckdeschel JC, Lininger L, Bryzyski H, Miani M, Becker J (1979) Reanalysis of "in vitro" lymphocyte blastogenesis using the laser cytometry assay. In: Baum SJ, Ledney DG (eds) Experimental Hematology Today. Springer-Verlag, New York.

Ruckdeschel JC, Lininger L, Bryzyski H, Miani M, Becker J (1979) Serial quantitation of in vitro lymphocyte responsiveness of concanavallin A. Transplantation 38:203–206.

Shu S, Cimino EF, Mardiney MR Jr (1978) Light transmission of lymphocyte activation by mitogens: A new technique. J Immunol Methods 22:219–232.

Traganos F, Gorski AJ, Darzynkiewicz Z, Sharpless T, Melamed MR (1977) Rapid multiparameter analysis of cell stimulation in mixed lymphocyte culture reactions. J Histochem Cytochem 25:881–887.

Uzgiris EE, Cluxton DH (in press) A wide angle scattering configuration for laser Doppler measurements of electrophoretic mobility. Rev Sci Instrum.

Uzgiris EE, Kaplan JH (1974) Study of lymphocyte and erythrocyte electrophoretic mobility by laser Doppler spectroscopy. Anal Biochem 60:451–455.

Uzgiris EE, Kaplan JH (1976) Tuberculin-sensitized lymphocytes detected by altered electrophoretic mobility distributions after incubation with the antigen PPD. J Immunol 117:2165–2170.

Uzgiris EE, Kaplan JH, Cunningham TJ, Lockwood SH, Steiner D (1978) Laser Coppler spectroscopy in experimental and clinical immunology. In: Catsimpooles T (ed) Electrophoresis '78. Elsevier North Holland, Amsterdam, pp. 427–440.

Uzgiris EE, Kaplan JH, Cunningham TJ, Lockwood SH, Steiner D (1979) Association of electrophoretic mobility with other cell surface markers of T cell subpopulations in normal individuals and cancer patients. Europ J Cancer 15:1275–1280.

Walsh RL, Coles ME, Geary TD (1979) Evaluation of two commercially available laser nephelometers and their recommended methods for measurement of serum immoglobulins G. Clin Chem 25:151–156.

Zlatev S, Yanev E, Bozduganov A (1976) Immunocytogenesis and synthesis of antibodies after spleen laser irradiation. Folia Med 18:121–127.

# 24

# Laser Medical Technology for the Twenty-first Century

*Myron C. Muckerheide*

The ability of the laser to vaporize minute quantities of material may result, in the twenty-first century, in a controlled, subatomic tool. It is certainly feasible at the present time to vaporize single cells or portions of cells with a broad range of laser devices and wavelengths, and certain characteristics of laser vaporization are analogous to cosmic-particle penetration.

The characteristic that is perhaps most similar is the ability to produce channels such as those evidenced in astronaut environments and produced by cosmic particles. In the macroscopic region, the spallation techniques are of interest. Particles moving back from the laser-bombarded target are often at extremely high temperatures and can produce minute cell damage. The spallation particles can, indeed, actually cauterize fragments of cells. Some spallation can be magnetically attenuated and thus create a highly reproducible phenomenon.

## IMPROVEMENTS OF MENTAL DISORDERS

The destruction of small targets in the micron range, by controlling both the pulse width and the energy of the laser, offers the field of neurology a truly new instrument for application in the area of mental disorders. The probability of utilizing the particles generated by laser bombardment in neurosurgical applications appears to still be some distance off, but the technology for guiding laser-generated particles, which are both macroscopic and microscopic in size, is presently available.

Never before in all of man's existence on the planet has there been a device that can penetrate, in a needlelike fashion, with the diameter of a bundle of photons. As the technology advances and surgeons extend themselves beyond the brute

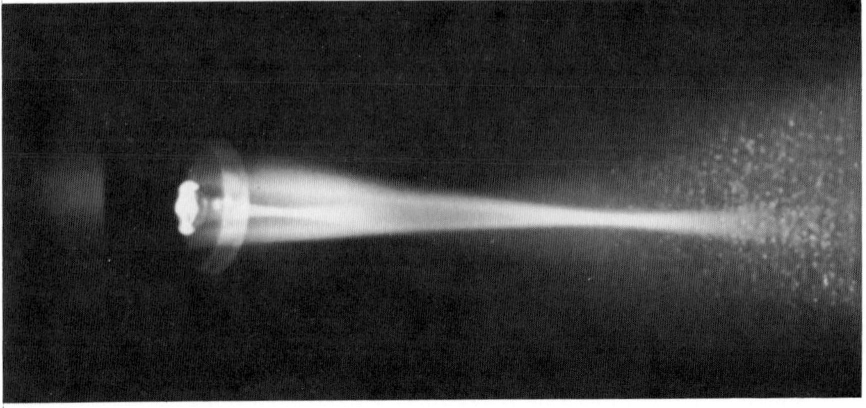

**Fig. 24.1.** Beam shaped by annular lens, producing particle breakup in air *(at right)*.

force of surgical machines into the realm of the atomic and subatomic, one may certainly envision an improved condition for those who suffer from mental disorders.

## Laser Chemistry and Physics

Besides the actual vaporization of cells, there is also the vast field of laser chemistry in which reactions occur in billionths of a second and create an entirely new environment. Who is to say what characteristics the brain may exhibit in the twenty-first century after being modified by laser-produced surgical, particle, and chemical interactions. Certainly humankind stands to benefit from this new technology in the field of mental disorders.

An interesting phenomenon was created in our laboratory by a laser beam which was shaped by an annular lens to produce a strange breakup of particles in room air (Fig. 24.1). Continuing investigation of such a phenomenon shows frequency shifting along with acceleration of various particles. Experiments relating to the reproduction of such interactions should be undertaken with caution, and as always in all laser technology, proper eye protection is a must. Extreme caution is recommended.

Spallation, particle generation, thermal and vaporization techniques, along with chemical conditioning, offer man a new dawn in his fight to overcome mental disorders.

# THE LASER'S ROLE IN THE RELIEF OF PAIN

The laser offers another unique and extremely exciting technology—that for the relief of human pain. There are strong electrical fields generated by laser pulses, which have been focused in various gases.

The laser-generated spark phenomenon, which has been in evidence for the past decade, is of interest in producing fields around nerve fibers. The transmission and collision states that occur when ions are produced in the spark are directed at nerve-fiber material to inhibit or accelerate electron transmission. This ionization of air surrounding the high-density plasma creates a corona (Fig. 24.2).

The very hot plasma contains strong magnetic and electrical fields that may be of interest to the physician of the twenty-first century for the treatment of painful conditions by blocking the transmission of electrical signals in nerve fibers or by amplifying the signals in nerve fibers. The distribution appears to be gaussian, and the controlled plasma envelope may offer some structural relief by actually interfering with nerve electrical transmission.

## Photon Penetration

The photons that escape the very hot plasma can create other conditions of interest, especially in air where ultraviolet (UV) frequencies are ample in themselves to create new transmission phenomena in the nerve bundles. The predictability of producing the breakdown phenomenon was indicated when breakdown was induced with a pulse of 1.06-$\mu$m radiation, a pulse width of 30 ns, and an energy of 90 J sharply focused to a point suspended within the palm of the hand (Fig. 24.3).

The demonstration was to merely emphasize the simplicity of creating the spark and the predictability of locating it over a desired area. It must be remembered that the energy deposition at the point of focus can be totally destructive of tissue, and extreme caution should be observed in any attempt to reproduce such an

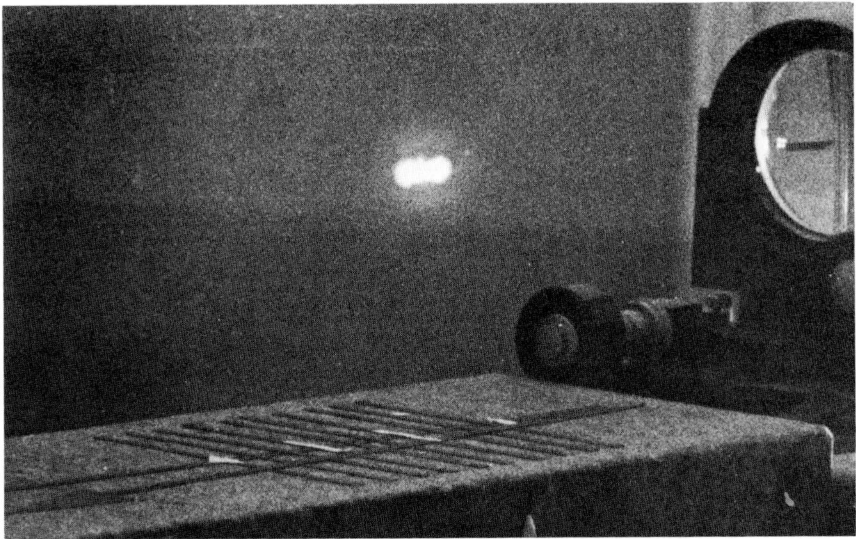

**Fig. 24.2.** Laser-generated spark with high-density plasma and accompanying corona.

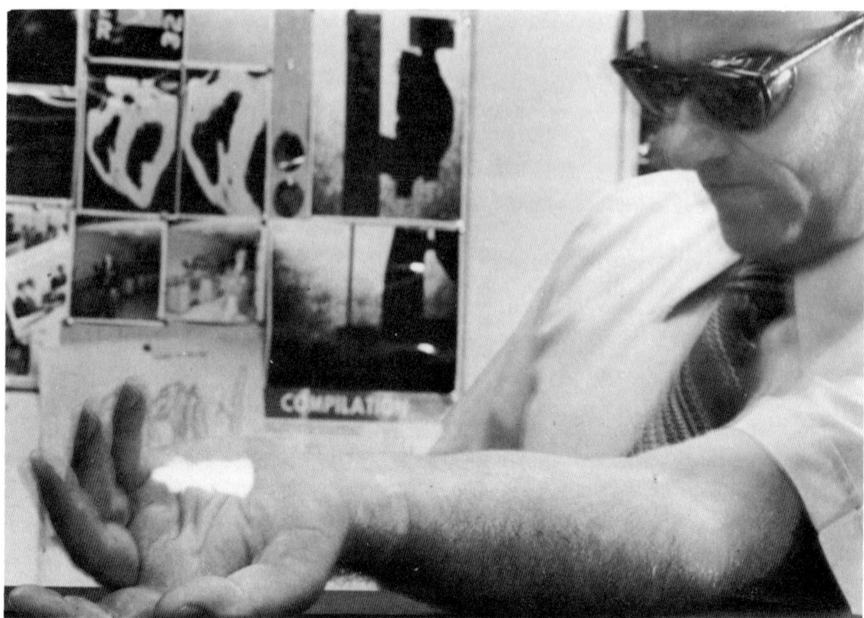

**Fig. 24.3.** Laser-generated plasma suspended within palm of the hand. Time exposure was used because of narrow pulse width; therefore some evidence of motion may be noted in face and hand.

event. Under no circumstances should any person not familiar with the technology attempt to undertake the experiment described.

In addition to the harmful effect of focused laser radiation on the hand, the intense reflections of the plasma can create a serious eye hazard unless extraordinary precautions are undertaken to protect the eyes. In air there is also the possibility of creating UV radiation from the intense plasma.

## THE LASER AND ARTIFICIAL-ORGAN PRODUCTION

Certainly upon us is the period in evolution when genetics are under scrutiny beneath the searching beam of the laser.

### Cell Modification

Studies indicate that cell modification can be effected by knocking off or fragmenting the DNA that is intrinsic to cell behavior. If DNA sensitivity to laser light is construed to create a risk of inducing strange anomalies or mutations, then the positive side of the issue is the use of the various laser frequencies to create new and desirable effects. The concept that light may be absorbed by specifically colored material is certainly a proper approach to the modification of the cell. Add to the light-absorption potential the ability of the laser to modify by intense shock waves, and another new tool for the twenty-first century is in the process of being created. Perhaps the proximity of one cell to another and the atomic bonding which exists will be strongly altered during the next century.

Several other reasons point to the need for a positive approach to such prospects. Present concerns with ecology should foreshadow a new era in the maintenance of the fragile balance needed for sustaining healthy organs in human beings. The transplant, too, certainly is characteristic of conservation efforts. Yet there seems to be resistance to or lack of interest in producing artificial organs.

## Microbonding Techniques

I would like to venture into the realm of the extremely microscopic world of laser-etched circuits and the probability that organ production may be totally feasible in this fantastic world of microcircuits and microbonding techniques.

Minute bonding techniques to produce new filters and fibers by using laser technology may implement a totally new concept in kidney replacement. The lung as an absorber of oxygen to saturate the blood may be found to be totally replaceable by tiny lattices, produced by the laser, which have the ability to exchange gases. Even such organs as the brain may be replaced by tiny chemical fluidics that will be chemically enhanced and produced by laser beams. Fluidics may create various reservoir phenomena to release the presently unknown chemistry of thought.

Entry into the realm of artificial organs came upon the human subject in a startling array of new heart valves, vessel-replacement materials, and tissue-replacement plastics. Perhaps the new organs will not be recognized as structured objects, as we know the organs, but merely small modalities where the laser has performed its chemical magic to produce new substances that might replace the organ entirely as we perceive it. No wonder can be too great for the fast chemical processes that the laser can already produce. Indeed, man is entering a new era of physics and chemistry that is due to the laser.

## Replication and Modification

Besides the true artificial organs, man may be able to replicate and modify existing organs by the restructuring of the chromosomes through fast-laser chemistry. There will be new substances generated by the laser chemist that will both alter present organs and perhaps raise them to a more efficient level. There will be a chemistry of continuing improvement rather than deterioration. The production of new organ substances and chromosome alteration may produce for man a longevity of unknown dimensions.

The food supply for man may well be solved by adjustments of the new organs to very high workload conditions, in which the body needs very little food. With organs that are artificial and replaceable, there will be a total altering of man's life-style and existence. The laser's light may be the key to this new threshold of longevity with highly tuned organs that function on totally new principles.

## THE LASER'S SOLUTION TO BLINDNESS

The laser's ability to adjust itself with ease to every technology will, in turn, certainly be responsible for creating a new series of element combinations. These new systems will, in actuality, be signal generators.

Mosaics that can produce excellent resolution will make man's eye virtually replaceable. The tiny microcircuits, which will be energized by the chemicals of the body and activated by light striking their elaborate interfaces, are the eye replacements for tomorrow. The laser can bond and form new textures in even today's most exotic structures. There will be sensors of great quality and minuteness. Laser microetching and vaporization techniques will produce a new generation of logic systems. Even small lasers within the body structure itself may be able to retrosense by beams directed from the area within the artificial eye, not unlike side-looking radar or other excellent sensing systems of today.

The ability of light to be the fastest means of signal transmission may find application by enhancing the normal sight too. Rapidity of function may be increased by adding the laser as a sensor to the present eye, so that image persistence is more rapidly enhanced and certain profiles are held constant on the retina of the eye. Actual freezing of images might be possible. For instance, the retinal image could be stored from a received signal. Then the memory of man would have greater recall, especially if the chip could call up random images. Such miniature systems are well within the realm of possibility when one considers the technology available even today.

The eye of man, at present, is a sensor of great capability. With laser assistance, images will certainly be more vivid. There could be sight into other parts of the spectrum, and, in fact, man's present eyes, which are very blind to an array of frequencies, will be able to see in another dimension.

It is not improvement of sight for only the blind that is at stake, but improvement of all of our evolution-structured "blindness" which will be helped by the laser in the twenty-first century. The form such systems take may be implants or merely fixtures to the body, such as eyeglasses. Man will no longer be blind to the beauty that is around him in other frequencies.

The ability to see has already been greatly increased with the aid of infrared lights. The curiosity exhibited for such a phenomenon can be satisfied only by total laser-enhanced viewing in the twenty-first century.

## THE ANALYSIS OF HUMAN PATHOLOGY BY THE LASER

Despite all human experience, it has not been possible to visualize problems as they develop in the diseases people are prone to. Early warning, however, is possible beyond the stages of modern microscopy, radiology, and chemistry.

The infrared imaging of human pathology is new to the laser field and, therefore, a mere infant, but the laser and its ancillary systems will be the new warning of disease. The ability, for instance, of neodymium laser light to pass through tissue to produce images is but a start in the battle to produce a new enhancement quality to pathologic conditions. The ability of the laser's light to scatter through certain plasmas in varying degrees may certainly indicate a time is upon us when daily analysis of our health may be available at home.

The computer's linkage to the laser in the recognition of significant profiles in blood and lymph conditions signals changes to come in laser analysis of pathologic conditions. The linkage of small microprocessors to the laser interface is without precedent in its possibilities for analyzing the ills that continue to beset human beings.

### Scanning

The computer laser interface has another fantastic analytic potential for the twenty-first century. The scanning capability of the laser and the analysis of the computer makes the marriage one of infinite consequence. The intelligence that will be acquired by laser scanners, linked to computers, will exceed all that has been acquired in the past in determining pathologic conditions. The ability to have data acquisition at the speed of light and to search all past information at speeds near that of light will alter the world of diagnosis and produce a new technological entity.

### Holography

Besides the scanning techniques, there will be holographic presentations of information for the viewer to analyze in three dimensions. The scanner will have acquisition to the third dimension, and therefore it is natural that its imaging and analysis will take place in the reconstruction of the third dimension.

Laser radiographic analysis will take on scanning concepts in holographic dimensions and, when linked to the computer, will produce images of such clarity that they will compete with the real. Holography, in combination with the computer laser scanner, will facilitate the study of moving organs, with the dynamics involved in each axis of presentation.

Cross sections with holographic rotation will make reconstruction of pathology a science of great sophistication. The laser will be the reason for this new adventure in diagnosis.

## THE NONCONTACT TRANSMITTAL OF PHYSIOLOGIC DATA FROM THE HUMAN SUBJECT

There will be diagnostic tools employing the laser in the twenty-first century that will make use of noncontacting data acquisition. The reflection of beams from the body will call up information for analysis, and the various frequencies will make possible the acquisition of data from many parameters.

The condition of the blood and skin will be easily accessible to the prying eye of the laser. Dynamics of the skin will exhibit warnings of coming disease, and chemical evaluation can be made by the interference of two or more beams on the surface of the body. The laser will probe the location of the internal organs and will be able, by transmission and interference, to predict coming problems of health. The simplicity of diagnostic techniques will be astounding.

Abstraction of information from real-time image and its comparison with past imaging will give sensing capability unlike anything known today. Remote sensing and noncontacting transmittal are not well established in the health fields today. The technology of the Vietnam War, in which a light signal indicated true range, indicated the direction the laser would take in the development of noncontacting systems. The combination of laser sensing for surface and depth conditions will also lend a new dimension to the quality of an evaluation. Both acquisitions will use the common denominator of light frequencies for supplemental display reasons.

The pulsed laser and the continuous-wave laser will find common ground in the manner of data acquisition for sensing. Because both will interact at the same speed, which is that of light, there will be an added time feature never before explored.

The hazards encountered in contacting transducer technology will not exist with low-energy laser modalities, and the problems of tissue destruction will not be present in such systems. Noncontacting systems will be especially important in the analysis of the brain during surgical procedures, and the laser will be able to transmit information never before obtainable. The heart will also be scrutinized by the laser, and there will be no interference with the electrical system of the heart during time of transmittal.

It is not difficult to envision a total system obtaining data at rates of speed near that of light and a computer analysis a few seconds later.

## THE LASER AND WOUND HEALING

For the maximum impact in the area of wound healing, the laser may well begin to make its impression in the twenty-first century. The work that presently continues in the area of new physics, involving the interaction of laser light on tissue for purposes of granulation, is making new advances. Probing into the bonds that control the affinity of atom for atom, technology will devise molecular and atomic means for rapidly healing wounds.

It is not difficult to foresee a device that will heal a wound instantaneously, once the cellular concepts of photon interaction with tissue are better understood. The effect the photon has upon atomic structure in periods at and near the speed of light has advanced the time base for healing. The production of free radicals and cellular modification by photon bombardment opens a panorama of new techniques. The rapid chemical reactions now occurring in the chemistry laboratory are an indication of the new and wonderful technology that is near.

Once the laser was used for healing, a vast barrier was obliterated. Since the first appearance of humankind on earth, the light of the sun has aided in the disinfection process and reduced the potential for infection. It is a natural next step that the intense beam of the laser, with its high brightness, be used to implement wound healing.

The field of medicine has merely attained, at its very best, the approximation of tissue masses, so that the process of cellular bonding may occur at a precise and rapid rate. What the laser can do in the twenty-first century is assist in the approximation of the microscopic and even the submicroscopic. Once cellular modification is well understood in the world of the laser, it will be a simple step to use laser "sutures" in approximating microcellular masses. Retinal welding by laser heralded the brave penetration of medicine into microsurgery.

Cellular modification began, for many reasons still not well defined, once the brilliant flash of the laser found its path through the optics of the microscope. The rewards of the new adventure would appear to be as close as the twenty-first century.

## LASER-GENERATED PHENOMENA IN PATHOLOGIC STATES

Laser visualization of pathologic states was addressed in earlier comments on laser scanning procedures. However, the visualization of pathologic conditions by laser-generated phenomena reaches beyond the mere interplay of laser light for purposes of analysis. Visualization is also possible by the production of highly ionizing forms of radiation and the myriad combinations of neutrons and x rays generated by laser.

Intense fields of neutrons can be created by the interaction of the laser beam with very miniscule amounts of specially selected matter. The emissions can be directed, or their velocity slowed, for reasons essential to the new generators of electrooptic enhancers.

There is a new potential in the creation of x rays that may be manifest in the twenty-first century. Present x-ray generation from laser plasmas signals the advent of very small laser x-ray systems and the immediate availability, in medicine, of highly sophisticated x-ray generators on a mobile basis.

The need for very small and very intense short-duration, high-resolution x-ray units at the site of accidents has long been understood. The movement of a patient after an accident would be made much safer if a flash laser x-ray unit were available for instantaneous evaluation and computer read-out of the condition.

The fields generated by light interactions with other incident light quanta may produce high enhancement of visualization on a real-time or stored basis. The ability to introduce, for instance, an immediate visualization prior to movement from an accident scene, and the storage of the same data for field orientation in a select memory matrix, could affect the prognosis of accident-related injury.

At present, no real-time visualization techniques are really portable enough or adequate enough that the presence of a specialist is not required. The new laser phenomenon being experienced in laboratories all over the globe in relationship to x rays and other light quanta has revealed the promise that is not yet evident in practice. Hospitals and nursing homes all have records of paralysis and irreversible neurologic damage that occurred as a result of the inability of the ambulance team to cope technically with the movement of a patient at an accident site. The technology of the twenty-first century will alleviate such problems and ease the burden of the attending emergency teams.

## HEART REVASCULARIZATION BY THE LASER

It has been a well-known fact that the heart of the viper does not contain coronary arteries but is instead perfused by small channels from inside the heart which communicate with the thebesian vessels or pools located throughout the heart muscle. There have been some investigations into putting laser channels into heart muscles of animals to nourish the muscle after infarct. The experiments have met with good results.

If the muscle can be supplied with blood during the time of infarct, the result would be a continuing life-sustaining environment. No matter if the channels close after a few weeks or more. There will then be time to either do bypass procedures or implement other surgical techniques.

One can envision a portable laser device that will have the ability to localize the heart problem by imaging. The device will then vaporize very tiny channels in the heart muscle, which will temporarily bring life-giving blood to save the patient's life. There may even be, in the twenty-first century, systems adequately sophisticated to create channels in the heart muscle without opening the chest. Deep focusing of transmitted laser light through tissue, especially in the neodymium range, may be the system of choice. Concepts employing the $CO_2$ laser in the open chest have already been attempted and with a good degree of promise.

The profile of the beam for noninvasive penetration could be controlled with microprocessors or small chiplike computers that would employ a search technique using multiple frequencies. Once the search and display were oriented properly, the beam of choice could create the channel, bringing the life-giving blood to the muscle of the heart.

### Plasmas

Plasmas may well be the mode of producing the optical focusing of the main pulse so that optics that might be damaged can be eliminated from the system. There is also the possibility of using the shock phenomenon to produce the effects of mechanical force in the CPR environment. The same concepts employed at the present time to produce small channels in fluidics and to process industrial materials are certainly going to find their way into modern medical technology of the twenty-first century.

Today, while the ambulance life-support team depends upon drugs and mechanical manipulation of the infarcted heart, the insult to the muscle continues and becomes progressive. In the cardiac van of the future, there may well be a tiny laser device to produce the instantaneous channels needed to supply blood to the muscle, either by fiber-optic deployment or deposition of energy by deep focusing of the laser.

The viper will no longer have an edge on the human being who has, because of evolution, moved away from the simplistic into the sophisticated, thereby inhibiting the ability to cope with myocardial infarction. Small machines will exhibit fantastic power, and the advent of the eximer laser also offers new insight into the mechanisms of life support in the field of cardiology.

## LASER TREATMENT FOR ARTHRITIS

One of the challenges facing man today, treating or curing, is the riddle of arthritis. The laser has made some inroads in reducing the inflammation in tissue, probably as a result of the thermal gradients transmitted into the diseased area. However, there is a new possibility for the twenty-first century when one considers the application of the laser to treatment of arthritic conditions. A vast storehouse of knowledge is being accumulated in the laser chemistry laboratory of today. It is within the realm of possibility that certain frequencies of laser, when operating alone or in presence of other frequencies, can produce chemical reactions that might inhibit not only arthritis but other diseases such as cancer.

Perhaps the chemotherapeutic treatment of the future will be the interplay of the laser with chemicals already existent in the body. By altering the antigen interface or producing other effects not well understood at the present time, the laser may change the prognosis favorably.

Investigation into the illumination of diseased areas will rapidly expand in the twenty-first century and cross into the region of tunable lasers and mixed frequencies. Many of the machines that can play light upon diseased organs already exist, but there is legitimate restraint on their use, pending proper evaluation of their effects. Other disease models also may lend themselves more readily to the twenty-first century technology.

There are also other factors, however, which inhibit truly excellent technology from being used. Most manifest is the reluctance on the part of professional medical personnel to become involved. There is great safety traveling the well-established road and often a lack of true bravery in exploring the unknown or implementing the results obtained.

## SUMMARY

The improvement of mental disorders by laser-generated particles impinging upon the structure of the brain to produce modification by interaction or chemical modification replicates cosmic-particle reactions in the brain and offers an insight into future brain modification by laser. Electrical fields, magnetic fields, ions, and photons released from laser-generated plasmas show promise for blocking pain by producing new conditions in nerve-bundle structure.

Artificial-organ production by cell modification, chromosome alteration, DNA changes, and totally new modalities based upon laser-generated chemical interactions will offer greater freedom from disease and greater longevity.

Latent image retention and sensing of the total light spectrum with laser-modified optics, both inherent in the actual eye structure and external to it, will produce a new visual dimension and relief from blindness.

Laser infrared imaging and miniature x-ray units, combined with holography and computerized laser scanners for the analysis of pathology, will be significant in accurate analysis of disease. Laser noncontacting transmittal of physiologic data will offer remote sensing and a new dimension in diagnostic evaluation. The myriad combination of neutrons and x rays generated by the laser will produce portable visualization techniques and bring diagnosis to the scenes of accidents.

Alteration of the atomic structure by cellular reactions produced by laser-generated photons will introduce "sutures" of atomic light for rapid healing. New heart channels produced by the laser will offer relief from infarction and, perhaps, duplicate the manner of perfusion that exists in the heart of the viper, but has been lost in the sophisticated human heart. Arthritis conditions will be aided by deep laser-beam interactions in the inflamed joints, and chemical changes will be produced to give relief from, or cure, the disease.

The unique properties of the laser suggest such potential developments. As in all centuries past, the future is presently locked in the minds of men.

# 25

# Now and the Future: The Many Challenges to Laser Medicine and Surgery

*Leon Goldman*

In the preceding chapter, Muckerheide has ventured far into the future. Note also that in many instances initial pilot experiments have been started. These suggestions should continue to stimulate all who are interested in laser medicine and surgery.

What are some specific examples that call immediate attention to the need for cooperative work and endeavor? As the various sections in this book are reviewed, it is evident that all who are engaged in laser medicine and surgery need continued help for the development of instrumentation, adaptation of new laser systems, and monitoring programs, including adequate controls. So, at present, the laser biomedical engineer must continue to look over the shoulders of all who work in laser medicine and surgery. With knowledge of the laser in physics, optics, and instrumentation, the biomedical engineer can be of great help.

For laser biology as a prelude to clinical applications, there is a dream that has been called "molecular biomedical engineering," which comprises efforts to change the structure of a cell to promote more normal development and function, as Muckerheide suggests. The experiments on laser microsurgery of chromosomes show the possibility of altering the inherited pattern of the cell. This means continued laser micro- and scanning instrumentation for analysis of the individual cell, its structure and function, and the attempt to alter development by laser microsurgery. It may also be possible to extend laser microsurgery to the area of test tube fertilization in attempting to prevent congenital abnormalities. The cell-sorter techniques in immunology may be one of the first areas. The continued microirradiation research instituted by Bessis and continued by Rounds and Berns, as indicated in previous chapters, will make for great progress in this particular field. Only a beginning has been made in laser-induced fluorescence for clinical applications of early diagnosis and therapy of tumors.

## THE LASER'S WIDE RANGE OF APPLICATIONS

As the laser is applied to other areas of biology, its future is unlimited. In laser botany, the continued work on cytogenetics will improve hybrid seeds and crops. The initial experiments in China for silkworm production and rice have shown this. The initial developments in growth patterns from field exposure to the laser will also increase the practical application of the laser in agriculture. The use of the laser for the treatment of plant diseases is also a possibility. Chloroplasts continue to serve as excellent test models for studies of the effects of lasers on living cells. The dream of insect control by laser—in the field, in harvesting, and in processing—also continues. A whole new area of investigation is possible in that industry. According to Wood (1981), plant pathology offers a truly fertile field for studies on the suppression of tumorous growth. Lasers can be used in these test models to return cells to normal growth patterns.

The vast amount of progress in the various branches of laser spectroscopy now requires direct applications for analytic data in medicine, for the clinical laboratory, and for research. For example, the current research of infrared spectroscopy of Nils Kaiser, cited in previous chapters, suggests many applications for the developments in clinical medicine.

## CHALLENGES FOR LASER USE

Many challenges remain in the development of new instrumentation. As contributors to each discipline have suggested in their own particular fields, there is, as yet, no ideal type of laser, either as diagnostic or surgical instrument. The basic requirements continue to be reliability, flexibility, sterilizability, and suitable optics for transmission (infrared). Such infrared transmission fibers are just now being made for relatively short lengths. The laser manufacturer is interested in developing more markets for laser biomedical instrumentation. More government interest and support, and the encouragement of carefully controlled research protocols rather than overregulation by unlearned officials, along with the opening up of lines of communication by companies to research personnel and clinical investigators, all will help. Increased marketability for biomedical lasers will result in cheaper instrumentation.

The possibility of control of massive hemorrhage, such as in the liver with hepatectomy and in the lungs for pulmonary cancer, requires many basic and clinical studies. The gloomy statistics of cancer of the lung should stimulate tremendous research and development. As mentioned earlier, the use of laser-induced fluorescence to localize early cancer of the lung is indeed a great help. As Ascher and Heppner indicated for neurosurgery, precise instrumentation must be developed. Similar precise lasers ($CO_2$) are needed for cardiovascular surgery, as are Nd-YAG and argon lasers with fiber optics for blocking aneurysms and canalizing obstructed coronary vessels. As current studies indicate, there is now a new field: laser urologic surgery (Bülow et al., 1979a,b; Hoffstetter, 1979). There will also be increasing use of lasers for oral surgery and dentistry, and greater applications in veterinary medicine.

In addition to transmission for the $CO_2$ laser, fiber optics offer considerable advantage for laser surgery deep in viscera—for example, in the lungs, liver, and kidney—especially combined with laser-induced fluorescence for diagnosis. This is possible with developments in laser endoscopy combined with direct fiber-optic visualization. This can be supplemented by fiber optics for laser transillumination without the use of x rays. Then, more detailed surgery would be done without the need for so-called "open-field surgery." Furthermore, when all these types of instrumentation can be developed in the microsurgical phase, even more precise surgery can be accomplished without sacrifice of adjacent, noninvolved structures, especially, for example, in microneurosurgery. It will be difficult to establish precise controls for such types of microsurgical techniques. Therefore, microsurgery does not belong solely in the cloistered atmosphere of the research laboratory in biology and in cytogenetics. Further examples are the opening up of occluded fallopian tubes and, possibly, postvasectomy reopening.

Laser dentistry for diagnosis and treatment has lagged behind the other developments in laser medicine. However, as Stern (1972) indicated some time ago, efforts to prevent the tooth from becoming infected by applying a type of vitreous formation of the enamel probably would be the most common use of the laser in medicine. More investigations and investigators are needed, especially with techniques that can assure the complete surface treatment of the entire area of the tooth. The continued need for laser processing of fillings, diagnostics for circulation and cracks, the use of the UV laser for safe polymerization of plastics, and laser processing of dentures in the mouth all are projects to be pursued.

Fortunately, attention is being directed again to the possibilities of the laser in veterinary diagnostic medicine and surgery. The pulsed laser is being used to treat tendonitis in horses. One must not forget the history of laser cancer research in the early days of laser surgery with animal test models. Animal surgery is superior to tissue cultures for studies on the hyperthermia treatment of cancer with lasers and microwaves (Goldman and Dreffer, 1976). The laser has a brilliant future in all areas of cancer research.

For experiments in the development of the new instrumentation, it is obvious that suitable modality controls must be considered to determine the value and limitations of newly developed laser instrumentation. Often, unfortunately, what are offered as controls are usually the anecdotal experiences of the physician. A number of controls are available: the faithful scalpel, high-frequency electrosurgery, cryosurgery, and continued development of a safe and effective plasma scalpel. It is often difficult to develop adequate controls that parallel the energy and powerdensities of the laser. Here too, laser biology can help when the laser is used as adjunct therapy, such as cancer chemotherapy, surgery, and various modalities including magnetobiology (Polinsky et al., 1978). Then it becomes even more difficult to develop proper controls.

## NEED FOR FUNDAMENTAL STUDIES

It is necessary to emphasize again that one cannot have suitable progress in laser medicine without fundamental studies in laser biology. Laser biology now includes not only microirradiation studies, but also laser biophysics and laser chemistry and biochemistry. Increasing developments in laser holography and combinations with acoustic microscopy and holography are sorely needed. The emphasis in the past has been mainly on laser surgery but, as indicated in these chapters, it is possible to have further development in laser medical diagnosis, especially with laser UV and VUV.

Since laser biomedical engineering is still in its infancy, support for it must be developed, and also for laser medicine and surgery. It is true that governmental support is often influenced chiefly by the concern for laser safety. This can be provided by continued studies in laser biology and laser medicine. Unfortunately, the laser industry and the military do not often appreciate the need for such basic studies to develop effective programs for laser safety. Again, it is emphasized that true progress will be made when the support is given for basic investigations, as well as for applied studies. This is true at the present time, especially in Germany.

At present, the initiative for clinical research in the development of laser medicine and surgery is in Europe, Japan, China, and Russia. The traditional conservative position of medicine and the supposed need for "defensive medicine" suggested in the United States has interfered with continued research and development in laser medicine.

Again, the constant theme that should be part of all research and development in the application of the laser must be that oft-repeated cliche: If you don't need the laser, don't use it.

The specific properties of the laser as a diagnostic and therapeutic tool should always be emphasized: absolute precision, the potential for tremendous energy and power-densities, the color absorption of lasers in the visible-light range, and the significant effects on blood vessels in regard to hemorrhage. Moreover, the laser surgical operating instruments do not touch any tissues, especially blood vessels. Added to these is the study of other areas in the electromagnetic spectrum which have not yet been studied. The new wavelengths have great potential.

It is admitted that the current interest of the commercial market resides in the applications of the laser in industry, in the military, and in communications and information handling. These fields are more attractive to the manufacturer. The need is for manufacturers interested in various types of lasers "for the good of man"—those interested, of course, in laser medicine and surgery. In China, fortunately, both the manufacturer and the laser physicist are interested in biomedical applications of the laser. The Japanese government has also given substantial funds for laser medical research.

Often, in the past, especially for those with limited budgets, lasers that were available for other applications were seized upon and attempts made to develop and adapt "borrowed" instruments to medicine and surgery. From the initial experiments—which were carried out with lasers on the optical bench—to the flexible and mobile self-contained units of the present, it is evident that there has been a tremendous advance in the development of laser medical instrumentation. As the various chapters of this book indicate, more flexible, more reproducible, reliable results are necessary for the continued development of laser instrumentation.

These chapters also show a continued emphasis on the cooperation of the biomedical engineer and the biologist, physician and surgeon concerned. It is hoped that the increasing developments in electrooptical technology will improve the lines of communication and give rise to more continued sympathetic understanding and helpful cooperation. In this connection, additional training programs are needed not only for technicians, but also at undergraduate and graduate levels for biomedical engineers and laser experts in medicine and surgery.

It is hoped that with the industrial education version of the video disks (MCA Disco Vision and Pioneer Laserdiscs), this technique can be expanded to education and training in the fields of biology, medicine, and surgery. The great potential of these systems for providing better health care is obvious. There is also the challenge to the optoelectronic engineer to change the video disks into three-dimensional vision.

These are but brief, superficial remarks to stimulate interest so that there will be continued development and progress. For all this, it is necessary again to have open lines of communication so that all who are engaged in laser technology understand what physicians and surgeons are attempting to do, and can help. The International Laser Surgery Society, the Laser Gynecological Society, and the American Society for Laser Medicine and Surgery should coordinate their efforts and cooperate in developing educational programs. Then laser biology, laser medicine, and laser surgery will truly be for the good of man.

## REFERENCES

Bülow H, Levene S (1979) Development of a carbon dioxide laser endoscope without a mobile arm system. J Urol 121:1979.

Bülow H, Bülow U, Frohmuller HG (1979a) Laser investigations of the structured dog urethra. Investigative Urology 16:403.

Bülow H, Bülow U, Frohmuller HG (1979b) Transurethral laser urethrotomy in man, preliminary report. J Urol 121:286.

Goldman L, Dreffer R (1976) Microwaves, magnetic iron particles and lasers as a combined test model for investigation of hyperthermia treatment of cancer. Arch Derm Res 257:227.

Hofstetter, F (1979) A new laser endoscope for irradiation of bladder tumors. Fortschr Med 97:232.

Polinsky AK, et al. (1978) Traitment par le laser et un champ magnetic des ulcers cutanes chronique des plaies infectee. Rev Med Tours 12(5):612–616; Abst Excerpta Medica Dermatologica 33:2109.

Stern RH (1972) Laser inhibition of dental caries suggested by first test in vitro. JADA 85:1087.

Wood, HN (1981) Suppression of the tumorous state. American Cancer Society's 23rd Science Writers Seminar, Daytona Beach, Florida.

# Index

## A



## B

# C

# D

## F



## G

## K



## L



## M

# N



# O

# P

# T